Measuring the Mind: Speed, Control, and Age

Measuring the Mind: Speed, Control, and Age

Edited by

John Duncan

Louise Phillips

Peter McLeod

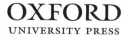

OXFORD

UNIVERSITY PRESS

OXFORD
UNIVERSITY PRESS

Great Clarendon Street, Oxford OX2 6DP

Oxford University Press is a department of the University of Oxford.
It furthers the University's objective of excellence in research, scholarship,
and education by publishing worldwide in

Oxford New York

Auckland Cape Town Dar es Salaam Hong Kong Karachi
Kuala Lumpur Madrid Melbourne Mexico City Nairobi
New Delhi Shanghai Taipei Toronto

With offices in

Argentina Austria Brazil Chile Czech Republic France Greece
Guatemala Hungary Italy Japan Poland Portugal Singapore
South Korea Switzerland Thailand Turkey Ukraine Vietnam

Oxford is a registered trade mark of Oxford University Press
in the UK and in certain other countries

Published in the United States
by Oxford University Press Inc., New York

British Library Cataloguing in Publication Data

Data available

Library of Congress Cataloging in Publication Data

Data available

Typeset by Newgen Imaging Systems (P) Ltd., Chennai, India
Printed in Great Britain
on acid-free paper by
Biddles Ltd, King's Lynn

ISBN 0–19–856641–7 (Hbk.)   978–0–19–856641–0
ISBN 0–19–856642–5 (Pbk.)   978–0–19–856642–7

10 9 8 7 6 5 4 3 2 1

Preface

On 28 and 29 June 2004, a group of friends, collaborators and acolytes met in Oxford to celebrate the career of Pat Rabbitt. This book is the result, reflecting his influence over the field of experimental psychology across almost 50 years of research. Organizing this meeting was an effortlessly positive experience—we simply listed the 16 contributors we would most like to attend, and these are the 16 people whose work appears here. Their eagerness in itself speaks of the respect and affection that Pat has inspired with his experiments, his wisdom, and his mastery of the scientific epigram (examples here quoted from memory and with no promise of accuracy).

The sections of the book reflect some of the many topics that Pat's experiments have illuminated—in early years in Cambridge, Oxford, Durham, and Newcastle, since 1983 as Director of the University of Manchester's Age and Cognitive Performance Research Centre, and since 1991 also as Adjunct Professor at the University of Western Australia in Perth. When Pat entered the field in the late 1950s, the concepts of information processing were first being applied to experimental psychology. One of the key results was increase of reaction time (RT) with the number of stimulus/response alternatives, and in the early part of his career, Pat worked extensively on choice reaction time and its components. Early on he realised the limitations of static performance models and took up his lifelong interest in change—in the flattening of the RT function with practice ("With the passage of time this proud function detumesces . . ."), and in RT increases in old age ("As you watch elderly people deliberating over whether to cross the street you might be tempted to think that the time taken reflects a natural cautiousness. But . . . you can't be anthropomorphic about old people . . ."). An interest in speed and change has remained central to much of what he has done, and the first section of the book picks up several of Pat's favourite themes—basic mechanisms of speeded decision, changes with age, and their relationship to the broader question of differences between one person and another.

In the early years, Pat's theoretical leaning was distinctly spartan, with a preference for the well-defined concepts of 1950s information processing over the sudden, chaotic flowering of the cognitive revolution. ("I still think of myself as an old-style human experimental psychologist rather than a modern cognitive psychologist. The difference is that the human experimental psychologist picks some point of method so detailed that nobody could possibly care to defend it, and subjects it to a merciless attack; the cognitive psychologist picks some theoretical position so vague that nobody could possibly think of attacking it, and offers a heroic defence.") But an interest in errors and their correction led soon to a rather complex view of performance control in reaction time experiments, with subjects engaging in a continuous hunt for the optimal balance between speed and accuracy. By the late 1970s, Pat had generalized this idea to propose that the simplest laboratory tasks involve a complex structure of internal control processes—estimating optimal speed and decision criteria, determining where and when information should be acquired, adjusting expectations and preparation, and so on. Such ideas fit well with doubts over static performance models, and with an interest in processes of change. Soon Pat was studying age-related changes in control processes, and the role of frontal lobe functions. Among his telling conclusions was that age indeed has strong effects on dynamic control processes—but that these are only poorly reflected in conventional frontal lobe tests. In the second section of the book, we pick up this theme of executive or control processes, their importance in explaining normal individual differences and changes with age, and the neuropsychology and neurophysiology of the frontal lobe.

Perhaps the central issue in aging research has been differentiation of cognitive changes: whether age declines in cognition are general, or instead reflect more specific mechanisms of information-processing. In Durham, Newcastle, and Manchester, Pat set up studies of aging with sample sizes sufficiently large to examine this question, with a series of striking results. On the one hand, he showed the remarkable degree to which age changes can be captured by a simple test of fluid intelligence. Often he found that, once fluid intelligence was partialled out, little additional age decrement remained. To some extent, the results showed that a simple measure of choice reaction time can behave in much the same way, capturing much or most age-related change. At the same time, the data also showed some more specific age effects. One example was memory decline (though intriguingly, Pat also found that old people's own estimates of memory change might be more related to depression than to objective performance loss.) In the third section of the book we take up this question of age and memory.

Trained originally at the MRC Applied Psychology Research Unit, Pat, throughout his career, has maintained a firm eye on what cognition is for—not for laboratory experiments, and not to provide us with rich mental experience, but to control effective, adaptive behaviour. ("An experienced macaque would soon show that it knows exactly what to *do* with a madeleine.") Indeed, real-world problems repeatedly emphasize some of Pat's central ideas—flexibility of control, the importance of change, and the way cognition is shaped by skill, knowledge and ability. His own work has addressed the performance of Post Office workers—complex tasks for personnel selection and training—driving safety—the effects of alcohol—health status in old age and cognitive changes with approach to death. In the final section of the book we consider real-world cognition, and the richness of behaviour outside the laboratory.

We are tremendously grateful to the contributors who have given unstintingly of their time and enthusiasm to make this book an appropriate tribute to Pat's career. We are also grateful for the hospitality of the University Department of Experimental Psychology and Queen's College in Oxford—where Pat worked from 1968 to 1982 as University Lecturer and College Fellow, and where our meeting was held. Finally, we were fortunate to receive generous financial support from the Experimental Psychology Society, the British Psychological Society, and the British Academy. Thanks to all these individuals and organizations we are able to thank our friend and mentor for a lifetime of guidance, entertainment, and fascinating ideas.

J.D.   March 2005
L.P.
P.M.

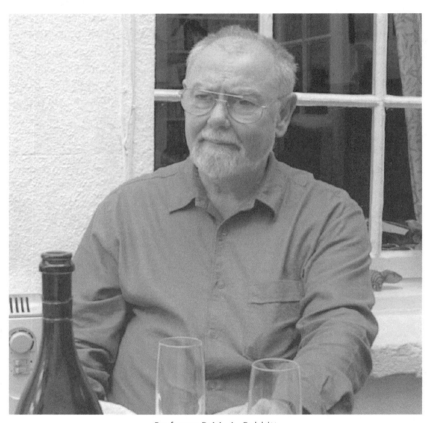

Professor P. M. A. Rabbitt

Contents

Contributors

Mike Anderson
School of Psychology,
The University of Western Australia
Crawley, Australia

Alan Baddeley
Department of Psychology,
University of York,
York, UK

Hilary Baddeley
Department of Care of the Elderly,
University of Bristol,
Bristol, UK

Elina Birmingham
Department of Psychology,
University of British Columbia,
Vancouver, Canada

Walter F. Bischof
Department of Computing Science,
University of Alberta,
Edmonton, Canada

Paul W. Burgess
Institute of Cognitive Neuroscience
and Department of Psychology,
University College London,
London, UK

Dave Cameron
Department of Psychology,
University of British Columbia,
Vancouver, Canada

Dino Chincotta
Department of Experimental
Psychology,
University of Bristol,
Bristol, UK

Fergus Craik
Rotman Research Institute,
Baycrest Centre,
Toronto, Canada

Ian J. Deary
Department of Psychology,
University of Edinburgh,
Edinburgh, UK

Geoff Der
MRC Social and Public Health
Sciences Unit,
Glasgow, UK

Iroise Dumontheil
Institute of Cognitive Neuroscience
and Department of Psychology,
University College London,
London, UK

John Duncan
MRC Cognition and Brain
Sciences Unit,
Cambridge, UK

Sam J. Gilbert
Institute of Cognitive Neuroscience
and Department of Psychology,
University College London,
London, UK

Julie D. Henry
School of Psychology,
University of New South Wales,
Sydney, Australia

G. Robert J. Hockey
Department of Psychology,
University of Sheffield,
Sheffield, UK

David F. Hultsch
Centre on Aging,
University of Victoria,
Victoria, Canada

Michael A. Hunter
Centre on Aging,
University of Victoria,
Victoria, Canada

Alan Kingstone
Department of Psychology,
University of British Columbia,
Vancouver, Canada

Simona Luzzi
Department of Neuroscience,
University of Ancona,
Ancona, Italy

Stuart W. S. MacDonald
Aging Research Center,
Karolinska Institute,
Stockholm, Sweden

Elizabeth A. Maylor
Department of Psychology,
University of Warwick,
Coventry, UK

Gail McKoon
Department of Psychology,
The Ohio State University,
Columbus, OH, USA

Peter McLeod
Department of Experimental
Psychology,
Oxford University,
Oxford, UK

Christobel Meikle
Department of Experimental
Psychology,
University of Bristol,
Bristol, UK

Stephen Monsell
School of Psychology,
University of Exeter,
Exeter, UK

Helen C. Moon
School of Psychology,
University of Plymouth,
Plymouth, UK

Jeff Nelson
School of Psychology,
The University of Western Australia,
Crawley, Australia

Timothy J. Perfect
School of Psychology,
University of Plymouth,
Plymouth, UK

Louise Phillips
School of Psychology,
University of Aberdeen,
Aberdeen, UK

Roger Ratcliff
Department of Psychology,
The Ohio State University,
Columbus, OH, USA

Nick Reed
Department of Experimental
Psychology,
Oxford University,
Oxford, UK

Jon S. Simons
Institute of Cognitive Neuroscience
and Department of Psychology,
University College London,
London, UK

Daniel Smilek
Department of Psychology,
University of Waterloo,
Waterloo, Canada

Philip L. Smith
School of Behavioural Science,
University of Melbourne,
Melbourne, Australia

Peter Sommerville
Department of Experimental
Psychology,
Oxford University,
Oxford, UK

Esther Strauss
Centre on Aging,
University of Victoria,
Victoria, Canada

Anjali Thapar
Department of Psychology,
Bryn Mawr College,
Bryn Mawr, PA, USA

Derrick G. Watson
Department of Psychology,
University of Warwick,
Coventry, UK

John H. Wearden
Department of Psychology,
Manchester University,
Manchester, UK

Section 1

Reaction time and mental speed

Chapter 1

Aging and response times: a comparison of sequential sampling models

Roger Ratcliff, Anjali Thapar,
Philip L. Smith, and Gail McKoon

Abstract

Ratcliff and colleagues have examined the effects of aging on cognitive processes in a number of two choice tasks. They fit the diffusion model to the response time and accuracy data for each task and interpreted the effects of aging in terms of the components of processing identified by the model. The question addressed in this chapter is whether the interpretations are specific to the diffusion model. To address this question, we fit two other models, the accumulator model and the leaky competing accumulator model of Usher and McClelland, to the data from young and older subjects for six experiments. We found that, although the diffusion model fit the data better than the other models for most of the experiments, the models' explanations of how aging affects components of processing do not differ significantly.

Introduction

A central finding in the literature on aging is that people's response times in cognitive tasks increase with age. Along with the increase in response times, performance sometimes shows a decrease in accuracy. Recently, Ratcliff, Thapar, and McKoon (2001, 2003, 2004), Ratcliff, Thapar, Gomez, and McKoon (2004), and Thapar, Ratcliff, and McKoon (2003) examined the effects of aging on performance in a number of two-choice decision tasks: signal detection-like tasks, a masked brightness discrimination task, a recognition memory task, a lexical decision task, and a masked letter discrimination

Preparation of this article was supported by NIA grant R01-AG17083, NIMH grants R37-MH44640 and K05-MH01891.

task. These tasks were chosen because they span a range of cognitive processes that might be expected to show deficits, including perceptual processing, lexical processing, and memory, with the signal detection task representing a case where only general deficits might occur. Ratcliff and his colleagues applied a sequential sampling model, the diffusion model (Ratcliff, 1978, 1981, 1985, 1988; Ratcliff, Van Zandt, & McKoon,1999; Ratcliff & Rouder, 1998, 2000), to the data to identify the effects of aging on several of the components of processing that determine performance, separating from each other such factors as the quality of stimulus information available to the processing system and the amount of information required before making a decision.

The older subjects in these studies adopted more conservative criteria for their decisions than the young subjects and they were also slower in components of processing outside the decision process (e.g. encoding and response execution). In all of the tasks except letter discrimination, the quality of the stimulus evidence driving the decision process was not significantly lower for the older subjects than the young ones. For the brightness and letter discrimination tasks, the deficits occurred exactly as would be predicted from psychophysical research on the effects of aging on visual discrimination (Coyne, 1981; Fozard, 1990; Owsley, Sekuler, & Siemsen, 1983; Spear, 1993): a deficit occurred with the high spatial frequencies of letters in the letter discrimination task but not with the low spatial frequencies of the stimuli in the brightness discrimination task.

The advantage of models like the diffusion model is that they provide insights into performance that allow the response time (RT) and accuracy data from two-choice tasks to be decomposed into components of processing. This theoretical approach also has the advantage that it deals with all aspects of the data: correct and error RTs and their relative speeds, the shapes of the RT distributions for correct and error responses, and accuracy values.

This chapter has two aims. First, we fit two other sequential sampling models to the 12 sets of data from Ratcliff et al. (2001, 2003, 2004), Ratcliff et al. (2004), and Thapar et al. (2003) in order to determine whether the conclusions from the diffusion model about the components of processing that differ between young and older subjects are the same for the other models. The two other models, reviewed by Ratcliff and Smith (2004), are the accumulator model (Smith & Vickers, 1988; Vickers, 1970, 1979; Vickers, Caudrey, & Willson, 1971) and the leaky competing accumulator model (the LCA model, Usher & McClelland, 2001). Second, the relative qualities of the fits across the three models allows a moderately comprehensive comparison of them that serves to extend the comparisons in Ratcliff and Smith.

The diffusion model

The diffusion model is a model of the cognitive processes involved in making simple twochoice decisions. It separates the quality of evidence entering the decision from the decision criteria and from other, nondecision processes such as encoding the stimulus and response execution. The diffusion model, like the other two models as they are considered here, applies only to relatively fast two-choice decisions (mean RTs less than about 1000 to 1500 ms) and only to decisions that are a single-stage decision process (as opposed to the multiple-stage processes that might be involved in, for example, reasoning tasks or card sorting tasks). Other models in the class of diffusion models have been applied to other types of decision making (Busemeyer & Townsend, 1993; Diederich, 1995, 1997; Roe, Busemeyer, & Townsend, 2001) and to simple RT (Smith, 1995).

The diffusion model assumes that decisions are made by a noisy process that accumulates information over time from a starting point toward one of two response criteria or boundaries, as in Figure 1.1, where the starting point is labeled z and the boundaries are labeled a and 0. When one of the boundaries is reached, a response is initiated. The rate of accumulation of information is called the drift rate (v), and it is determined by the quality of the information extracted from the stimulus. There is noise (variability) in the process of accumulating information from the starting point toward the boundaries so that processes with the same mean drift rate do not always terminate at the same time (producing RT distributions) and do not always terminate at the same boundary (producing errors). This source of variability is called within trial variability. Empirical RT distributions are positively skewed and in the

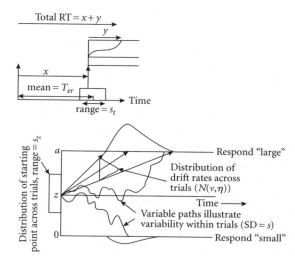

Fig. 1.1 An illustration of the diffusion model. The top panel shows the combination of the nondecision component of RT, x, and the decision component, y. The bottom panel shows the diffusion decision process.

diffusion model, this is naturally predicted by simple geometry (see figure 1.1, Ratcliff & Rouder, 1998).

Components of processing are assumed to be variable across trials. From a theoretical perspective, one would not expect subjects to be able to achieve identical settings of the various components of processing from trial to trial (e.g. Van Zandt & Ratcliff, 1995). From a practical perspective, the assumption of across-trial variability allows the model to account for differences in RTs between correct and error responses (Luce, 1986). Variability in drift rate across trials leads to slow errors and variability in starting point leads to fast errors (Ratcliff et al. 1999; Ratcliff & Rouder, 1998), and the relative values of the two control the pattern of error compared to correct RTs that is obtained in an experiment. Drift rate is assumed to be normally distributed with standard deviation η and starting point is assumed to be uniformly distributed with range s_z. In addition, the nondecision components, which are combined into one component with mean T_{er}, are assumed to have variability across trials that is uniformly distributed with range s_t (Ratcliff, Gomez, & McKoon, 2004; Ratcliff & Tuerlinckx, 2002).

In four of the six experiments discussed in this chapter, subjects are sometimes instructed to respond as quickly as possible and sometimes to respond as accurately as possible. Speed-accuracy tradeoffs are modeled by altering the boundaries of the decision process—wider boundaries require more information before a decision can be made and this leads to more accurate and slower responses.

For each stimulus condition in an experiment, it is assumed that the rate of accumulation of evidence is different and so each has a different value of drift, v. A zero point, the drift criterion, separates stimuli into those with positive drift rates and those with negative drift rates, functioning in the same way as the criterion in signal detection theory. Like the signal detection criterion, the value of the drift criterion can vary with experimental manipulations such as payoffs or the proportions of stimuli for which one versus the other of the responses is correct (Ashby, 1983; Link, 1975; Link & Heath, 1975; Ratcliff, 1978, 1985, 2002; Ratcliff et al. 1999). Changing the drift criterion from one block of trials to another is equivalent to adding or subtracting a constant to the drift rates for all stimuli in one block relative to another (Ratcliff, 2002).

In sum, the parameters of the diffusion model correspond to the components of the decision process as follows: z is the starting point of the accumulation of evidence, a is the upper boundary and the lower boundary is set to 0; η is the standard deviation in drift rate across trials; s_z is the range of the starting point across trials; T_{er} is the mean time taken up by the nondecision components of processing, and s_t is the range of the values of T_{er} across trials. For each stimulus condition in an experiment, there is a different value of drift, v. Within-trial variability in drift rate (s) is a scaling parameter for the diffusion process (i.e. if it were doubled, other parameters could be multiplied or divided by two to produce exactly the same fits of the model to data). s is set to 0.1 in fits to the data as it has been in other applications of the model to data.

The accumulator model

The accumulator model (Smith & Vickers, 1988; Vickers, 1970, 1978, 1979; Vickers et al. 1971) assumes that evidence in favor of one response is accumulated in one accumulator, evidence in favor of the other response is accumulated in a second accumulator, and the decision is determined by the first accumulator to reach its criterion (see Figure 1.2). Evidence is accumulated at discrete time steps. The amount of evidence accumulated on each step is variable, normally distributed with standard deviation 1.0 and a mean, μ, that depends on the quality of the information from the stimulus. With this variability, information in the wrong accumulator can reach its criterion first, leading to an error. A criterion, termed the "sensory referent," is set on the underlying evidence dimension such that if the amount of evidence sampled at a time step falls above the criterion, an amount equal to the difference between that amount and the criterion is added to one accumulator. If the amount falls below the criterion, the difference is added to the other accumulator. Like the drift criterion in the diffusion models, this criterion represents a point of zero stimulus information. Because evidence is accumulated at discrete time steps, a parameter, λ, is required to converts time steps to continuous time.

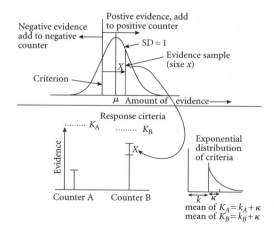

Fig. 1.2 An illustration of the accumulator model.

Ratcliff and Smith (2004) assumed that there is variability across trials in three components of the accumulator model (*cf.* Smith & Vickers, 1988) for the same reasons as for the diffusion model. First, the means of the evidence distributions are assumed to vary randomly across trials according to a normal distribution with mean μ and standard deviation σ_μ. This variability is the counterpart to variability in drift rates across trials in the diffusion model. Second, the nondecision component of RT varies across trials with a rectangular distribution with mean T_{er} and range s_t, exactly as in the diffusion model. Third, the values of the response criteria vary across trials. The values of the criteria on each trial (Figure 1.2) are calculated by adding a value obtained from an exponential with mean κ to two base values, k_A and k_B (the same value added to each), to obtain the values of K_A and K_B for each trial (i.e. the mean values of the criteria are $k_A + \kappa$ and $k_B + \kappa$). Without this variability, RT distributions are not skewed enough to match empirical data. Also, in order to accommodate differences in performance, it is necessary for the mean of the exponential to be larger when subjects are instructed to respond accurately than when they are instructed to respond quickly.

This model produces error responses that are slower than correct responses, a pattern that is often found in experimental data, but not always. An important problem for the model is that no way has been found for it to produce errors faster than correct responses, a pattern often obtained experimentally especially in paradigms such as choice RT (Ratcliff & Smith, 2004). The problem arises because the evidence sample is larger for evidence added to the positive accumulator (in Figure 1.2) than evidence added to the negative accumulator, because the average amount of evidence above the criterion is larger (e.g. above μ) than the average amount below (e.g. just a little below the criterion).

The leaky competing accumulator model

The LCA model (Usher & McClelland, 2001) was developed as an alternative to the diffusion model with the aim of implementing neurobiological principles that the authors felt should be incorporated into RT models, especially mutual inhibition mechanisms and decay of information across time.

The LCA model is similar to the accumulator model in that evidence is accumulated in separate accumulators for the two responses (see Figure 1.3), but the accumulation processes themselves are modeled as diffusion processes. Evidence is continuously distributed and accumulates in continuous time, just as in other diffusion process models. The rate of accumulation is a combination of three components. The first is the input from the stimulus, v, with a different value of v for each experimental condition. If the input to one of the

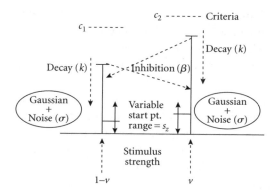

Fig. 1.3 An illustration of the leaky competing accumulator model.

accumulators is v, the input to the other is $1 - v$ so that the sum of the two rates is 1. The second component is decay in the amount of accumulated information, k, with decay growing as the amount of information in the accumulator grows, and the third is inhibition from the other accumulator, β, with the amount of inhibition growing as the amount of information in the other accumulator grows. Combining the three components, the equivalent of drift rate in the diffusion model for accumulator i (where j is the competing accumulator) is $v - kx_i - \beta x_j$, where x_i and x_j is the amount of evidence already accumulated in accumulator i and j respectively.

If the amount of inhibition is large, the model exhibits features similar to the diffusion model because an increase in accumulated information for one of the response choices produces a decrease for the other choice. The assumption of inhibition between accumulators makes the model similar to an earlier, discrete-time model proposed by Heuer (1987).

The rate of accumulation of information is variable; the amount of evidence added to an accumulator on each trial includes Gaussian variability with standard deviation σ. Because of this variability, accumulated information can reach the wrong criterion, resulting in an error. Because of the decay and inhibition in the accumulation rates, the tails of RT distributions are longer than would be produced without these factors (*cf.* Vickers, 1970, 1979; Vickers et al. 1971), which leads to good matches with the skewed shape of empirical RT distributions.

The expression for the increment to the amount of accumulated information at time t in accumulator i, is:

$$dx_i = \left[v_i - kx_i - \beta \sum_{j \neq i} x_j \right] \frac{dt}{\tau} + \sigma \sqrt{\frac{dt}{\tau}},$$

where dt/τ is set to 0.1 to correspond to 10 ms steps as in Usher and McClelland (2001). The amount of accumulated information is not allowed to take on values below zero, so if it is computed to be below zero, it is reset to zero; this constraint is written as $x_i \rightarrow \max(x_i, 0)$ and it introduces nonlinearity into the model.

The LCA model without across-trial variability for any of its components predicts errors slower than correct responses. To produce errors faster than correct responses, Usher and McClelland assumed variability in the accumulators' starting points, just as is assumed for the diffusion model. Also, we made the same assumption about nondecision components of processing as for the diffusion and accumulator models, that they vary with a rectangular distribution with range s_t and mean T_{er} (Ratcliff & Smith, 2004).

Displaying data and fitting the models to the data

In fits of any model to RT data, there are two dependent variables to consider, accuracy and RT. The proportions of correct and error responses and the relationships between their RTs, as well as the distributions of the RTs, must all be considered when assessing the fit of a model. Traditionally, accuracy, mean RTs, and RT distributions have all been plotted separately as a function of experimental condition. Here, we display them all together in quantile probability functions (QPFs). This method of displaying the data has the advantage that the joint behaviors of the dependent variables can be more easily examined. The QPF derives from the latency probability function (LPF), which was used to display the joint behavior of mean RT and accuracy in early work on sequential sampling models by Audley and Mercer (1968), Audley and Pike (1965), LaBerge (1962), Pike (1973), Pike and Ryder (1973), and others.

A QPF is constructed by plotting the quantiles of the distribution of RTs for each experimental condition on the y-axis and the probability of the response on the x-axis. For the data presented in this chapter, we used five quantiles, with the plotted quantile points representing the RTs below which fall 0.1, 0.3, 0.5, 0.7, and 0.9 of the total probability mass in the distribution. The lines that connect the quantiles across experimental conditions, as in Figures 1.4 and 1.5, form the QPF, and the shape of this function must be explained by the models. For each experimental condition, the quantile points plotted on the y-axis show the shape of the RT distribution. Because there is 0.2 probability mass between each pair of quantiles (e.g. the 0.1 and 0.3 quantiles), equal area rectangles can be constructed between the quantiles and these approximate the RT histograms that conventional analyses would produce (see Ratcliff & Smith, 2004, figure 1.5).

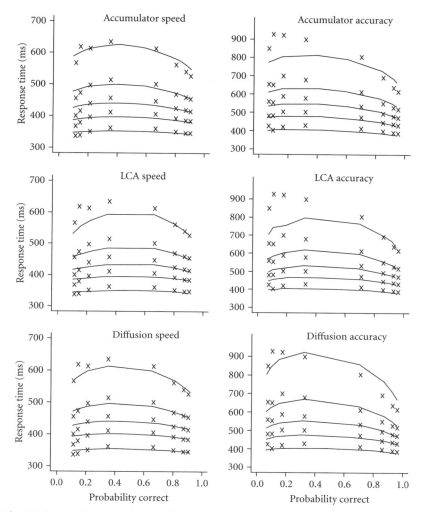

Fig. 1.4 Sample fits for the accumulator, LCA, and diffusion models to data from the letter discrimination experiment with young subjects. X^2 values are 22.4, 15.7, and 7.5, respectively. (a) Letter discrimination: young subjects; (b) diffusion model recognition memory older subject data; (c) LCA model recognition memory older subject data.

A full representation of the data from an experiment requires two QPFs, one for each response, as were plotted for the data from Experiments 4, 5, and 6 below. However, if the data are symmetric for the two responses (i.e. RTs and accuracy values for the two choices are about the same), they can be averaged across responses to give a single QPF with error responses plotted to the left of 0.5 and correct responses to the right. Experiments 1, 2, and 3 below yielded symmetric data of this kind.

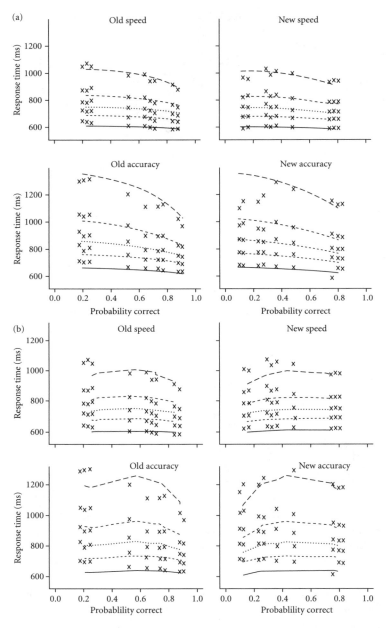

Fig. 1.5 Sample fits for the accumulator, LCA, and diffusion models to data from the recognition memory experiment with older subjects. X² values are 60.9, 151.9, and 64.9, respectively. (a) Letter discrimination: young subjects; (b) diffusion model recognition memory older subject data; (c) LCA model recognition memory older subject data.

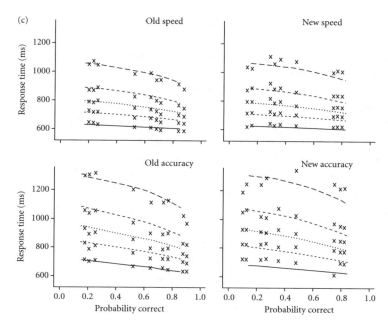

Fig. 1.5 (*Continued*)

When difficulty is varied across experimental conditions in such a way that subjects cannot know at the time a stimulus is presented which condition it is in (e.g. when high and low frequency words are presented in random order in a lexical decision experiment), there are two important constraints on the models. First, the effects of difficulty are determined by only one parameter, the rate of accumulation of evidence: drift rate in the diffusion model and accumulation rate in the accumulator and LCA models. With only drift or accumulation rate varying, accuracy rates plus mean RTs and RT distributions for both correct and error responses must be explained.

The second constraint is that the shape of the QPFs is determined by only a few parameters of the models. For example, in the diffusion model with starting point equidistant from the two boundaries, the form of the QPF is determined by three parameters: a (boundary separation), η (across-trial variability in drift rate), and s_z (across-trial variability in starting point). With starting point half way between the decision boundaries, then: When η and s_z are zero, RTs for correct and error responses for each experimental condition are equal and the QPF is symmetric with an inverted U shape. When η is high and s_z is low, error responses are slower than correct responses and the QPF has a peak to the left of the 0.5 probability point. When η is low and s_z is high, error responses are faster than correct responses and the QPF has a peak to the right of the 0.5 probability point. Thus the shape of the QPF allows the relative speeds of correct and error responses to be determined by visual inspection. The vertical location of the QPF is determined by the nondecision component of response time, T_{er}.

We chose to evaluate the models against group data obtained by averaging quantiles of the RT distributions and response probabilities across subjects (Ratcliff, 1979; Thomas & Ross, 1980). Fits to individual subjects and fits to quantile-averaged group data exhibit very similar features and the parameter values obtained from group fits are in good agreement with the average parameter values obtained from fits to individual subjects (see Ratcliff, Thapar & McKoon, 2001, 2003, 2004; Ratcliff, Thapar, Gomez & McKoon, 2004; and Thapar et al. 2003, for examples with about 40 subjects per group, and Smith, Ratcliff, & Wolfgang, 2004, with six subjects). Fitting individual subjects would have required months of computer time for the LCA and accumulator models.

We used a minimum χ^2 statistic to assess how well a model fit experimental data. For N observations grouped into six bins between the five quantile RTs and outside the two extreme quantiles, this statistic has the form

$$\chi^2 = \Sigma\, N\, (p_i - \pi_i)^2 \,/\, \pi_i,$$

where p_i is the observed proportion of responses in the ith bin, π_i is the theoretical (expected) proportion of responses in the ith bin, and N is the number of observations per condition.

Because our fits were carried out on group data, obtained by averaging quantiles across subjects, it was not appropriate to weight the observed and predicted proportions in the χ^2 statistic by the total sample size N as is done in the usual Pearson χ^2 test. Instead, we calculated the statistic from the observed and predicted proportions instead of frequencies and multiplied the values by 100 for readability. We use this statistic as a relative rather than absolute measure of fit and denote it by the symbol X^2 to emphasize that it is not a proper χ^2 because it has been calculated from quantile-averaged data. In order to compare the models, later we divide the X^2 values by the number of experimental conditions in each experiment to provide X^2 values that are approximately in the same range across the experiments (e.g. Experiments 5 and 6 had 4 conditions whereas Experiments 3 and 4 had 18 conditions).

The diffusion model was fit to the experimental data by minimizing the X^2 value with a general Simplex minimization routine that adjusts the parameters of the model to find the parameters that give the minimum X^2 value (see Ratcliff & Tuerlinckx, 2002, for a full description of the methods). The data entered into the minimization routine for each experimental condition were the RTs for each of the five quantiles for correct and error responses and the accuracy values. The quantile RTs and the diffusion model were used to generate the predicted cumulative probability of a response occurring at or before the given quantile RT. Subtracting the cumulative probabilities for each successive quantile from the next higher quantile gives the proportion of responses between each quantile. These expected values are compared to the observed proportions of responses between the quantiles and the observed proportions of responses for each quantile are the proportions of the distribution between successive quantiles (i.e. the proportions between 0, 0.1, 0.3, 0.5, 0.7, 0.9, and 1.0 are 0.1, 0.2, 0.2, 0.2, 0.2, and 0.1).

The expected (theoretical) values of the probabilities were generated from the models in two different ways. For the diffusion model, an explicit expression for the cumulative distribution function is available (Ratcliff, 1978; Ratcliff et al. 1999). This involves an infinite series that must be summed numerically, with numerical integration over the distributions of drift rate, starting point, and the nondecision component of RT that represent across-trial variability in these components of processing. This combination was used to produce the cumulative probabilities at the quantile RTs. From these, the proportions between successive quantiles needed for X^2 can be computed.

For the accumulator model, a simulation method was used to compute accuracy and RT distributions. Because we wished to allow independent variability in criteria, it was more efficient to generate predictions by simulation than to use the exact numerical methods used by Ratcliff and Smith (2004) Smith and Vickers (1988). Exact methods require an additional numerical integration for each new source of parameter variability, which appreciably slows program execution. In contrast, simulations make it easy to add sources of across trial variability in parameters of the models because all that is required is for a random value to be selected from the appropriate distribution on each trial. The simulation method allowed us to avoid the need to do extensive checking on the four numerical integrations that are needed to handle variability across trials in accumulation rate, the nondecision component of RT, and the two decision criteria. One hundred thousand simulations of the accumulator process for each experimental condition were used, which provided highly accurate predictions (repeated runs provided the same values of all the quantile RTs except the 0.9 quantile for errors that varied by a few ms from run to run).

No explicit expressions have yet been obtained for the RT distributions predicted by the LCA model when the amount of accumulated evidence is constrained to be positive. Because of this, Usher and McClelland (2001) obtained predictions from the model by simulation and we followed their method. In the fits of the model to the data described here, 20,000 simulations of the decision process per condition were used to compute the accuracy values and the RT distributions for the two responses (fewer simulations were used than for the accumulator model because the fitting program took 4 to 6 h for the larger data sets for one fit).

Each of the models was fit to the data using a Simplex algorithm (Nelder & Mead, 1965) along with a set of starting values that were a reasonable guess based on other fits. The Simplex algorithm is given ranges (we used 0.1 times the parameter values) for each of the starting values and the algorithm evaluates the χ^2 function for a range of values of the parameters based on these initial points and ranges. One hundred iterations of the Simplex algorithm were run and then the final parameters were used as initial points with the same ranges around these values. This was repeated for five sets of runs of the Simplex algorithm with the last set running for 400 iterations. If the fits were moderately poor, new starting values were tried and the fitting procedure run again until different and better fits could not be found.

Experiments

The data against which the models were tested came from six experiments each with one data set for young subjects and one data set for older subjects, previously published by Ratcliff and colleagues. The experimental tasks, all two-choice tasks, were chosen to allow comparison of the performance of young and older subjects across several different kinds of cognitive processing. In two of the tasks, one with high spatial frequency letters and one with low spatial frequency brightness arrays, the stimuli were masked in order to look at the effect of limited availability of stimulus information. Another of the tasks was recognition memory, chosen to investigate the availability of newly learned information, and another was lexical decision, chosen to investigate the availability of well-known information. For the first five experiments, there was a speed-accuracy manipulation: In half the blocks of trials, subjects were instructed to respond quickly, while in the other half of the trials, subjects were instructed to be as accurate as possible. For all the experiments, sufficient data were collected per subject to provide reliable estimates of the differences in components of processing between young and older subjects. The young subjects were all Bryn Mawr or Northwestern University students and the older subjects were all between the ages of 60 and 75 and they were matched to the young subjects on standard characteristics.

Experiment 1: Signal detection

In this experiment (Ratcliff et al. 2001), two vertically-aligned dots were displayed on each trial and subjects were asked to decide whether the separation between them was "large" or "small." Stimulus difficulty was varied via the amount of separation: There were 32 possible separations, labeled 1 through 32 with 1 being the smallest separation, ranging from 1.75 cm to 3.33 cm in equal intervals. After each trial, subjects were given feedback such that the response was designated as "correct" or "error." The response classification was probabilistic, so it was not possible for subjects to be perfectly correct. Feedback was determined by a probability associated with each stimulus: For stimuli 1–7, "small" was designated correct with probability 0.999. For stimuli 8–16, "small" was designated correct with probabilities 0.913, 0.888, 0.856, 0.819, 0.774, 0.722, 0.664, 0.601, and 0.534, respectively. For stimuli 26–32, "large" was designated correct with probability 0.999, and for stimuli 25 through 17, "large" was correct with the same probabilities as for "small" for stimuli 8 through 16. Subjects understood that they could not be completely accurate, that for separations in the middle of the range, either response might be designated as correct, and that their task was to give their best judgment. There were 12 blocks of stimuli in each session, with 3 presentations of each of the 32 stimuli in each block. In 6 of the blocks, subjects were given accuracy instructions and in the other 6, they were given speed instructions. Speed versus accuracy instructions alternated between blocks. Subjects were asked either to respond as quickly as possible or to make as few errors as possible. In the speed blocks, responses longer than 700 ms were followed by a "Too slow" message. In the accuracy blocks, "large" responses to stimuli 1–6 and "small" responses to stimuli 26–32 were followed by a "Bad error" message. There were 17 young and 13 older subjects, and each participated in two 45 min sessions.

The data were grouped into four conditions such that high probability responses were grouped together ("large" responses to large separations and "small" responses to small separations) and low probability responses were grouped together ("small" responses to large separations and "large" responses to small separations). Specifically, the stimulus groupings were: "small" responses to distances 1–8 were grouped with "large" responses to distances 21–32; "small" responses to distances 9 and 10 were grouped with "large" responses to distances 19 and 20, "small" responses to distances 11 and 12 were grouped with "large" responses to distances 17 and 18, and "small" responses to distances 13 and 14 were grouped with "large" responses to distances 15 and 16.

Experiment 2: Letter discrimination with masking

In this experiment (Thapar et al. 2003), subjects were presented on each trial with a letter that was masked after 10, 20, 30, or 40 ms. The task was to decide whether the masked letter was one of two target letters, which were presented in the top corners of the display screen and changed after every block of

96 trials. The mask consisted of a square outline, larger than the letter stimuli, filled with randomly placed horizontal, vertical, and diagonal lines that were different on every trial. Subjects participated in six blocks of speed trials alternating with six blocks of accuracy trials in each session for either two or three sessions each. There were 40 young and 38 older subjects.

For the speed blocks, subjects were instructed to respond as quickly as possible. Responses longer than 650 ms were followed by a "Too slow" message, and responses faster than 250 ms were followed by a "Too fast" message. For the accuracy blocks, subjects were instructed to respond as accurately as possible. Incorrect responses were followed by an "Error" message. No feedback was provided for correct responses.

Experiment 3: Brightness discrimination with masking

The task in this experiment (Ratcliff, Thapar, & McKoon, 2003) was to decide whether 64 × 64 arrays of black and white pixels were "bright" or "dark." On each trial, an array was presented for 50, 100, or 150 ms, then masked by four different checkerboard patterns, each 64 × 64 pixels, presented sequentially for 17 ms each. There were six brightness conditions, determined by the probability of a pixel being white equal to 0.350, 0.425, 0.475, 0.525, 0.575, or 0.650. Thirty six young and 35 older subjects participated in two or three sessions each, with five blocks of speed trials alternating with five blocks of accuracy trials (144 trials per block) in each session. In accuracy blocks, if a response was an error, the word "Error" was displayed and in speed blocks, there was no accuracy feedback. In speed blocks, if a response was longer than 700 ms, "Too slow" was displayed.

Experiment 4: Recognition memory

In this experiment (Ratcliff et al. 2004), subjects studied lists of single words. Each list had 9 words presented once and 9 words presented 3 times for a study list of 36 words, presented at a rate of 1 s per word. Immediately following each study list, subjects were presented with 36 single test words, deciding for each word whether it had been in the study list or not (half of the 36 had been in the study list, half had not). Within lists, accuracy was manipulated by varying the number of times a word appeared in the study list (one or three) and by using high, low, and very low frequency words (mean frequency values of 325, 4.4, and 0.37, Kucera & Francis, 1967).

Subjects received alternating speed and accuracy blocks of trials. In accuracy blocks, if a response was incorrect, the word "Error" was displayed before the next test word was presented. In speed blocks, there was no accuracy feedback, and if a response was longer than 800 ms for young subjects and 900 ms for older subjects, "Too slow" was displayed.

In each session, there were 10 blocks of accuracy trials and 10 blocks of speed trials. A minimum of two sessions per subject were used in data analyses.

Thirty nine young adults and 41 older adults participated in the experiment.

Experiments 5 and 6: Lexical decision

On each trial of these experiments (Ratcliff et al. 2004), a letter string was presented and subjects were asked to judge whether it was a word or a non-word. In each session, there were 70 blocks of 30 trials each, half words and half nonwords. In each block, there were equal proportions of high, low, and very low frequency words, the same pools of words as in Experiment 4. In Experiment 5, the nonwords were constructed from words by randomly replacing all the vowels in each word with other vowels and in Experiment 6, the nonwords were random letter strings. Subjects were instructed to respond quickly and accurately and error feedback was given.

Fifty four young adults and 44 older adults participated in Experiment 5 and 54 young adults and 40 older adults participated in Experiment 6.

Components of processing

When the models were fit to the data from the six experiments, the diffusion model fit 30% better on average than the accumulator and LCA models, as is shown in the next section. Despite this difference in the qualities of the fits, the differences in performance between the young and older subjects were generally ascribed to the same sources by all three models. The parameter values corresponding to each component of processing are shown in the Tables 1.1–1.6 for the three models. Sample fits for Experiments 2 and 4 are presented in Figures 1.4 and 1.5. Here, the main findings are reviewed.

Rates of accumulation of information

Figure 1.6 (bottom right panel) shows the differences in average drift and accumulation rates between young and older subjects for the three models for each experiment. The rates of accumulation of evidence for the older subjects were substantially lower than those for the young subjects only for masked letter discrimination, for which the stimuli are high spatial frequency. For all the other tasks, the rates for older subjects were at least as high as those for the young subjects; in other words, the quality of the information they obtained from the stimuli was not measurably worse than for the young subjects. (The

Table 1.1 Diffusion model parameters for fits to the 12 experiments

Experiment	a speed	a accuracy	z speed	z accuracy	T_{er}	η	s_z	s_t
SDT young	0.082	0.146	0.041	0.073	305	0.151	0.004	122
SDT older	0.097	0.181	0.048	0.090	358	0.151	0.017	173
Letter young	0.074	0.111	0.037	0.056	337	0.119	0.004	121
Letter older	0.109	0.178	0.054	0.089	403	0.244	0.009	132
Bright young	0.073	0.137	0.036	0.066	409	0.142	0.044	179
Bright older	0.072	0.126	0.036	0.063	456	0.167	0.040	163
Recogn young	0.076	0.140	0.040	0.065	488	0.172	0.053	181
Recogn older	0.100	0.135	0.046	0.062	589	0.203	0.004	213
Lex pseud young	—	0.126	—	0.064	439	0.101	0.062	159
Lex pseud older	—	0.190	—	0.096	518	0.090	0.032	171
Lex rand young	—	0.154	—	0.086	406	0.183	0.115	140
Lex rand older	—	0.199	—	0.108	458	0.137	0.078	96

Table 1.2 Drift rates for the diffusion model for the 12 experiments

Experiment	v_1	v_2	v_3	v_4	v_5	v_6	v_7	v_8	v_9
SDT young	0.370	0.230	0.128	0.051	—	—	—	—	—
SDT older	0.397	0.217	0.123	0.048	—	—	—	—	—
Letter young	0.328	0.283	0.211	0.095	—	—	—	—	—
Letter older	0.260	0.185	0.096	0.033	—	—	—	—	—
Bright young	0.322	0.205	0.089	0.373	0.248	0.098	0.375	0.265	0.083
Bright older	0.320	0.198	0.065	0.371	0.229	0.075	0.384	0.244	0.093
Recogn young	−0.185	−0.240	−0.256	0.003	0.122	0.161	0.168	0.304	0.398
Recogn older	−0.190	−0.200	−0.220	−0.003	0.081	0.126	0.152	0.267	0.313
Lex pseud young	0.442	0.249	0.161	−0.231	—	—	—	—	—
Lex pseud older	0.374	0.242	0.173	−0.218	—	—	—	—	—
Lex rand young	0.573	0.454	0.396	−0.409	—	—	—	—	—
Lex rand older	0.475	0.372	0.306	−0.363	—	—	—	—	—

Note: Drift criteria for the brightness discrimination experiments are for young subejcts: −0.058, 0.004, and 0.048, and for older subjects: −0.039, 0.023, and 0.061. Order of conditions for experiments. Dot separation, extreme to intermediate separation. Letter discrimination: large stimulus presentation to small. Brightness discrimination, intermediate brightness, long to short stimulus presentation; moderate brightness long to short stimulus presentation, extreme brightness long to short stimulus presentation. Recognition memory, H, L, VL frequency new words, H, L, VL once presented words, and H, L, VL three times presented words. Lexical decision, H, L, VL frequency words and nonwords.

Table 1.3 Accumulator model parameters for fits to the 12 experiments

Experiment	Crit 1 speed	Crit 2 speed	Crit 1 acc	Crit 2 acc	T_{er}	σ	λ	κ speed	κ acc	s_t
SDT young	0.565	0.565	1.594	1.594	315	0.481	0.058	0.960	2.317	90
SDT older	0.894	0.894	1.936	1.936	352	0.491	0.068	1.079	3.193	78
Letter young	0.609	0.609	1.370	1.370	340	0.377	0.052	0.818	1.281	83
Letter older	0.807	0.807	2.085	2.085	411	0.698	0.053	1.904	3.010	65
Bright young	0.487	0.487	1.804	1.804	405	0.469	0.054	0.835	1.901	164
Bright older	0.657	0.657	1.968	1.968	443	0.426	0.046	1.013	1.540	129
Recogn young	0.480	0.513	1.863	1.452	475	0.583	0.092	0.314	0.698	163
Recogn older	0.978	0.630	1.600	1.010	596	0.907	0.126	0.317	0.592	160
Lex pseud young	—	—	1.406	0.976	419	0.450	0.074	—	1.745	101
Lex pseud older	—	—	1.153	1.114	577	0.660	0.113	—	2.787	125
Lex rand young	—	—	1.450	0.413	389	0.286	0.083	—	1.502	105
Lex rand older	—	—	1.212	0.775	510	0.298	0.073	—	3.506	76

Table 1.4 Accumulation rates for the accumulator model for the 12 experiments

Experiment	v_1	v_2	v_3	v_4	v_5	v_6	v_7	v_8	v_9
SDT young	1.177	0.708	0.368	0.074	—	—	—	—	—
SDT older	1.258	0.690	0.377	0.002	—	—	—	—	—
Letter young	0.884	0.775	0.555	0.142	—	—	—	—	—
Letter older	0.773	0.543	0.263	0.120	—	—	—	—	—
Bright young	0.926	0.546	0.193	1.020	0.712	0.260	0.981	0.695	0.229
Bright older	0.971	0.435	0.178	1.034	0.644	0.272	1.020	0.628	0.243
Recogn young	−0.581	−0.760	−0.820	0.092	0.345	0.474	0.534	0.917	1.054
Recogn older	−0.783	−0.882	−0.944	−0.004	0.306	0.462	0.614	1.056	1.243
Lex pseud young	1.441	0.953	0.626	−0.772	—	—	—	—	—
Lex pseud older	2.095	1.514	1.056	−1.393	—	—	—	—	—
Lex rand young	1.460	1.188	0.997	−0.813	—	—	—	—	—
Lex rand older	1.718	1.341	1.011	−1.389	—	—	—	—	—

Note: Accumulation rate criteria for the brightness discrimination experiments are for young subjects: −0.174, 0.012, and 0.134 and for older subjects: 0.010, 0.029, and 0.048. Order of conditions for expts. Dot separation, extreme to intermediate separation. Letter discrimination: large stimulus presentation to small. Brightness discrimination, intermediate brightness, long to short stimulus presentation; moderate brightness long to short stimulus presentation, extreme brightness long to short stimulus presentation. Recognition memory, H, L, VL frequency new words, H, L, VL once presented words, and H, L, VL three times presented words. Lexical decision, H, L, VL frequency words and nonwords.

Table 1.5 LCA model parameters for fits to the 12 experiments

Experiment	crit 1 speed	crit 2 speed	crit 1 acc	crit 2 acc	T_{er}	k	β	σ	s_z	s_t
SDT young	1.642	1.642	2.562	2.562	278	4.127	0.188	0.595	0.754	86
SDT older	1.806	1.806	2.745	2.745	323	4.967	0.234	0.618	0.583	121
Letter young	1.431	1.431	2.137	2.137	326	2.680	0.125	0.667	0.560	112
Letter older	1.726	1.726	2.245	2.245	360	8.931	0.245	0.509	0.507	110
Bright young	1.073	1.073	1.709	1.709	372	3.693	0.331	0.433	0.281	166
Bright older	1.091	1.091	1.638	1.638	414	3.061	0.296	0.397	0.329	139
Recogn young	1.329	1.251	2.020	2.002	492	3.194	0.521	0.989	0.441	197
Recogn older	1.506	1.432	1.658	1.755	611	3.808	1.008	1.106	0.008	213
Lex pseud young	—	—	1.807	1.896	315	0.447	0.087	0.537	1.105	158
Lex pseud older	—	—	2.281	2.563	413	0.577	0.113	0.602	1.135	177
Lex rand young	—	—	1.957	1.755	308	0.433	0.082	0.534	0.992	76
Lex rand older	—	—	3.313	3.161	423	0.560	0.127	0.642	1.073	92

Table 1.6 Accumulation rates for the LCA model for the 12 experiments

Experiment	v_1	v_2	v_3	v_4	v_5	v_6	v_7	v_8	v_9
SDT young	0.884	0.746	0.623	0.550	—	—	—	—	—
SDT older	0.885	0.706	0.616	0.547	—	—	—	—	—
Letter young	0.615	0.729	0.811	0.878	—	—	—	—	—
Letter older	0.523	0.573	0.641	0.694	—	—	—	—	—
Bright young	0.716	0.639	0.552	0.732	0.670	0.568	0.727	0.665	0.563
Bright older	0.741	0.640	0.552	0.757	0.666	0.557	0.751	0.669	0.564
Recogn young	0.724	0.808	0.813	0.456	0.312	0.258	0.269	0.054	0.071
Recogn older	0.699	0.729	0.760	0.401	0.314	0.226	0.219	0.000	0.008
Lex pseud young	0.035	0.234	0.342	0.767	—	—	—	—	—
Lex pseud older	0.065	0.213	0.308	0.784	—	—	—	—	—
Lex rand young	0.086	0.157	0.229	0.822	—	—	—	—	—
Lex rand older	0.140	0.232	0.298	0.784	—	—	—	—	—

Note: Accumulation rate criteria for the brightness discrimination experiments are for young subjects: −0.041, 0.002, and 0.033 and for older subjects: −0.035, 0.016, and 0.039. Order of conditions for expts. Dot separation, extreme to intermediate separation. Letter discrimination: large stimulus presentation to small. Brightness discrimination, intermediate brightness, long to short stimulus presentation; moderate brightness long to short stimulus presentation, extreme brightness long to short stimulus presentation. Recognition memory, H, L, VL frequency new words, H, L, VL once presented words, and H, L, VL three times presented words. Lexical decision, H, L, VL frequency words and nonwords.

difference for the lexical decision task with random letter strings appears to be large, but this task has very high drift and accumulation rates and their estimates have much higher variability than those for the other tasks.)

For the diffusion model, for the signal detection, masked brightness discrimination, recognition memory, and lexical decision tasks, we were able to perform significance tests between the 4–9 drift rates for young and older subjects. But we could not do this for other parameters because only one value was computed. There were no significant differences in drift rates between the older and young subjects. The difference for masked letter discrimination was significant ($t(3) = 6.84$, $p < 0.05$ for all t-tests reported in this chapter unless otherwise stated). For lexical decision with nonwords random letter strings, accuracy rates were very high so drift rates we high and quite variable.

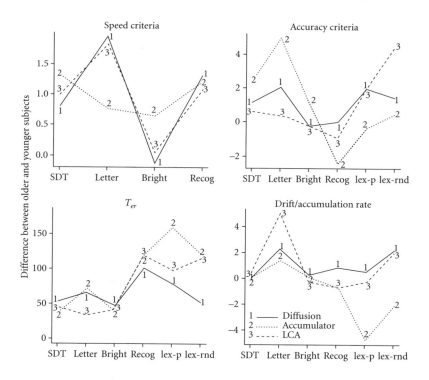

Fig. 1.6 Differences in parameter values between older and young subjects. SDT represents the signal detection task, "letter" represents the letter discrimination task with masking, "bright" represents the brightness discrimination task with masking, "recog" represents the recognition memory task, and "lex" represents the lexical decision task where "lex-p" is the experiment with pseudoword nonwords and "lex-rnd" is the experiment with random letter string nonwords.

Thus, although the difference was close to two in Figure 1.6, it was not significant. For the LCA model, the results were the same ($t(3) = 7.41$ for the letter discrimination task). For the accumulator model, the results were also the same except that the rate of accumulation was larger in the lexical decision task for the older than the young subjects ($t(7) = 4.82$ for lexical decision, $t(3) = 2.71, p = 0.073$, significant by 1-tailed test for masked letter discrimination). However, the accumulator model did not fit the lexical decision experiments particularly well because it was unable to accommodate error response times shorter than correct response times.

Response criteria

Figure 1.6 (top two panels) shows the differences in response criteria between older and young subjects with speed instructions in the left-hand panel and accuracy instructions in the right-hand panel. There were both speed and accuracy instructions in the first four experiments. The criteria for the last two experiments, lexical decision experiments, are shown on the right-hand panel along with accuracy criteria for the other experiments because subjects tend to more conservative criteria in the lexical decision task without speed instructions.

For the diffusion model, boundary separation was larger for older than young subjects except with both speed and accuracy instructions in the brightness discrimination task and accuracy instructions in the recognition memory task. For the accumulator model, the decision criteria were higher for older than young subjects with both speed and accuracy instructions in the signal detection, letter discrimination, and brightness discrimination experiments, and with speed instructions in the recognition memory experiment. With accuracy instructions in the recognition memory experiment, the decision criteria were lower for older than young subjects. The differences in criteria were small for the lexical decision experiments, with the older subjects criteria higher in one experiment and lower in the other than the young subjects.

For the LCA model, the decision criteria behaved similarly to the criteria for the diffusion model. The only exceptions were a small difference between the two models for the recognition memory task with accuracy instructions and the much higher criteria for older compared to young subjects in the lexical decision experiment with random letter strings as the nonwords.

Nondecision component of RT

The bottom left panel of Figure 1.6 shows how much slower older subjects were than young subjects in the nondecision components of RT. The estimates of T_{er} averaged 69, 91, and 78 ms longer for older subjects for the diffusion, accumulator, and LCA models, respectively. The estimate of the nondecision components is a measure of the same quantity for each of the models (unlike the estimates of decision criteria and drift or accumulation rates), and correlations between the models' estimates across the six experiments can show the extent to which a large value of T_{er} for one model corresponds to a large value of T_{er} for another model. Tables 1.1, 1.3, and 1.5 provide the results that were used to compute the correlations. The correlation between the T_{er} values for the diffusion and accumulator models was 0.96, between the diffusion and LCA models 0.88, and between the accumulator and LCA models, 0.84. Correlations were also computed between the ranges of the nondecision component (s_t); they were 0.81, 0.77, and 0.59, for the three comparisons, respectively. Larger values of T_{er} would be expected to have larger values of s_t and hence larger correlations, so the correlations between s_t and T_{er} were also computed; they were 0.62, 0.52, and 0.72 for the diffusion, accumulator, and LCA models, respectively. Thus, the models produce qualitatively similar accounts of the duration of the nondecision components of processing (and therefore the duration of the decision process) across experiments.

Summary

Within the frameworks of the models, the main effects of aging on cognitive processes were that decision criteria were higher for older subjects in most experiments and that the nondecision components of RT were somewhat longer. However, despite the more conservative decision criteria and slower nondecision processes, there was little difference between the older and young subjects in the rate of accumulation of information, that is, little difference in the quality of information available from the stimuli, except with masked letter stimuli that contain high spatial frequency information. Although there were differences in the parameter values that represent the components of processing across the three models, the differences occurred in only a few cases and they were only minor. In general, the behavioral differences in RT and accuracy between young and older adults had the same sources in all three models.

Goodness of fit

When the models were fit to the experimental data, the chi-square values used as the criteria for goodness of fit used the same weights for each experimental condition because the data were averaged over experiments (see above and Ratcliff & Smith, 2004). The minimum X^2 values are shown in Table 1.7 for each model for each experiment. To more easily compare the models across experiments, the X^2 values in Table 1.7 were divided by the number of conditions in an experiment so that they were adjusted to approximately the same range (Experiment 1: 8; Experiment 2: 8; Experiment 3: 18; Experiment 4: 18; Experiment 5: 4; Experiment 6: 4) and the results are shown in Figure 1.7. The means of the adjusted X^2 values in Figure 1.7 are 2.95, 3.94, and 3.91, for the diffusion, accumulator, and LCA models, respectively. The diffusion model fit 7 of the 12 data sets best, the accumulator model fit 1 best, and the LCA model fit 4 best (see Table 1.7 and Figure 1.7). As mentioned above, no one model fit the data best in every case and every model fit the data best in at least one case.

To show samples of the qualities of the fits, Figure 1.4 shows fits of all three models to the QPFs for young subjects for the letter discrimination experiment and Figure 1.5 shows fits for older subjects for the recognition memory experiment.

For the letter discrimination experiment with speed instructions, each of the models fit well with the accumulator model missing a little in the 0.9 quantile for correct responses and the LCA model missing a little for error RTs for the 0.9 quantile. For accuracy instructions, the diffusion model fit the error RT distributions better than the other models and it fit the RT distributions for correct responses in the 0.9 quantiles a little worse than the other models. The accumulator model missed the 0.9 quantile RTs for both errors and correct responses, and the LCA model fit correct response RTs better than the diffusion model but fit error RTs worse than either of the other models.

For the recognition memory experiment, the diffusion model captures the leading edges of the RT distributions (the 0.1 quantile RTs) and misses only in the 0.9 quantiles for "new" responses. The accumulator model misses all the quantiles for "new" responses with accuracy instructions, especially the 0.1 quantile. The LCA model misses the 0.1 quantiles for "new" responses (and for "old" responses to a lesser extent) with accuracy instructions, and the model

Table 1.7 X^2 values for diffusion, accumulator, and leaky competing accumulator models for signal detection, letter discrimination, brightness discrimination, recognition memory, and lexical decision experiments for older and young subjects

	SDT young	SDT older	Letter young	Letter older	Bright young	Bright older	Recogn young	Recogn older	Lex pseud young	Lex pseud older	Lex rand young	Lex rand older
Diffusion	13.70	13.28	7.47	5.34	84.33	119.14	85.25	64.90	16.66	11.59	7.94	6.81
Accumulator	11.31	32.02	22.38	12.99	70.97	110.41	97.76	60.92	22.64	16.21	22.38	12.74
LCA	9.25	17.09	15.70	13.59	59.98	55.12	150.44	151.90	13.91	20.09	14.15	18.96

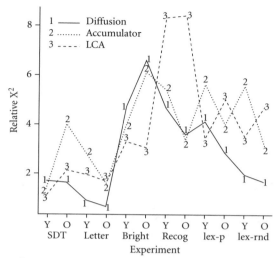

Fig. 1.7 Relative X^2 values for the accumulator, LCA, and diffusion models. The X^2 values in Table 7 were divided by the number of conditions in each experiment and plotted as a function of experiment. Y = young subjects, O = older subjects, and SDT represents the signal detection task, "letter" represents the letter discrimination task with masking, "bright" represents the brightness discrimination task with masking, "recog" represents the recognition memory task, and "lex" represents the lexical decision task where "lex-p" is the experiment with pseudoword nonwords and "lex-rnd" is the experiment with random letter string nonwords.

fits the higher quantiles for "new" responses but misses them for "old" responses.

Ratcliff and Smith (2004) provided similar comparisons across three experiments using young subjects only. One was Experiment 1 from this chapter (signal detection for young subjects), the second was a lexical decision experiment with speed and accuracy instructions, and the third was a recognition memory experiment that manipulated the proportion of old and new items. They found similar results: the diffusion model fit somewhat better on average than the accumulator and LCA models.

General discussion

Theoretical development in the domain of models for two-choice decisions has matured over the last few years. Existing models have been augmented so that they can now overcome some of the seemingly insurmountable theoretical problems of the past. Also, new models have been developed. In parallel with theoretical development, large data sets have become available against which the models can be tested. In this chapter, we applied three models to 12 sets of data from five different tasks, the first comparison of sequential sampling models for two-choice decisions with such a large number of data sets. In past studies, usually only a single model has been evaluated, fit to only one or two sets of data.

What we found is that the diffusion model gave the best overall account of the data. The LCA and accumulator models fit the data about equally well, about 30% worse than the diffusion model (in terms of the χ^2 measure we used). Even though the accumulator model fit about as well as the LCA model, no way has yet been found to allow it to predict RTs for errors shorter than RTs for correct responses. Based on this qualitative problem, it can be rejected. In contrast, even though the LCA model fit worse on average than the diffusion model, there are no qualitative grounds for choosing one over the other.

One concern that might have been raised about the application of the diffusion model to aging data is that any conclusions about the effects of aging on cognitive processes might be specific to the diffusion model. By fitting all three models, we have shown that the general conclusions are the same from all three. For all three models, in five of the six experiments, there was no difference in the rate of accumulation of evidence from the stimuli between young and older subjects. In most cases, the decision criteria were set more conservatively by the older subjects than the young subjects, and this was largely responsible for the longer RTs for the older subjects. There was also an increase in the duration of the nondecision component of processing for older subjects that was quite consistent across the models.

Models for simple two choice decisions have reached a degree of maturity that is rare in modeling in cognitive psychology. The models address most of the phenomena within their domains of study and they fit the phenomena quite accurately. It is now possible to critically test them against each other (Ratcliff & Smith, 2004) and they can be used to interpret the effects of aging, as studied here, and the effects of head injury on cognitive processes (e.g. Ratcliff, Perea, Coleangelo & Buchanan, 2004). In addition to these psychological investigations, the models are also being tested in computational neuroscience as simultaneous accounts of neural processes and behavioral data (e.g. Glimcher, 2003; Gold & Shadlen, 2001; Platt, 2002; Ratcliff, Segraves, & Cherian, 2003; Roitman & Shadlen, 2002; Smith & Ratcliff, 2004). At this point in the evolution of the models, they offer an explanation of processing that encompasses applications to group and individual differences as well as to the neurophysiological underpinnings of cognition.

References

Ashby, F. G. (1983). A biased random walk model of two choice reaction times. *Journal of Mathematical Psychology*, **27**, 277–97.

Audley, R. J., & Mercer, A. (1968). The relation between decision time and the relative response frequency in a blue-green discrimination. *British Journal of Mathematical and Statistical Psycology*, **21**, 183–92.

Audley, R. J., & Pike, A. R. (1965). Some alternative stochastic models of choice. *The British Journal of Mathematical and Statistical Psychology*, **18**, 207–225.

Busemeyer, J. R., & Townsend, J. T. (1993). Decision field theory: A dynamic–cognitive approach to decision making in an uncertain environment. *Psychological Review*, **100**, 432–459.

Coyne, A. C. (1981). Age difference and practice in forward visual masking. *Journal of Gerontology*, **36**, 730–732.

Diederich, A. (1995). Intersensory facilitation of reaction time: Evaluation of counter and diffusion coactivation models. *Journal of Mathematical Psychology*, **41**, 260–274.

Diederich, A. (1997). Dynamic stochastic models for decision making under time constraints. *Journal of Mathematical Psychology*, **41**, 260–274.

Fozard, J. L (1990). Vision and hearing in aging. In J. E. Birren & K. W. Schaie, (Eds.), *Handbook of the psychology of aging* (pp. 150–170). San Diego, CA: Academic Press.

Glimcher, P. W. (2003). The neurobiology of visual-saccadic decision making. *Annual Review of Neuroscience*, **26**, 133–179.

Gold, J. N., & Shadlen, M. N. (2001). Neural computations that underlie decisions about sensory stimuli. *Trends in Cognitive Science*, **4**, 10–16.

Heuer, H. (1987). Visual discrimination and response programming. *Psychological Research*, **49**, 91–98.

Kucera, H., & Francis, W. (1967). *Computational analysis of present-day American English*. Providence, RI: Brown University Press.

LaBerge, D. A. (1962). A recruitment theory of simple behavior. *Psychometrika*, **27**, 375–396.

Link, S. W. (1975). The relative judgement theory of two choice response time. *Journal of Mathematical Psychology*, **12**, 114–35.

Link, S. W., & Heath, R. A. (1975). A sequential theory of psychological discrimination. *Psychometrika*, **40**, 77–105.

Luce, R. D. (1986). *Response times*. New York: Oxford University Press.

Nelder, J. A., & Mead, R. (1965). A simplex method for function minimization. *Computer Journal*, **7**, 308–13.

Owsley, C., Sekuler, R., & Siemsen, D. (1983). Contrast sensitivity through adulthood. *Vision Research*, **23**, 689–699.

Pike, R. (1973). Response latency models for signal detection. *Psychological Review*, **80**, 53–68.

Pike, R., & Ryder, P. (1973). Response latencies in the yes/no detection task: An assessment of two basic models. *Perception & Psychophysics*, **13**, 224–32.

Ratcliff, R. (1978). A theory of memory retrieval. *Psychological Review*, **85**, 59–108.

Ratcliff, R. (1979). Group reaction time distributions and an analysis of distribution statistics. *Psychological Bulletin*, **86**, 446–461.

Ratcliff, R. (1981). A theory of order relations in perceptual matching. *Psychological Review,* **88**, 552–572.

Ratcliff, R. (1985). Theoretical interpretations of speed and accuracy of positive and negative responses. *Psychological Review,* **92**, 212–225.

Ratcliff, R. (1988). Continuous versus discrete information processing: Modeling the accumulation of partial information. *Psychological Review,* **95**, 238–255.

Ratcliff, R. (2002). A diffusion model account of reaction time and accuracy in a brightness discrimination task: Fitting real data and failing to fit fake but plausible data. *Psychonomic Bulletin and Review,* **9**, 278–91.

Ratcliff, R., Gomez, P., & McKoon, G. (2004). Diffusion model account of lexical decision. *Psychological Review,* **111**, 159–182.

Ratcliff, R., Perea, M., Coleangelo, A. & Buchanan, L. (2004). A diffusion model account of normal and impaired readers. *Brain & Cognition,* **55**, 374–82.

Ratcliff, R., & Rouder, J. F. (1998). Modeling response times for two-choice decisions. *Psychological Science,* **9**, 347–356.

Ratcliff, R., & Rouder, J. F. (2000). A diffusion model account of masking in two-choice letter identification. *Journal of Experimental Psychology: Human Perception and Performance,* **26**, 127–140.

Ratcliff, R., Segraves, M., & Cherian, A. (2003). A comparison of macaque behavior and superior colliculus neuronal activity to predictions from models of simple two-choice decisions. *Journal of Neurophysiology,* **90**, 1392–1407.

Ratcliff, R., & Smith, P. L. (2004). A comparison of sequential sampling models for two-choice reaction time. *Psychological Review,* **111**, 333–367.

Ratcliff, R., Thapar, A., Gomez, P., & McKoon, G. (2004). A diffusion model analysis of the effects of aging on lexical decision. *Psychology and Aging,* **19**, 278–89.

Ratcliff, R., Thapar, A., & McKoon, G. (2001). The effects of aging on reaction time in a signal detection task. *Psychology and Aging,* **16**, 323–341.

Ratcliff, R., Thapar, A., & McKoon, G. (2004). A diffusion model analysis of the effects of aging on recognition memory. *Journal of Memory and Language,* **50**, 408–424.

Ratcliff, R., Thapar, A., & McKoon, G. (2003). A diffusion model analysis of the effects of aging on brightness discrimination. *Perception and Psychophysics,* **65**, 523–535.

Ratcliff, R., & Tuerlinckx, F. (2002). Estimating the parameters of the diffusion model: Approaches to dealing with contaminant reaction times and parameter variability. *Psychonomic Bulletin and Review,* **9**, 438–481.

Ratcliff, R., Van Zandt, T., & McKoon, G. (1999). Connectionist and diffusion models of reaction time. *Psychological Review,* **106**, 261–300.

Roe, R. M., Busemeyer, J. R., & Townsend, J. T. (2001). Multialternative decision field theory: A dynamic connectionist model of decision-making. *Psychological Review,* **108**, 370–392.

Roitman, J. D., & Shadlen, M. N. (2002). Responses of neurons in the lateral interparietal area during a combined visual discrimination reaction time task. *Journal of Neuroscience,* **22**, 9475–9489.

Smith, P. L. (1995). Psychophysically principled models of visual simple reaction time. *Psychological Review,* **102**, 567–91.

Smith, P. L., & Ratcliff, R. (2004). The psychology and neurobiology of simple decisions. *Trends in Neuroscience,* **27**, 161–168.

Smith, P. L., & Vickers, D. (1988). The accumulator model of two-choice discrimination. *Journal of Mathematical Psychology,* **32**, 135–168.

Spear, P. D. (1993). Minireview: Neural bases of visual deficits during aging. *Vision Research,* **33**, 2589–2609.

Thapar, A., Ratcliff, R., & McKoon, G. (2003). A diffusion model analysis of the effects of aging on letter discrimination. *Psychology and Aging,* **18**, 415–429.

Thomas, E. A. C., & Ross, B. H. (1980). On appropriate procedures for combining probability distributions within the same family. *Journal of Mathematical Psychology,* **21**, 136–152.

Usher, M., & McClelland, J. L. (2001). The time course of perceptual choice: The leaky, competing accumulator model. *Psychological Review,* **108**, 550–592.

Van Zandt, T., & Ratcliff, R. (1995). Statistical mimicking of reaction time distributions: Mixtures and parameter variability. *Psychonomic Bulletin and Review,* **2**, 20–54.

Vickers, D. (1970). Evidence for an accumulator model of psychophysical discrimination. *Ergonomics,* **13**, 37–58.

Vickers, D. (1978). An adaptive module of simple judgements. In J. Requin (Ed.), *Attention and performance, Part* VII. (pp. 599–618). Hillsdale, NJ: Erlbaum.

Vickers, D. (1979). *Decision processes in visual perception.* New York: Academic Press.

Vickers, D., Caudrey, D., & Willson, R. J. (1971). Discriminating between the frequency of occurrence of two alternative events. *Acta Psychologica,* **35**, 151–172.

Chapter 2

Inconsistency in response time as an indicator of cognitive aging

David F. Hultsch, Michael A. Hunter,
Stuart W. S. MacDonald,
and Esther Strauss

Abstract

In this chapter, we consider the proposition that intraindividual variability in speed of performance is a useful indicator of cognitive aging. In particular we review recent research that examines both group differences and longitudinal changes in performance inconsistency on reaction time tasks. This literature suggests that: (a) Greater inconsistency in physical and cognitive performance is observed for older compared with younger adults; (b) Greater inconsistency is observed for individuals with neurological disorders, even at the preclinical stages of the illness, compared with neurologically intact adults; (c) There are consistent and stable individual differences in inconsistency across tasks and time intervals, respectively; (d) There are cross-domain links between inconsistency on cognitive tasks and both level and variability of physical performance; (e) Greater inconsistency is associated with poorer levels of performance on cognitive tasks and measures of intelligence; (f) Greater inconsistency is associated with proximity to death, particularly for older adults and individuals who will ultimately die of cardiovascular illnesses;

Research from our laboratory reported in this chapter was supported by grants to David Hultsch from the Canadian Institutes of Health Research, to Esther Strauss from the Alzheimer Society of Canada, and to Roger Dixon from the National Institute on Aging. Stuart MacDonald was supported by a research fellowship from the Canadian Institutes of Health Research. Preparation of this chapter and travel to the related conference was also supported by a Research Unit Infrastructure Grant to the University of Victoria Center on Aging by the Michael Smith Foundation for Health Research.

(g) Longitudinal evidence indicates that inconsistency increases with age, and changes in inconsistency covary with changes in cognition; (h) Longitudinal evidence also shows that inconsistency increases as the individual approaches death; and (i) Individual differences in inconsistency are predictive of level of cognitive performance and mortality over and above mean level influences. We conclude that measures of intraindividual variability may be plausible behavioral indicators of cognitive aging.

Introduction

Researchers examining aging-related changes in cognition have often used average response time (RT) on relatively simple laboratory tasks to index performance. Normal aging is characterized by slowing in the rate of information processing; indeed such slowing represents the most prominent and well-replicated manifestation of cognitive aging (Birren & Fisher, 1995). Some theorists, notably Salthouse (1996), have argued that information processing speed is a basic resource of the cognitive system, and that age changes in processing speed mediate aging-related declines in performance on more complex cognitive tasks (see also Cerella, 1990; Myerson, Hale, Wagstaff, Poon, & Smith, 1990). Other theorists, notably Rabbitt (2000), have critiqued such global accounts of cognitive aging, arguing that measures of RT index the efficiency of the cognitive system rather than representing its fundamental building blocks (see also Fisk & Fisher, 1994; Mayr & Kliegl, 1993). Moreover, it has been shown that important aspects of RT data are not captured by measures of average speed (Ratcliff, 1978; Ratcliff, Spieler, & McKoon, 2000). In particular, several writers have argued recently that intraindividual variability of RT and other measures carries information independent of level of performance and should be considered in constructing theories of cognitive aging (e.g. Dixon & Hertzog, 1996; Hultsch & MacDonald, 2004; Lindenberger, Li, & Brehemer, 2002; Rabbitt, 2000).

Intraindividual variability in this context refers to relatively rapid and transient shifts in behavior that may be distinguished from relatively enduring changes such as learning or development (Nesselroade & Featherman, 1997). More specifically, in the cognitive domain, Hultsch and colleagues (Hultsch, MacDonald, Hunter, Levy-Bencheton, & Strauss, 2000; Hultsch, MacDonald, & Dixon, 2002) have labeled the phenomenon *inconsistency* and operationally defined it as within-person fluctuations in RT performance across trials within a session or across multiple sessions spanning somewhat longer intervals (e.g. hours, days, weeks). Although intraindividual variability in performance over short intervals has been considered traditionally to indicate unreliability of measurement, recent evidence suggests that it represents a stable characteristic of individuals that shows consistent differences across groups as well as associations with other cognitive and physical measures (Hultsch & MacDonald, 2004; Rabbitt, 2000).

Intraindividual variability may be of particular relevance to researchers interested in cognitive aging because several theorists have proposed that performance inconsistency at the behavioral level may be an indicator of central nervous system (CNS) functioning. For example, it has been suggested that inconsistency in RT could be caused by random errors or neural "noise" in the transmission of signals in the CNS (Hendrickson, 1982). This view maps onto hypotheses in the gerontological literature that propose aging-related cognitive declines are a function of increased information loss due to neural noise (Crossman & Szafran, 1956; Myerson et al. 1990; Welford, 1965) or random breaks in neural networks (Cerella, 1990). More recently, Li and her colleagues have suggested that the signal-to-noise ratio of neural information processing may be regulated by the functioning of catecholaminergic neurotransmitters such as epinephrine, norepinephrine, and dopamine (Li & Lindenberger, 1999; Li, Lindenberger, & Sikström, 2001). At the psychological level, theorists have suggested that RT inconsistency may be a function of lapses of attention (e.g. Bunce, Warr, & Cochrane, 1993), failures of executive control (e.g. West, Murphy, Armillio, Craik, & Stuss, 2002), or more conservative settings of response criteria (Ratcliff, Thapar, & McKoon, 2001). We take no position on the potential neurobiological or psychological mechanisms that may determine or influence behavioral inconsistency in performance. Similarly, we do not propose that inconsistency reflects some fundamental performance characteristic of the CNS that accounts for all or most of the aging-related variance in cognitive functioning. Rather, following Rabbitt (2000), we suggest that it is more prudent at this stage of investigation into the phenomenon to view performance inconsistency as an indicator of processing efficiency. To the extent that this is the case, it may be a potentially useful indicator of cognitive aging. In this chapter, we review empirical evidence in support of this modest proposal.

We begin by examining evidence for group differences in performance variability across trials on RT tasks. In introducing this section, we discuss issues related to the measurement of intraindividual variability in performance, and in particular, the need to address potential confounds related to group differences in level of performance and systematic time-related changes associated with practice, fatigue, and the like. We then examine associations between performance inconsistency and chronological age, neurological status, and physical functioning. The next section examines individual differences in inconsistency. We review evidence indicating that inconsistency shows a pattern of relative consistency across tasks and stability over time, suggesting that the magnitude of within-person variability appears to be a characteristic of the individual. The next three sections focus on the extent to which inconsistency is related to various outcomes. Specifically, we examine the association of inconsistency with cognitive performance and mortality. We focus on longitudinal evidence which addresses the critical question of whether changes in inconsistency are associated with changes in cognition or distance to death. In the last of these sections, we examine whether measures of variability are predictive of outcomes independent of overall level (speed) of performance. The final section of the chapter summarizes the evidence reviewed and presents our conclusion that inconsistency is an important indicator of cognitive aging.

Age differences

If intraindividual variability in RT is an indicator of either neural or information processing efficiency, we would obviously expect to observe greater inconsistency for older adults compared with younger adults. Indeed, several studies have shown that inconsistency across trials on RT tasks increases with age (Anstey, 1999; Fozard, Vercruyssen, Reynolds, Hancock, & Quilter 1994; Salthouse, 1993), although some researchers have suggested that this increase can be accounted for by individual differences in mean-level performance (Salthouse, 1993; Shammi, Bosman, & Stuss, 1998). In addition to inconsistency across trials within a session, intraindividual variability may be observed across multiple testing occasions. For example, Li, Aggen, Nesselroade, and Baltes (2001) examined intraindividual variability for a set of sensorimotor and memory variables across 13 biweekly sessions in a sample of adults aged 64–86 years. They found that variability in performance was positively correlated with age for most of the sensorimotor measures and one of the memory measures.

One issue that has not been adequately addressed in many studies examining age differences in performance inconsistency is the impact of age differences in overall speed of performance and systematic changes in speed related to practice and other time-related processes. The simplest and most frequently used index of intraindividual variability is the intraindividual standard deviation (ISD) computed across time (trials or occasions). However, computation of ISDs using raw-score responses (e.g. reaction time latencies) is problematic. Performance inconsistency is defined as intraindividual variability that is unrelated to between-subject effects as well as systematic within-subject time-related effects (Hultsch & MacDonald, 2004; Nesselroade & Featherman, 1997). Group differences in average level of performance as well as systematic changes over time (e.g. across trials or occasions) associated with practice or different materials therefore represent potential confounds for the analysis of intraindividual variability. For example, older adults may exhibit increased ISDs computed on raw RT scores simply as a function of their slower average response latencies (i.e. higher mean RTs are typically associated with higher standard deviations). Similarly, practice often markedly reduces response times and may do so at a differential rate for different age groups.

There are multiple ways to address these potential problems (Hultsch & MacDonald, 2004). For example, the problem of practice effects could be addressed by examining performance following performance asymptote (i.e. computing ISDs only for trials or sessions over which no further improvement in performance is discernable; for example, Rabbitt, Osman, Moore, & Stollery, 2001). Similarly, the problem of group differences in average performance could be addressed if it was possible to identify a task on which younger and older adults' average level of performance was equivalent. Although these approaches are useful, a more practical solution to the problem is to statistically remove the effects of potential confounds. A procedure proposed by Hultsch and his colleagues (Hultsch & MacDonald, 2004; Hultsch et al. 2000) removes overall group and time-related effects from subjects' performance data prior to computing ISDs. Using a person by time data matrix, split-plot analysis of variance (ANOVA) is used to partial age group, gender, and occasion effects and all their interactions by regressing each dependent measure on these potential confounding variables. This approach to investigating inconsistency amounts to analyzing the residuals from a Groups by Occasions mixed-model ANOVA where all group and occasion effects and their interactions are partialed from subjects' scores prior to computing ISDs. If several performance tasks are included in a study, the resulting residual or purified scores are first converted to T-scores to permit comparisons across tasks in the same metric. Notably, it has been demonstrated that even though all systematic effects are partialed from the data using this technique (i.e. $M = 50$ for groups averaged over occasions, occasions averaged over groups, and each group by occasion cell), substantial individual differences in intraindividual variability remain to be explained. (e.g. see Hultsch et al. 2000, Figure 2.2).[1]

---

[1] All analyses from our laboratory reported in this chapter used this approach to computing ISD scores which was developed by our collaborator Michael Hunter.

In a recent analysis using this approach, Hultsch et al. (2002) examined age differences in RT inconsistency for younger adults (19–36 years, $n = 99$) and three groups of older adults (Young-old, 54–64 years, $n = 178$; Mid-old, 65–74 years, $n = 361$; and Old-old, 75–94 years, $n = 224$). Participants completed two basic nonverbal RT tasks (SRT and CRT) and two more complex verbal RT tasks (lexical decision and semantic decision). ISDs were computed across trials for each task according to the described procedure. As shown in Figure 2.1, greater inconsistency was observed for older compared with younger adults on all tasks, particularly for individuals over age 75. Participants in this group showed greater inconsistency than all other age groups on all tasks. Effect sizes associated with the age group differences ranged from medium to large in most case. These results, along with those from other studies, point to robust age differences that are consistent with the argument that performance inconsistency is a potential indicator of processing efficiency (even when controlling for group differences in speed and practice). However, many questions remain. Age, of course, is not an explanatory variable, and even the demonstration of age differences is not very meaningful theoretically (Perfect & Maylor, 2000). However, examination of other group and individual difference patterns of performance inconsistency can help shed more light on the issue.

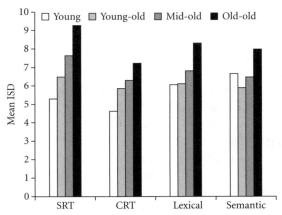

Fig. 2.1 Mean trial-to-trial intraindividual standard deviation (ISD) *T*-scores for four RT tasks by age group. SRT = simple reaction time; CRT = choice reaction time. Young = 19–36 years, Young-old = 54–64 years, Mid-old = 65–74 years, Old-old = 75–94 years. From figure 2.3, Hultsch, D. F., MacDonald, S. W. S., & Dixon, R. A. (2002). Variability in reaction time performance of younger and older adults. *Journal of Gerontology: Psychological Sciences*, 57B, P101–P115. Copyright © The Gerontological Society of America. Reproduced by permission of the publisher.

Neurological status

To support the hypothesis that short-term fluctuations in performance represent an indicator of CNS functioning, it is necessary (but not sufficient) to demonstrate associations between measures of inconsistency and neurological status. In support of this condition, there is an accumulating body of empirical work that shows inconsistency in cognitive performance is prevalent in individuals with various types of neurological disturbance including epilepsy (Bruhn & Parsons, 1977), mental retardation (Wade, Newell, & Wallace, 1978), traumatic brain injury (Collins & Long, 1996; Stuss, Pogue, Buckle, & Bondar, 1994), Parkinson's disease (Burton, Strauss, Hultsch, Moll, & Hunter, in press), and dementia (Gordon & Carson, 1990; Hultsch et al. 2000; Knotek, Bayles, & Kaszniak, 1990).

In an initial study examining this issue, Hultsch et al. (2000) contrasted healthy adults with individuals who were neurologically impaired but otherwise healthy (mild dementia patients) and individuals who were neurologically intact but experiencing significant somatic disturbance (adults with arthritis). This comparison was used to help determine whether inconsistency is primarily a CNS phenomenon, or whether it is also driven by other transient somatic conditions. A total of 45 adults ranging in age from 57–87 years of age participated in the study. In addition to demographic and benchmark cognitive status measures, the participants completed two basic RT tasks (SRT and 2-CRT) and two more complex recognition memory tasks (word and story recognition). Participants were tested on these tasks on four separate occasions separated by about one week. ISDs were computed both across trials within sessions (for each of the four sessions) and across the four sessions (based on the average RT for each session). Figure 2.2 shows the mean trial-to-trial ISD score on the four tasks for each of the three groups. For each task, the dementia group showed more inconsistency in performance than the healthy and arthritic groups, which did not differ. The same pattern of results was observed for the week-to-week ISD scores, although the magnitude of inconsistency across occasions was only about half that seen across trials. These results suggest that inconsistency may be a feature of neurological disturbance rather than somatic conditions such as pain (although a wider range of somatic conditions and accompanying levels of severity remain to be explored).

Many neurological disturbances manifest over an extended transitional or preclinical phase. This phase has been variously defined and labeled (e.g. mild cognitive impairment, MCI; cognitive impairment no dementia; preclinical Alzheimer's disease). Nevertheless, in all cases, the phase is characterized by detectable performance deficits in the context of generally preserved global

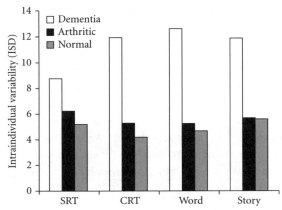

Fig. 2.2 Mean trial-to-trial intraindividual standard deviation (ISD) *T*-scores by group and task. SRT = simple reaction time; CRT = 2-choice reaction time. From figure 2.2, Hultsch, D. F., MacDonald, S. W. S., Hunter, M. A., Levy-Bencheton, J., & Strauss, E. (2000). Intraindividual variability in cognitive performance in older adults: Comparison of adults with mild dementia, adults with arthritis, and healthy adults. *Neuropsychology*, 14, 588–598. Copyright © 2000 by the American Psychological Association. Reprinted with permission.

cognitive functioning and functional abilities (Palmer, Fragtigloni, & Winblad, 2003). An important question is whether greater performance inconsistency is also observed during this preclinical phase, or whether it is only apparent once the disturbance has progressed to the point that diagnosis is possible. In a recent examination of this question, Lentz, Strauss, Hultsch, and Hunter (2003) assessed performance inconsistency for two age groups (64–73 years, $n = 170$ and 74–92 years, $n = 135$) of community-dwelling adults varying in cognitive status. Although none of the participants was diagnosed with any neurological condition, two MCI groups were identified: Participants were classified as MCI-mild if they scored one or more standard deviations (SD) below their age and education group mean on one of five cognitive reference measures indexing perceptual speed, fluid reasoning, episodic memory, verbal fluency, and vocabulary. Participants were classified as MCI-moderate if they scored one or more SD below their group mean on two or more of the reference tasks. The remaining participants were considered not cognitively impaired (NCI). Participants completed three RT tasks of varying difficulty: SRT, 4-CRT, and 4-CRT in which they had to respond to the stimulus from the previous trial (CRT-1Back task). ISDs were computed across trials for each of the three tasks. The results indicated that inconsistency varied with cognitive status. For all tasks, the MCI-moderate group was more variable than the MCI-mild group, which in turn, was more variable than the NCI group. For two of the tasks (SRT and CRT-1Back), age and cognitive status interacted such that the cognitive status differences were exacerbated in the older group compared with the younger group. Specifically, increased inconsistency was observed for the MCI-mild group relative to the NCI group in the older adults but not the younger adults. The interaction for the CRT-1Back task is shown in Figure 2.3. These results suggest that performance inconsistency may be associated with very mild levels of cognitive impairment, particularly in late life.

In a more differentiated look at this issue, Christensen et al. (in press) recently examined trial-to-trial variability in RT performance for individuals meeting various definitions of preclinical cognitive impairment compared with individuals not meeting such criteria. The age range in this study was restricted (60–64 years), and the subsample meeting diagnostic criteria ($n = 68$) was small relative to the nondiagnosed group ($n = 2671$). Nevertheless, the results showed that participants with a diagnosis of cognitive impairment had slower RT and increased intraindividual variability. For the diagnostic subgroups, this finding was observed for participants classified as MCI as specified by Petersen et al. (1999) and Age Associated Cognitive Decline as defined by Levy (1994), but not Age Associated Memory Impairment (Crook et al. 1986).

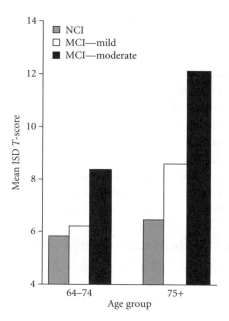

Fig. 2.3 Mean trial-to-trial intraindividual standard deviation (ISD) *T*-scores for CRT 1-Back task by age and cognitive status group. NCI = not cognitively impaired; MCI = mild cognitive impairment.

Physical functioning

Markers of physical functioning also represent useful proxies of CNS integrity. In keeping with the variability hypothesis, it follows that measures of inconsistency in physical performance should (a) show increased within-task inconsistency with increasing age, (b) share systematic negative associations with measures of level of cognitive performance, and (c) show a pattern of positive correlations with measures of inconsistency in cognitive performance. Li et al. (2001) examined intraindividual variability across multiple biweekly sessions for sensorimotor measures of balance and gait and reported findings consistent with the first two expectations. Variability in sensorimotor performance increased as a function of age and was negatively correlated with mean text and spatial memory performance. Similarly, Strauss, MacDonald, Hunter, Moll, and Hultsch (2002) found that individuals who fluctuated more from week-to-week on measures of diastolic blood pressure and nondominant hand finger tapping speed performed worse on measures of word and story recall. In a related finding, Anstey (1999) reported that level of performance for select sensory (vision, hearing, and vibration sense) and physical (grip strength, peak expiratory flow) measures was associated with age-related increases in intraindividual variability for several cognitive measures. Informing the last expectation, Strauss et al. (2002) observed that inconsistency in physical performance was related to variability in cognitive functioning. However, in most cases, these cross-domain relations were observed for participants diagnosed with dementia but not for an arthritic group (non-neurological somatic disturbance) and a healthy control group. Importantly, the cross-domain links observed between increased inconsistency in physical and cognitive performance did not generalize to comparisons of variability between cognitive performance and self-perceived affect and beliefs. This dissociation between patterns of inconsistency for physical versus affect measures lends further support to claims that sources of inconsistency may differentially reflect endogenous as opposed to exogenous factors. Moreover, the positive manifold of correlations between inconsistency in the cognitive and physical domains serves to buffer against criticisms that inconsistency reflects mere error variance in the psychometric sense. Rather, measures of both cognitive and physical variability may serve as important behavioral markers of neurological integrity (Strauss et al. 2002).

Individual differences in inconsistency

If inconsistency in performance is the result of relatively general neurobiological influences, one would expect to observe relative stability of individual differences in inconsistency over time and positive associations among different measures of inconsistency. Three patterns of results in line with this view have been observed in several studies (e.g. Fuentes, Hunter, Strauss, & Hultsch, 2001; Hultsch et al. 2002; Rabbitt et al. 2001). First, measures of inconsistency computed for a given task across different time intervals (e.g. trials versus weeks) are positively correlated (Hultsch et al. 2000; Rabbitt et al. 2001). Second, individuals who are more inconsistent on one RT task are also more inconsistent on other RT tasks. Table 2.1 shows an example of intercorrelations among measures of inconsistency in performance for four different tasks performed by a sample of older adults (Hultsch et al. 2000). The top panel of the table shows intercorrelations of trial-to-trial inconsistency averaged across four testing occasions. The last three columns of the bottom panel show intercorrelations of week-to-week inconsistency, and the first four columns of the bottom panel show the correlations of trial-to-trial and week-to week inconsistency. All but two of these correlations are significant and all are positive. Finally, there appear to be cross-domain links suggesting that greater inconsistency in cognitive functioning is associated with greater inconsistency in physical functioning, at least in individuals with neurological compromise (Strauss et al. 2002).

Thus, the magnitude of within-person variability appears to be somewhat characteristic of the individual. This is what one would expect if such variability were substantially influenced by relatively stable endogenous mechanisms

Table 2.1 Intercorrelations among measures of intraindividual variability in latency

Variable	(1)	(2)	(3)	(4)	(5)	(6)	(7)	(8)
			ISD across-trials					
(1) SRT	—							
(2) CRT	0.76[b]	—						
(3) Word	0.69[b]	0.73[b]	—					
(4) Story	0.69[b]	0.79[b]	0.90[b]	—				
			ISD across-occasions					
(5) SRT	0.58[b]	0.60[b]	0.52[b]	0.49[b]	—			
(6) CRT	0.42[b]	0.75[b]	0.51[b]	0.53[b]	0.33[a]	—		
(7) Word	0.54[b]	0.60[b]	0.71[b]	0.63[b]	0.18	0.54[b]	—	
(8) Story	0.46[b]	0.64[b]	0.62[b]	0.68[b]	0.15	0.62[b]	0.84[b]	—

[a] $p < 0.05$.   [b] $p < 0.01$.

From table 2.3, Hultsch, D. F., MacDonald, S. W. S., Hunter, M. A., Levy-Bencheton, J., and Strauss, E. (2000). Intraindividual variability in cognitive performance in older adults: Comparison of adults with mild dementia, adults with arthritis, and healthy adults. *Neuropsychology*, 14, 588–598. Copyright © 2000 by the American Psychological Association. Reprinted with permission.

such as neurological integrity rather than relatively labile exogenous influences such as pain, fatigue, and stress. Nevertheless, it is not completely clear that measures of inconsistency across different time periods and tasks reflect the same underlying determinants. For example, although Rabbitt et al. (2001) observed that measures of within- and between-session variability were positively and significantly correlated, additional analyses suggested that individual differences in within-session variability did not account for all of the variance in between-session variability. This suggests that in addition to trial-to-trial fluctuations, performance variability must also have been influenced by changes in state from one week to the next. It seems plausible that the inconsistency observed across the very short interval of trial-to-trial processing might best reflect fluctuations associated with the neurological mechanisms posited by some theorists. In contrast, inconsistency observed across longer intervals of days or weeks might also include variability related to exogenous sources of influences such as changes in pain, mood state, sleep deprivation, and stress.

Similarly, because all of the existing analyses have been conducted at the zero-order level, many questions relevant to the structure of inconsistency remain. Central among these is the question of whether it is possible to identify one or more inconsistency variables at the latent level. If inconsistency is a general phenomenon, it is possible that multiple measures of inconsistency obtained from tasks varying in difficulty and underlying processes may load on a single common inconsistency factor. Alternatively, it is possible that the structure of inconsistency is more adequately described by multiple factors reflecting variations in task complexity or processing requirements.

Predicting cognitive performance

Significant increases in performance variability are seen with increasing age and appear to be moderated by neurological dysfunction and sensorimotor decline. Not surprisingly, then, greater intraindividual variability is associated with lower levels of general intelligence (Jensen, 1982; Rabbitt et al. 2001) and poorer level of performance on multiple cognitive tasks (e.g. Anstey, 1999; Hultsch et al. 2002; Li et al. 2001; Rabbitt et al. 2001; Salthouse, 1993; West et al. 2002). For example, Rabbitt et al. (2001) computed both shorter- (trial-to-trial) and longer-term (week-to-week) measures of inconsistency for a letter identification task in a sample of older adults. Results indicated that greater variability was associated with poorer performance on the Culture Fair Intelligence Test for both inconsistency measures. Similarly, Hultsch et al. (2002) reported that poorer cognitive performance for measures of perceptual speed, working memory, episodic memory, and crystallized abilities was associated with greater trial-to-trial inconsistency for four different RT measures. Table 2.2 reports the correlations for the youngest (17–36 years) and oldest (75–94 years) age groups in this study, showing that significant relationships were more widespread for the older compared with the younger group.

The association of concurrent measures of inconsistency in RT and level of performance on a range of other cognitive measures is consistent with the view that performance variability might be an important indicator of cognitive aging. However, it is not very compelling evidence. A key issue is not simply whether inconsistency predicts concurrent level of cognitive performance, but whether it also predicts changes in level of cognitive performance. MacDonald, Hultsch, and Dixon (2003) recently provided a more stringent longitudinal test of the relationship between inconsistency and level of cognitive performance. This study examined whether age differences and change in inconsistency were related to changes in multiple cognitive abilities. Data were available from 446 participants from two samples of the Victoria Longitudinal Study (VLS) tested on three occasions over 6 years. Participants were divided into three age groups based on age at initial testing (55–64 years, $n = 135$; 65–74 years, $n = 225$; 75–89 years, $n = 86$). Trial-to-trial inconsistency scores for a single occasion were computed from four RT tasks: two basic nonverbal RT tasks (SRT and CRT) and two more complex verbal RT tasks (lexical decision and semantic decision). Cognitive performance was assessed using a

Table 2.2 Age-specific correlations of intraindividual variability (ISD across trials) on four RT tasks with mean performance on other cognitive measures

Cognitive measure	RT-ISD (trials)			
	SRT	CRT	Lexical	Semantic
		Young		
Perceptual speed	−0.15	−0.20[a]	−0.41[b]	−0.33[b]
Working memory	−0.02	−0.09	−0.16	−0.11
Episodic memory	−14	−0.15	−0.31[b]	−0.48[b]
Crystallized ability	−0.11	−0.04	−0.13	−0.14
		Old-old		
Perceptual speed	−0.35[b]	−0.34[b]	−0.42[b]	−0.27[b]
Working memory	−0.23[b]	−0.15[a]	−0.31[b]	−0.28[b]
Episodic memory	−0.21[b]	−0.21[b]	−0.29[b]	−0.24[b]
Crystallized ability	−0.24[b]	−0.13	−0.28[b]	−0.28[b]

[a] $p < 0.05$.   [b] $p < 0.01$.

continuum of measures spanning processes to products of cognition, including indicators of perceptual speed (identical pictures), working memory (computation span), fluid reasoning (letter series), episodic memory (word recall and story recall), and crystallized verbal ability (vocabulary).

Three related analyses shed light on the linkage between inconsistency and cognitive change. First, there were associations between inconsistency at the first wave of measurement and subsequent cognitive change over the 6 years. Significant declines in cognitive performance were observed for all six measures. However, a repeated measures analysis of covariance revealed that longitudinal declines were no longer significant after controlling for Time 1 level of inconsistency. Up to 96% of the variance associated with wave and 42% of the variance associated with the age by wave interaction was attenuated. As expected, the inconsistency covariate significantly predicted cognitive change for all six measures.

Second, there were significant within-person increases in inconsistency over the longitudinal interval, as implied by previous cross-sectional comparisons of younger and older adults (e.g. Hultsch et al. 2002). As shown in Figure 2.4, increases were observed for the oldest age group in contrast to the two younger groups, which showed relatively little change. Although SRT exhibited the most inconsistency per individual wave, 6-year changes in inconsistency as a function of age were greater for the verbal (lexical, semantic) compared with the nonverbal (SRT, CRT) tasks. This interaction may reflect a diminished ability of the oldest age group to compensate on these verbal RT tasks as crystallized abilities begin to decline in late life (Schaie, 1996). Interestingly, Deary and Der (in press) recently reported longitudinal increases in intraindividual variability in simple and choice RT for both middle-aged and older adults. Their population-based sample was probably less select than the VLS samples which may account for the observation of significant changes at younger ages.

Finally, in the most stringent test of the link between inconsistency and cognitive change, MacDonald et al. (2003) used hierarchical linear modeling to examine covariation between inconsistency and cognitive performance. As expected, they found that individuals had lower cognitive performance for waves on which they were more inconsistent relative to those on which they were less inconsistent. Over three waves of testing, increasing inconsistency was associated with declining cognitive performance for five of the six measures (all but vocabulary). Notably, these observed covariations were independent of the average linear trend across waves. For example, for the identical pictures test, the average individual identified 28.08 correct match-to-targets for Wave 1 at the sample mean on inconsistency and subsequently declined 0.57 matches for

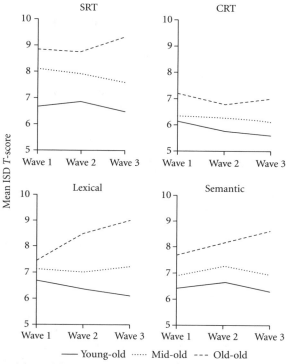

Fig. 2.4 Mean trial-to-trial intraindividual standard deviation (ISD) *T*-scores for four RT tasks by age group and longitudinal wave of testing. Young-old = 54–64 years, Mid-old = 65–74 years, Old-old = 75–94 years at Wave 1. From figure 2.3, MacDonald, S. W. S., Hultsch, D. F., and Dixon, R. A. (2003). Performance variability is related to change in cognition: Evidence from the Victoria Longitudinal Study. *Psychology and Aging*, 18, 510–523. Copyright © 2003 by the American Psychological Association. Reprinted by permission.

each increment in inconsistency. This covariation between changes in inconsistency and changes in cognition implies that the association of inconsistency and performance is not an artifact of initial level, and further supports the view that performance variability represents a useful marker of cognitive aging.

Predicting mortality

At a more global level, recent evidence suggests that inconsistency may foreshadow impending death. There is substantial evidence in the literature for an association between accelerated cognitive decline and proximity to death in older adults (Bosworth & Schaie, 1999; Johansson & Zarit, 1997; Kleemeier, 1962).

Research has also suggested that this pattern of terminal decline may be associated both with general CNS disturbances (Berg, 1996) and specific causes of death such as cardiovascular disease (MacDonald, 2003). Given this, it is plausible to expect that inconsistency in performance might be associated with proximity to death, and possibly with specific causes of death. MacDonald (2003) recently examined this question using data from the VLS. The sample consisted of a total of 707 older adults (aged 59 to 95 years at final testing), including 442 survivors who completed all waves of testing and 265 decedents who participated on at least one occasion. Decedents' date and cause of death information were obtained from Vital Statistics records of the province of British Columbia. Participants were grouped by age (59–79 years and 80–95 years) and presence or absence of cardiovascular and cerebrovascular conditions (CVD; current diagnosis for survivors and cause of death for decedents). Measures of trial-to-trial response time inconsistency were available for two speeded verbal decision tasks (lexical decision and semantic decision).

As expected, greater inconsistency at the last wave of testing was observed for older adults, individuals with CVD, and decedents. However, for both RT measures, these factors interacted. Figure 2.5 shows the results for the lexical decision task. For the younger group, inconsistency across trials was relatively comparable across mortality status and disease classification. Decedents with CVD were more variable than both survivor groups, but no other comparisons were significant. In contrast, for the older group, all pairwise comparisons were significant with the exception of the two survivor groups. These results suggest that, in addition to general neurological disturbances, specific disease processes may magnify differences in inconsistency late in life.

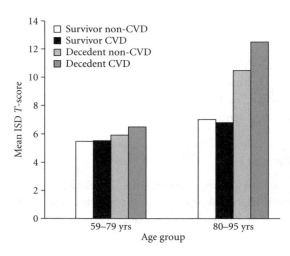

Fig. 2.5 Mean trial-to-trial intraindividual standard deviation (ISD) *T*-scores for lexical decision RT by age group, disease classification, and mortality status.
CVD = cardiovascular and cerebrovascular disease.

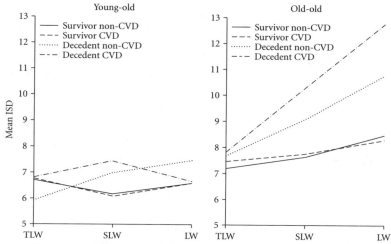

Fig. 2.6 Six-year change in mean trial-to-trial intraindividual standard deviation (ISD) *T*-scores for lexical decision RT by age group, disease classification, and mortality status. CVD = cardiovascular and cerebrovascular disease. TLW = third last wave, SLW = second-last wave, LW = last wave.

As with the previously reported analyses predicting cognition, these cross-sectional results are intriguing, but limited. More compelling evidence comes from longitudinal analyses which also indicated differential increases in performance inconsistency over time as a function of age, disease condition, and mortality status. As shown in Figure 2.6, increases in inconsistency over 6 years were observed for older individuals, and these increases were particularly notable for individuals who died of CVD-related causes. Finally, hierarchical linear modeling was used to examine the time-varying covariation between changes in inconsistency and time to death. The results showed that performance inconsistency increased per each additional year closer to death. Rates of change in inconsistency were significantly higher for older adults and for decedents. Similar to the results for cognition, these analyses point to a predictive relationship between inconsistency in RT and proximity to death.

But does it tell us anything new?

Although measures of intraindividual variability in RT are predictive of cognitive performance and proximity to death, an important question is whether measures of inconsistency predict performance independent of overall level of performance. Although our analyses partialed group differences in speed, it is still the case that variability and level of performance are correlated at the individual level. Therefore, it is important to examine the unique and shared contributions of intraindividual variability and average level estimates of performance as predictors. To the extent that inconsistency represents an influential and independent indicator of cognitive functioning, intraindividual variability estimates (ISDs) should account for a significant proportion of variance in cognitive performance over and above average level estimates (mean RT).

In one approach to this question, Hultsch et al. (2002) examined unique and shared contributions of ISD estimates and mean estimates of RT as predictors of cognitive performance. They used partial set correlation (Cohen, 1982) to examine the unique and shared influences of unpurified intraindividual mean and purified ISD estimates for two groups of RT tasks (nonverbal and verbal) as predictors of cognition, including measures of perceptual speed, working memory, episodic memory, and crystallized ability. Three set correlations were computed: regression of cognitive measures onto mean RT without partialing any variables, regression of cognitive measures onto ISD partialing out mean RT performance, and regression of cognitive measures onto mean RT performance partialing out ISD. Not surprisingly, mean and variability estimates shared a considerable amount of overlapping variance as indexed by R^2. However, mean and variability estimates also made unique predictive contributions. For both categories of RT measures, mean-level performance significantly predicted cognitive performance independent of variability. Of particular interest, inconsistency estimates (unique ISD) for nonverbal estimates (based on SRT and CRT tasks) significantly predicted variance in cognitive performance over and above mean-level influences for all four cognitive domains. Specifically, ISDs for nonverbal RT uniquely accounted for 16% (perceptual speed), 11% (working memory), 12% (episodic memory), and 20% (crystallized ability) of total R^2. Other studies have also reported that estimates of intraindividual variability predict outcome measures over and above measures of average level of performance. For example, Li et al. (2001) found that fluctuations in physical performance (walking steps) made more of a unique contribution to accounting for individual differences in text and spatial memory than the level score (number of walking steps).

Given that inconsistency is associated with specific neurological disturbances, another approach to this question is to ask whether measures of inconsistency predict group membership independent of measures of average level of performance. For example, Hultsch et al. (2000) used discriminant function analysis to estimate the extent to which dementia and nondementia groups could be differentiated by measures of inconsistency and level of performance. Separate analyses were run for four tasks using multiple indicators of inconsistency (across trials, across occasions) and level of performance (average accuracy, average latency). For all tasks, the combined performance and variability information differentiated the dementia from the nondementia groups, correctly classifying from 87% to 100% of participants depending on the task. Across-trial latency ISD was the most consistent independent predictor overall, making a significant independent contribution to classification on all four tasks. In contrast, average speed did not make a unique contribution, although it approached significance for the CRT task. Measures of average accuracy also uniquely contributed to group classification for the word and story recall tasks.

In a similar approach, MacDonald, Hultsch, and Dixon (2004) used Cox regression models to evaluate whether inconsistency provides unique predictive information about impending death beyond that contributed by mean level performance. Table 2.3 presents the results from a survival analysis predicting mortality status as a function of covariates entered in five hier-archical blocks. Demographic variables (age, education, self-reported health) and indicators of cardiovascular disease (presence of CVD, number of CVD medications) were entered in Blocks 1 and 2, respectively. Mean level cognitive performance was entered in Block 3, with separate models computed for indicators of working memory (computation span, listening span, sentence construction), episodic memory (word recall, story recall), semantic memory (fact recall), and verbal ability (vocabulary). Next, each of two indicators of average RT (lexical decision speed, semantic decision speed) were entered separately in Block 4, followed by individual entry of the corresponding RT inconsistency indicators (e.g. lexical level followed by lexical ISD) for Block 5. Not surprisingly, the results demonstrated that age, number of CVD medications, and performance inconsistency all shared significant associations with mortality status. Examination of the Block 3 results shows that no measures of mean level cognitive performance significantly predicted increased risk of mortality; the odds ratios were all approximately 1, indicating that mortality risk was unrelated to mean performance. Examination of the results from Blocks 4 and 5 indicated that both level and variability indicators were predict-ive of mortality independent of demographic indicators, CVD measures, and mean level cognitive performance. Importantly, the contrasting patterns of significance between Blocks 4 and 5 indicated that response speed level was not uniquely significant for any models that included response speed inconsistency, whereas inconsistency predicted mortality independent of level.

The results summarized above indicate that, in many cases, indicators of inconsistency predict performance or group membership above and beyond

Table 2.3 Cox regressions predicting mortality status as a function of demographic and cognitive covariates ($n = 707$)

Covariates	∃	Odds Ratio	95% CI	p
Block 1				
Age	0.026	1.026	1.008–1.045	0.005
Education	0.024	1.024	0.989–1.061	0.173
Relative health	0.013	1.013	0.864–1.188	0.870
Block 2				
CVD conditions	−0.033	0.967	0.808–1.158	0.717
CVD medications	0.229	1.257	1.065–1.483	0.007
Block 3				
Computation span[a]	−0.004	0.996	0.981–1.011	0.582
Block 4: RT level semantic	−0.020	0.981	0.967–0.994	0.006
Block 4: RT level lexical	−0.018	0.982	0.971–0.994	0.002
Block 5: RT ISD semantic	0.119	1.127	1.044–1.216	0.002
Block 5: RT ISD lexical	0.088	1.092	1.035–1.153	0.001
Listening span[a]	−0.007	0.993	0.978–1.009	0.412
Block 4: RT level semantic	−0.019	0.982	0.968–0.995	0.009
Block 4: RT level lexical	−0.017	0.983	0.971–0.994	0.004
Block 5: RT ISD semantic	0.118	1.126	1.043–1.214	0.002
Block 5: RT ISD lexical	0.088	1.092	1.035–1.152	0.001
Sentence construction	−0.003	0.997	0.985–1.008	0.592
Block 4: RT level semantic	−0.011	0.989	0.977–1.001	0.079
Block 4: RT level lexical	−0.013	0.987	0.977–0.998	0.024
Block 5: RT ISD semantic	0.068	1.070	1.001–1.145	0.048
Block 5: RT ISD Lexical	0.034	1.034	0.987–1.034	0.156
Story recall	−0.001	0.999	0.985–1.014	0.919
Block 4: RT level semantic	−0.013	0.987	0.974–1.000	0.052
Block 4: RT level lexical	−0.013	0.987	0.976–0.998	0.018
Block 5: RT ISD semantic	0.070	1.072	1.002–1.147	0.042
Block 5: RT ISD lexical	0.035	1.035	0.988–1.035	0.145
Word recall	−0.002	0.998	0.986–1.011	0.813
Block 4: RT level semantic	−0.012	0.988	0.976–1.001	0.065
Block 4: RT level lexical	−0.013	0.987	0.976–0.998	0.021
Block 5: RT ISD semantic	0.069	1.071	1.001–1.146	0.046
Block 5: RT ISD lexical	0.034	1.034	0.987–1.083	0.158

Table 2.3 (Continued)

Covariates	Ǝ	Odds Ratio	95% CI	p
Fact recall	−0.003	0.997	0.983–1.010	0.626
Block 4: RT level semantic	−0.012	0.988	0.974–1.001	0.072
Block 4: RT level lexical	−0.013	0.987	0.976–0.998	0.024
Block 5: RT ISD semantic	0.069	1.071	1.001–1.146	0.046
Block 5: RT ISD lexical	0.034	1.035	0.988–1.084	0.149
Vocabulary	0.008	1.008	0.996–1.020	0.185
Block 4: RT level semantic	−0.019	0.982	0.969–0.994	0.005
Block 4: RT level lexical	−0.016	0.984	0.973–0.994	0.003
Block 5: RT ISD semantic	0.066	1.068	1.000–1.141	0.050
Block 5: RT ISD lexical	0.047	1.048	0.999–1.099	0.055

Note: Statistical models were computed separately for each cognitive and RT measure. Results represent parameters for a given regression block controlling for the influence of all predictors on previous blocks. Mortality status was coded as either 0 (survivor) or 1 (decedent). CI = confidence interval; CVD = cardiovascular disease; RT = response time. Subjects rated their health relative to same-aged peers on a 5-point scale ranging from (0) very good to (4) very poor. CVD conditions represent self-reported presence of four cardiovascular diseases (heart disease, stroke, arteriosclerosis, and high blood pressure) for any wave of testing. CVD medications reflect self-reported use of medications prescribed to treat cardiovascular symptoms and disease (heart, chest, high blood pressure, and anticoagulants). ISD = intraindividual standard deviation. [a]N = 707 for all measures except computation span and listening span (n = 635).

indicators of mean level performance. Not all studies have found this result. For example, Christensen et al. (in press) reported that although RT variability was greater for individuals classified as MCI, it did not contribute uniquely to group membership over and above mean RT. However, the age range of this study was relatively restricted (60–64 years). Given, that we have repeatedly seen that inconsistency effects appear to be particularly robust after approximately age 75, it may be the case that effects were attenuated in this relatively young sample.

Conclusions

The results reviewed above are relatively consistent and suggest several preliminary conclusions:

1 Greater inconsistency in physical and cognitive performance is observed for older compared with younger adults;

2 Greater inconsistency is observed for individuals with neurological disorders, even at the preclinical stages of illness, compared with neurologically intact adults;

3 There are consistent and stable individual differences in inconsistency across tasks and time intervals, respectively;

4 There are cross-domain links between inconsistency on cognitive tasks and both level and variability of physical performance;

5 Greater inconsistency is associated with poorer levels of performance on cognitive tasks and measures of intelligence;

6 Greater inconsistency is associated with proximity to death, particularly for older adults and individuals who will ultimately die of cardiovascular illnesses;

7 Longitudinal evidence indicates that inconsistency increases with age, and changes in inconsistency covary with changes in cognition;

8 Longitudinal evidence also shows that inconsistency increases as the individual approaches death;

9 Individual differences in inconsistency are predictive of level of cognitive performance and mortality over and above mean level influences.

This summary of research findings suggests that measures of intraindividual variability may be plausible behavioral indicators of aging-induced deterioration of neurobiological mechanisms which compromise the integrity of the brain across a wide range of areas and functional circuitry. For example, it has been suggested that older brains may need to recruit additional resources to manage executive functions of otherwise relatively simple tasks (Cabeza, 2002; Dixon & Bäckman, 1999). Thus, even localized neural deficits may be expressed as a generalized impairment (Raz, 2000). Such changes have been hypothesized as the common cause for aging-associated losses in cognitive capacity and plasticity (Baltes & Lindenberger, 1997, Lindenberger & Baltes, 1994).

At a methodological level, these findings argue that it is important to attend to both level and variability of performance. Each of these indices provides useful information that the other does not. Because a stability orientation tends to guide research, the current task is to supplement the dominant view by increasing attention to cycles, oscillations, and fluctuations in behavior and explore how these can contribute to the development of theories of cognitive aging. At the same time, it is important not to ascribe more significance to the concept of intraindividual variability than is warranted. For example, we do not wish to suggest that behavioral inconsistency represents some type of psychological "primitive" that will account for all or most of the age-related variance in cognitive performance. Rather, we suggest that this phenomenon is an integral part of cognitive functioning that needs to be considered both in theory development and in clinical assessment.

References

Anstey, K. J. (1999). Sensorimotor and forced expiratory volume as correlates of speed, accuracy, and variability in reaction time performance in late adulthood. *Aging, Neuropsychology, and Cognition, 6,* 84–95.

Baltes, P. B., & Lindenberger, U. (1997). Emergence of a powerful connection between sensory and cognitive functions across the adult lifespan: A new window to the study of cognitive aging? *Psychology and Aging, 12,* 12–21.

Berg, S. (1996). Aging, behavior, and terminal decline. In J. E. Birren & K. W. Schaie (Eds.), *Handbook of the psychology of aging* (4th ed., pp. 323–337). New York: Springer.

Birren, J. E., & Fisher, L. M. (1995). Aging and speed of behavior: Possible consequences for psychological functioning. *Annual Review of Psychology, 46,* 329–353.

Bosworth, H. B., & Schaie, K. W. (1999). Survival effects in cognitive function, cognitive style, and sociodemographic variables in the Seattle Longitudinal Study. *Experimental Aging Research, 25,* 121–140.

Bruhn, P., & Parsons, O. A. (1977). Reaction time variability in epileptic and brain damaged patients. *Cortex, 13,* 373–384.

Bunce, D. J., Warr, P. B., & Cochrane, T. (1993). Blocks in choice responding as a function of age and physical fitness. *Psychology and Aging, 8,* 26–33.

Burton, C. L., Strauss, E., Hultsch, D. F., Moll, A., & Hunter, M. A. (in press). Intraindividual variability as a marker of neurological dysfunction: A comparison of Alzheimer's disease and Parkinson's disease. *Journal of Clinical and Experimental Neuropsychology.*

Cabeza, R. (2002). Hemispheric asymmetry reduction in old adults: The HAROLD model. *Psychology and Aging, 17,* 85–100.

Cerella, J. (1990). Aging and information-processing rate. In J. E. Birren & K. W. Schaie (Eds.), *Handbook of the psychology of aging* (3rd ed., pp. 201–221). San Diego, CA: Academic Press.

Christensen, H., Dear, K. B. G., Anstey, K. J., Parslow, R. A., Sachdev, P., & Jorm, A. F. (in press). Within-occasion intra-individual variability and pre-clinical diagnostic status: Is intra-individual variability an indicator of mild cognitive impairment? *Neuropsychology.*

Cohen, J. (1982). Set correlation as a general multivariate data-analytic method. *Multivariate Behavioral Research, 17,* 301–341.

Collins, L. F., & Long, C. J. (1996). Visual reaction time and its relationship to neuropsychological test performance. *Archives of Clinical Neuropsychology, 11,* 613–623.

Crook, T., Bartus, R. T., Ferris, S. H., Whitehouse, P., Cohen, G. D., & Gershon, S. (1986). Age associated memory impairment: Proposed diagnostic criteria and measures of clinical change: report of a National Institute of Mental Health Work Group. *Developmental Neuropsychology, 2,* 261–276.

Crossman, E. R. F. W., & Szafran, J. (1956). Changes with age in the speed of information intake and discrimination. *Experientia Supplementum, 4,* 128–135.

Deary, I. J., & Der, G. (in press). Reaction time, age, and cognitive ability: Longitudinal findings from age 16 to 63 years in representative population samples. *Aging, Neuropsychology, and Cognition.*

Dixon, R. A., & Bäckman, L. (1999). Principles of compensation in cognitive neurorehabilitation. In D. T. Stuss, G. Winocur, & I. H. Robertson (Eds.), *Cognitive neurorehabilitation* (pp. 59–72). Cambridge University Press.

Dixon, R. A., & Hertzog, C. (1996). Theoretical issues in cognition and aging. In F. Blanchard-Fields & T. M. Hess (Eds.), *Perspectives on cognitive change in adulthood and aging* (pp. 25–65). New York: McGraw-Hill.

Fisk, A. D., & Fisher, D. L. (1994). Brinley plots and theories of aging: The explicit, muddled, and implicit debates. *Journal of Gerontology: Psychological Sciences, 49*, P81–P89.

Fozard, J. L., Vercruyssen, M., Reynolds, S. L., Hancock, P. A., & Quilter, R. E. (1994). Age differences and changes in reaction time: The Baltimore Longitudinal Study of Aging. *Journal of Gerontology: Psychological Sciences, 49*, P179–P189.

Fuentes, K., Hunter, M. A., Strauss, E., & Hultsch, D. F. (2001). Intraindividual variability in cognitive performance in persons with chronic fatigue syndrome. *The Clinical Neuropsychologist, 15*, 210–227.

Gordon, B., & Carson, K. (1990). The basis for choice reaction time slowing in Alzheimer's disease. *Brain and Cognition, 13*, 148–166.

Hendrickson, A. E. (1982). The biological basis of intelligence Part I: Theory. In H. J. Eysenck (Ed.), *A model for intelligence* (pp. 151–196). Berlin, Germany: Springer-Verlag.

Hultsch, D. F., & MacDonald, S. W. S. (2004). Intraindividual variability in performance as a theoretical window onto cognitive aging. In R. A. Dixon, L. Bäckman, & L-G. Nilsson (Eds.), *New frontiers in cognitive aging* (pp. 65–88). New York: Oxford University Press.

Hultsch, D. F., MacDonald, S. W. S., & Dixon, R. A. (2002). Variability in reaction time performance of younger and older adults. *Journal of Gerontology: Psychological Sciences, 57B*, 101–115.

Hultsch, D. F., MacDonald, S. W. S., Hunter, M. A., Levy-Bencheton, J., & Strauss, E. (2000). Intraindividual variability in cognitive performance in older adults: Comparison of adults with mild dementia, adults with arthritis, and healthy adults. *Neuropsychology, 14*, 588–598.

Jensen, A. R. (1982). Reaction time and psychometric g. In H. J. Eysenck (Ed.), *A model for intelligence* (pp. 93–132). Berlin, Germany: Springer-Verlag.

Johansson, B., & Zarit, S. H. (1997). Early cognitive markers of the incidence of dementia and mortality: A longitudinal population-based study of the oldest old. *International Journal of Geriatric Psychiatry, 12*, 53–59.

Kleemeier, R. W. (1962). Intellectual changes in the senium. *Proceedings of the American Statistical Association, 1*, 290–295.

Knotek, P. C., Bayles, K. A., & Kaszniak, A. W. (1990). Response consistency on a semantic memory task in persons with dementia of the Alzheimer type. *Brain and Language, 38*, 465–475.

Leutz, T., Strauss, E., Hultsch, D.F., & Hunter, M.A. (2003). *Intraindividual variability and severity of cognitive impairment.* Paper presented at International Neuropsychological Society, Honolulu, Hawaii.

Levy, R. (1994). Aging-associated cognitive decline. Working Party of the International Psychogeriatric Association in collaboration with the World Health Organisation. *International Psychogeriatrics, 6*, 63–68.

Li, S.-C., Aggen, S. H., Nesselroade, J. R., & Baltes, P. B. (2001). Short-term fluctuations in elderly people's sensorimotor functioning predicts text and spatial memory performance: The MacArthur successful aging studies. *Gerontology, 47*, 100–116.

Li, S.-C., & Lindenberger, U. (1999). Cross-level unification: A computational exploration of the link between deterioration of neurotransmitter systems and dedifferentiation of cognitive abilities in old age. In L.-G. Nilsson & H. Markowitsch (Eds.), *Cognitive neuroscience and memory* (pp. 103–146). Toronto, Canada: Hogrefe & Huber.

Li, S.-C., Lindenberger, U., & Sikström, S. (2001). Aging and cognition: From neuromodulation to representation. *Trends in Cognitive Science, 5,* 479–486.

Lindenberger, U., & Baltes, P. B. (1994). Sensory functioning and intelligence in old age: A strong connection. *Psychology and Aging, 9,* 339–355.

Lindenberger, U., Li, S.-C., & Brehmer, Y. (2002). Variabilité dans le vieillissement comportemental: Résultat et agent des changements ontogénétiques. In J. Lautrey, B. Mazoyer, & P. van Geert (Eds.), *Invariants et variabilités dans le sciences cognitives.* Paris, France: Presses de la MSH.

MacDonald, S. W. S. (2003). *Longitudinal profiles of terminal decline: Associations between cognitive decline, age, time to death, and cause of death.* Unpublished dissertation, Department of Psychology, University of Victoria, Victoria, BC, Canada.

MacDonald, S. W. S., Hultsch, D. F., & Dixon, R. A. (2003). Performance variability is related to change in cognition: Evidence from the Victoria Longitudinal Study. *Psychology and Aging, 18,* 510–523.

MacDonald, S. W. S., Hultsch, D. F., & Dixon, R. A. (2004). Intraindividual variability in neurocognitive performance predicts impending death. Manuscript under review.

Mayr, U., & Kliegl, R. (1993). Sequential and coordinative complexity: Age-based processing limitations in figural transformations. *Journal of Experimental Psychology: Learning, Memory, and Cognition, 19,* 1297–1320.

Myerson, J., Hale, S., Wagstaff, D., Poon, L. W., & Smith, G. A. (1990). The information-loss model: A mathematical theory of age-related cognitive slowing. *Psychological Review, 97,* 475–487.

Nesselroade, J. R., & Featherman, D. L. (1997). Establishing a reference frame against which to chart age-related changes. In M. A. Hardy (Ed.), *Studying aging and social change: Conceptual and methodological issues* (pp.191–205). Newbury Park, CA: Sage.

Palmer, K., Fratiglioni, L., & Winblad, B. (2003). What is mild cognitive impairment? Variations in definitions and evolution of nondemented persons with cognitive impairment. *Acta Neurologica Scandinavica, 107,* 14–20.

Perfect, T. J., & Maylor, E. A. (2000). Rejecting the dull hypothesis: The relation between method and theory in cognitive aging research. In T. J. Perfect & E. A. Maylor (Eds.), *Models of cognitive aging* (pp. 1–18). New York: Oxford University Press.

Petersen, R. C., Smith, G. E., Waring, S. C., Ivnik, R. J., Tangalos, E. G., & Kokman, E. (1999). Mild cognitive impairment: Clinical characterization and outcome. *Archives of Neurology, 56,* 303–308.

Rabbitt, P., Osman, P., Moore, B., & Stollery, B. (2001). There are stable individual differences in performance variability, both from moment to moment and from day to day. *The Quarterly Journal of Experimental Psychology A, 54,* 981–1003.

Rabbitt, P. M. A. (2000). Measurement indices, functional characteristics, and psychometric constructs in cognitive aging. In T. J. Perfect & E. A. Maylor (Eds.), *Models of cognitive aging* (pp. 160–187). New York: Oxford University Press.

Ratcliff, R. (1978). A theory of memory retrieval. *Psychological Review, 85,* 59–108.

Ratcliff, R., Spieler, D., & McKoon, G. (2000). Explicitly modeling the effects of aging on response time. *Psychonomic Bulletin and Review, 7,* 1–25.

Ratcliff, R., Thapar, A., & McKoon, G. (2001). The effects of aging on reaction time in a signal detection task. *Psychology and Aging,* 16, 323–341.

Raz, N., (2000). Aging of the brain and its impact on cognitive performance: Integration of structural and functional findings. In F. I. M. Craik & T. A. Salthouse (Eds.), *The handbook of aging and cognition* (2nd Edn., pp. 1–90). Mahwah, NJ: Erlbaum.

Salthouse, T. A. (1993). Attentional blocks are not responsible for age-related slowing. *Journal of Gerontology: Psychological Sciences,* 48, P263–P270.

Salthouse, T. A. (1996). The processing-speed theory of adult age differences in cognition. *Psychological Review,* 103, 403–428.

Schaie, K. W. (1996). *Intellectual development in adulthood: The Seattle Longitudinal Study.* New York: Cambridge University Press.

Shammi, P., Bosman, E., & Stuss, D. T. (1998). Aging and variability in performance. *Aging, Neuropsychology, and Cognition,* 5, 1–13.

Strauss, E., MacDonald, S. W. S., Hunter, M. A., Moll, A., & Hultsch, D. F. (2002). Intraindividual variability in cognitive performance in three groups of adults: Cross-domain links to physical status and self-perceived affect and beliefs. *Journal of the International Neuropsychology Society,* 8, 893–906.

Stuss, D. T., Pogue, J., Buckle, L., & Bondar, J. (1994). Characterization of stability of performance in patients with traumatic brain injury: Variability and consistency on reaction time tests. *Neuropsychology,* 8, 316–324.

Wade, M. G., Newell, K. M., & Wallace, S. A. (1978). Decision time and movement time as a function of response complexity in retarded persons. *American Journal of Mental Deficiency,* 83, 135–144.

Welford, A. T. (1965). Performance, biological mechanisms and age: A theoretical sketch. In A. T. Welford & J. E. Birren (Eds.), *Behavior, aging, and the nervous system* (pp. 3–20). Springfield, IL: Thomas.

West, R., Murphy, K. J., Armilio, M. L., Craik, F. I. M., & Stuss, D. T. (2002). Lapses of intention and performance variability reveal age-related increases in fluctuations of executive control. *Brain and Cognition,* 49, 402–419.

Chapter 3

Aging and the ability to ignore irrelevant information in visual search and enumeration tasks

Elizabeth A. Maylor[1] and Derrick G. Watson

Abstract

A classic study by Rabbitt (1965) demonstrated that older adults are particularly impaired by irrelevant distractors in a visual categorization task, a finding that has inspired many subsequent studies and theories of cognitive aging. In this chapter, we present some of our own recent experiments exploring age-related differences in the effects of irrelevant distractors in visual search and enumeration tasks. The first study shows that age differences in the effects of irrelevant distractors can vary depending on the perceptual load of relevant processing. The second study examines the ability to selectively facilitate the processing of new visual information by ignoring old irrelevant stimuli already present in the field (*visual marking*) and demonstrates age preservation for stationary stimuli but marked age decrements for moving stimuli. Finally, enumeration tasks again show that older adults' overall responses are disproportionately slowed by the presence of irrelevant distractors. Moreover, distractors have unexpected effects on age differences in enumeration rates that, together with investigations of eye movements, shed light on the specific task requirements of searching for versus enumerating visual stimuli.

Some of the research presented in this chapter was supported by Grant R000239180 from the Economic and Social Research Council of Great Britain. The authors are grateful to Friederike Schlaghecken and Nilli Lavie for helpful discussion.

[1] From 1984–92, I (Elizabeth A. Maylor) worked with Patrick Rabbitt as a postdoctoral researcher at the Age and Cognitive Performance Research Centre in Manchester. Our first project concerned the cognitive effects of alcohol and fatigue on young adults (see Maylor & Rabbitt, 1993, for a summary of some of this work). However, I was inevitably captured by Pat's enthusiasm for another factor associated with the slowing of behaviour (i.e. old age) and have continued to work in the area of cognitive aging ever since. My work has benefited considerably from Pat's insights and encouragement over many years and so I was delighted to be asked to contribute to this volume in his honour.

Introduction

The aim of this chapter is to illustrate Patrick Rabbitt's influence on the field of cognitive aging over the past 40 years, and on some of our own recent work, by a case study of one contribution in particular. The article we have chosen appeared in the *Journal of Gerontology* in 1965 and it showed an age decrement in a fundamental aspect of behaviour, namely, the ability to ignore irrelevant information. We discuss how this result has been interpreted and note its impact on subsequent theories of cognitive aging. We then present some of our own experiments exploring characteristics and boundary conditions of this age decrement. These include: (1) an investigation of the influence of perceptual load (Maylor & Lavie, 1998), (2) experiments exploring older adults' ability to ignore irrelevant information that appears prior to relevant information—an ability known as visual marking (Watson & Maylor, 2002), and (3) experiments in which the task is to enumerate multiple targets while ignoring irrelevant information (e.g. Watson, Maylor, & Manson, 2002). Finally, we return to Rabbitt (1965) to note some interesting parallels between our current explanations and Rabbitt's conclusions 40 years ago.

Ignoring irrelevant information (Rabbitt, 1965)

As noted by Scialfa and Joffe (1997), 1965 was "a watershed year for experimental gerontology" as it saw the publication of both "Rabbitt's seminal work in visual search and Brinley's generalized slowing analysis" (p. 227). These two articles have been cited almost identical numbers of times since 1981, and both were based on doctoral research (or shortly thereafter). However, as we shall see, their conclusions were rather different.

Rabbitt (1965) was one of the first studies of age differences in selective attention, that is, the ability to find information relevant to the current goal and to filter out all irrelevant information. A simple card-sorting task was employed in which participants were given packs of 48 visiting cards (similar in size to current credit cards) and were asked to sort them as quickly as possible into two piles according to whether there was a letter A (stencilled in india ink) on the card or a letter B. This target letter (A/B) appeared equally often in each of nine (3 × 3) possible locations on the card. There were four different packs of cards and these varied in terms of the number of irrelevant letters (chosen from the remaining letters of the alphabet) printed on each card (0, 1, 4, or 8 distractors).

The mean times to sort the 48 cards for 11 young and 11 old people (mean ages of 19 and 67 years, respectively) are shown in Figure 3.1. The old adults were slower than the young adults and both age groups took progressively longer as the number of irrelevant items on the cards increased. Crucially,

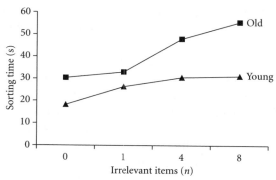

Fig. 3.1 Mean times (in seconds) to sort packs of 48 cards into two piles (A/B) as a function of number of irrelevant items for young and old adults. Data from table 1 of Rabbitt (1965), *Journal of Gerontology, 20*, 233–238. Copyright © The Gerontological Society of America. Adapted by permission of the publisher.

there was also an interaction such that this increase was steeper for the old adults, a result that was taken to indicate "an age-decrement in the ability to ignore irrelevant information" (Rabbitt, 1965, p. 233).

Rabbitt's (1965) interpretation was based on the localization approach to aging (see Salthouse, 1991, for discussion), which uses interactions between age and the treatment of interest to identify particular processes, or processing components, that are age sensitive—in this case, the ability to ignore irrelevant information. However, at least one problem with the localization approach has been that Age × Treatment interactions are so frequently observed across a wide range of cognitive tasks that, as Salthouse (1996a) noted, "either a large number of specific factors or a small number of general factors must be contributing to the age-related differences" (p. 287).

This suggests an alternative interpretation for the data in Figure 3.1. If they are considered in terms of the proportional increase in sorting times for old relative to young adults, this proportional increase was 1.7 for 0 irrelevant items and 1.8 for 8 irrelevant items. Thus, instead of a specific or localized age deficit in ignoring irrelevant information, this may be an example of general-ized slowing (e.g. Birren, 1965; Cerella, 1985, 1990; Cerella & Hale, 1994; Salthouse, 1985). In other words, regardless of the actual cognitive processes required by the task, older people may simply be slower than young people by a constant proportion.

Brinley (1965) recognized this possibility in his comparison of young and old adults (mean ages of 24 and 71 years, respectively) across 21 tasks, some of which required the same operation to be carried out on successive trials (nonshift tasks) whereas others required a different operation (shift tasks). Brinley then plotted the mean response times for the young adults on the *x*-axis and the mean response times for the old adults on the *y*-axis for each of the 21 tasks (see Figure 3.2). This first *Brinley plot* revealed that the "time of response in the old is simply and accurately described as a linear function of performance time in the young group . . . Consequently response times for both groups and for each type of task variation may be conceived as varying along a single dimension which might be termed 'task difficulty' " (p. 131). In other words, the data suggest that the critical determinant of age differences in performance is how much processing is required rather than which processing components.

Thus cognitive aging research over the last 20–30 years has seen a shift from local explanations (as illustrated in Figure 3.3(a) where age affects performance across different tasks through deficits in particular components of information processing) to global explanations (see Figure 3.3(b) where the effects of aging are attributable to a single common factor). Various candidates have been proposed as the single common factor (see Park, 2000; Salthouse, 2000, for discussion). One is reduced processing speed, or generalized slowing, as advocated most strongly by Salthouse (e.g. Salthouse, 1985, 1996b). Another that has been the subject of much recent research is reduced inhibition as proposed by Hasher and Zacks (1988) (see also Hasher, Zacks, & May, 1999). According to the inhibition deficit hypothesis of aging, age-related decline in cognition occurs largely as a result of age-related decline in the efficiency of inhibitory mechanisms

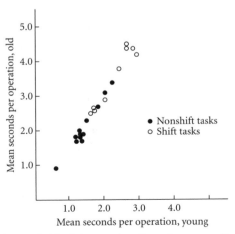

Fig. 3.2 Response times of old adults as a function of response times of young adults for nonshift and shift tasks. Reproduced from figure 2 of Brinley's (1965) chapter in A. T. Welford and J. E. Birren (Eds.), *Behaviour, aging and the nervous system*. Courtesy of Charles C Thomas Publisher, Springfield, IL.

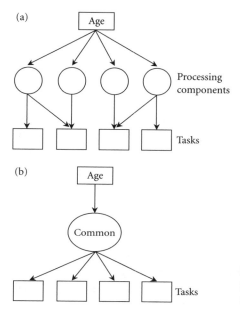

Fig. 3.3 Illustrations of (a) local and (b) global models of aging.

(see Maylor, Schlaghecken, & Watson, in press, for a summary), and these would include the ability to ignore irrelevant information. Rabbitt's (1965) study has therefore been an important influence on current theories of cognitive aging and also the subject of much debate concerning how to interpret cognitive aging data. In the sections that follow, we summarize some of our own studies investigating the ability to ignore irrelevant information in young and old adults in the context of some recent models of selective attention. In doing so, we are mindful of Plude, Enns, and Brodeur's (1994) conclusion that "Rabbitt's (1965) classic demonstration of an age decrement in visual search set the standard against which other visual search studies can be compared" (p. 247).

Perceptual load theory

The perceptual load theory of selective attention was first proposed in the mid-1990s by Nilli Lavie (Lavie, 1995; Lavie & Tsal, 1994). In her model, perceptual processing is viewed as a limited resource. Perceptual processing proceeds automatically from relevant to irrelevant items until it runs out of capacity. (Perception here includes all processes that lead to stimulus identification.) If perceptual load is high (i.e. relevant processing is relatively demanding), this should consume full capacity. The result is that irrelevant information is successfully ignored simply because it is not actually perceived.

On the other hand, if the perceptual load involved in processing relevant items is low, this should leave spare capacity to spill over and allow perception of irrelevant information.

Perceptual load theory has successfully resolved the early vs. late selection debate in the attention literature (Lavie & Tsal, 1994). Thus, evidence for early selection comes from studies in which perceptual load is high, whereas evidence for late selection comes from studies in which perceptual load is low. In addition, direct empirical support for the theory comes from studies in which perceptual load was experimentally manipulated (Lavie, 1995; Lavie & Cox, 1997; Lavie, Hirst, de Fockert, & Viding, 2004). Low perceptual load conditions resulted in interference from an irrelevant distractor whereas high perceptual load eliminated such interference.

Maylor and Lavie (1998) reasoned that perceptual load might also be an important factor in determining age differences in selective attention on the basis that perceptual capacity would be reduced in older adults. They therefore conducted a study in which perceptual load was manipulated as shown in Figure 3.4. In fact, a major component of the task was essentially a computerized version of Rabbitt (1965). Participants were instructed to press one of two keys as quickly as possible according to whether there was a letter X or a letter N present among the central items in the display, that is, those that appeared in an imaginary circle around the fixation point. The number of nontarget

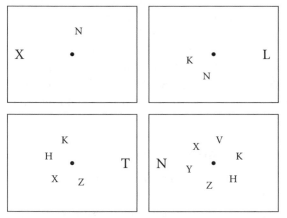

Fig. 3.4 Examples of the displays used in experiment 1 of Maylor and Lavie (1998). The target (X or N) was accompanied by 0, 1, 3, or 5 nontarget letters in a circle around fixation. In addition, a single distractor letter (X or N on incompatible trials; T or L on neutral trials) appeared either to the left or right of the central display. From figure 1 of Maylor and Lavie (1998), *Psychology and Aging, 13,* 563–573. Copyright © 1998 by the American Psychological Association. Adapted with permission.

letters in the circle varied between trials from 0 to 5 letters (i.e. low to high perceptual load).

In addition to these central items, there was also a larger distractor letter that appeared either to the left or to the right of the main display. These critical distractors were either incompatible with the target letter (i.e. associated with the other response) or they were neutral (i.e. the letters T and L). Participants were strongly encouraged to ignore this distractor letter because it would not help their performance if they attended to it.

Maylor and Lavie (1998) made the following predictions: (1) The neutral distractor condition was expected to replicate the results of Rabbitt (1965). (2) Response times (RTs) were expected to be slower when the single irrelevant distractor was incompatible rather than neutral with respect to the target. In other words, there should be a response compatibility effect (*cf.* Eriksen & Eriksen, 1974), at least when perceptual load was low. (3) In contrast, when perceptual load was high (i.e. a large number of nontarget letters accompanying the target), there should be no response compatibility effect (replicating Lavie, 1995). (4) Finally, the decrease in the response compatibility effect should occur at a lower perceptual load for the old than for the young because the processing of both relevant and irrelevant information was more likely to exceed the total available capacity of old adults than of young adults.

Figure 3.5 displays the results for the neutral distractor condition for 15 young and 15 old adults (mean ages of 23 and 73 years, respectively). The old adults were slower than the young adults, RTs increased with the number of nontargets in the search set, and there was a significant interaction between

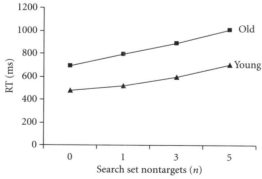

Fig. 3.5 Means of median response times (RTs) for the neutral distractor condition of experiment 1 of Maylor and Lavie (1998) as a function of the number of nontarget items in the search set for young and old adults. Data taken from table 1 of Maylor and Lavie (1998), *Psychology and Aging, 13*, 563–573. Copyright © 1998 by the American Psychological Association. Adapted with permission.

age group and set size. Also, the proportional increase in RTs for old relative to young adults was identical for 0 and 5 nontargets at 1.4, in accordance with generalized slowing. Thus Maylor and Lavie (1998) successfully replicated Rabbitt (1965) in finding age deficits in visual search that were consistent with generalized slowing such that old adults were proportionally slower than young adults in identifying a target surrounded by nontargets.

Differences between RTs in the incompatible and neutral distractor conditions are shown in Figure 3.6(a). As expected, participants were slower when the distractor was incompatible with the target at the three lowest levels

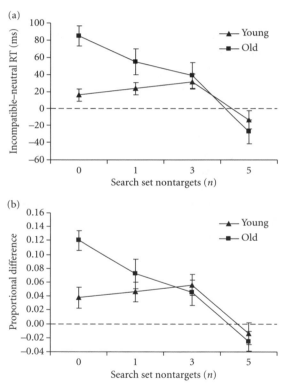

Fig. 3.6 (a) Mean response time (RT) differences (with standard error bars) between the incompatible and neutral conditions of experiment 1 of Maylor and Lavie (1998) as a function of the number of nontarget items in the search set and age group. (b) RT differences between the incompatible and neutral conditions of experiment 1 of Maylor and Lavie (1998) divided by RT in the neutral condition (with standard error bars) as a function of the number of nontarget items in the search set and age group. Data redrawn from figures 2 and 3 of Maylor and Lavie (1998), *Psychology and Aging, 13,* 563–573. Copyright © 1998 by the American Psychological Association. Adapted with permission.

of perceptual load but not at the highest level of perceptual load, thereby replicating Lavie (1995). Comparing the data for young and old adults, there are two findings to note. First, at the two lowest levels of perceptual load, there were larger distractor effects for the old than for the young. Second, for the young, the distractor effect did not decrease until there were five nontarget items, whereas it decreased significantly by three nontargets for the old (see Huang-Pollock, Carr, & Nigg, 2002, for a similar pattern of results in a study comparing young adults with children).

Why was the distractor effect larger for the old than for the young at low perceptual load? Obviously, one possibility is that because the old were slower overall than the young, then the RT differences would be correspondingly larger because of generalized slowing. This was tested by examining proportional rather than absolute RT differences, that is, (Incompatible RT—Neutral RT)/Neutral RT. As can be seen in Figure 3.6(b), the data were very similar. Thus at low levels of perceptual load, the old were less able to ignore the irrelevant distractor than the young and this could not be explained by generalized slowing. Interestingly, this finding may relate to Lavie et al.'s (2004) second mechanism of selective attention. In contrast to the passive effects of perceptual load, this is an active control mechanism that reduces interference from distractors when they are perceived (i.e. at low perceptual load) and which depends on higher cognitive functions, such as working memory, to maintain current processing priorities. The data in Figure 3.6 are at least consistent with the possibility of an age-related impairment in this active inhibitory control mechanism such that when distractors *are* processed, they have a greater detrimental effect on the efficiency of selective attention in old than in young adults.

With increasing perceptual load, the distractor effect decreased earlier for the old than for the young, which is also contrary to generalized slowing. However, this is exactly what was predicted on the assumption of an age reduction in perceptual capacity. It can be concluded that older adults are not always less able to "ignore" irrelevant information—at least one factor that should be considered is perceptual load. Thus, when relevant processing is demanding, irrelevant information may not even be perceived by older people.

Finally, we should mention a recent study by Madden and Langley (2003) that successfully replicated the main findings of both Rabbitt (1965)[2] and Lavie (1995)

---

[2] Madden and Langley (2003) attributed the Rabbitt (1965) effect of age on search efficiency to "general (relatively task-independent) changes in the speed of visual information processing" (p. 65).

but had mixed success in attempting to replicate Maylor and Lavie (1998). In their first two experiments, they made several methodological changes including the presentation of two rather than one irrelevant distractors always to the left and right of fixation and these were placed within the circle of items containing the target. In contrast to Maylor and Lavie, perceptual load effects were found to be similar for young and old adults. This could be regarded as consistent with evidence that age deficits can be minimized when the locations of irrelevant distractors are known in advance as in focused attention situations (for summaries, see Madden & Plude, 1993; Rogers, 2000).

Madden and Langley's (2003) third experiment used identical methodology to Maylor and Lavie (1998) and showed some similarities (e.g. distractor effects were significantly larger for the old than for the young at low levels of perceptual load) but also some differences (e.g. the compatibility effect did not decrease for either age group prior to the highest level of perceptual load). In fact, there is a suggestion in their data that the young showed a compatibility effect at all levels of perceptual load (i.e. 0, 1, 3, and 5 nontargets), whereas the compatibility effect for the old decreased from 3 to 5 nontargets. Thus the results of the equivalent experiments across the two studies are at least qualitatively similar and any discrepancies may be due to some general differences in visual stimuli leading to greater distractor effects or to Madden and Langley's use of more able participants (e.g. their old adults were seven years younger on average and their young adults were Duke University students). Clearly, additional work with this paradigm is required (see Madden & Whiting, 2004, for further discussion).

Visual marking

In many situations, a person is waiting for a target to appear such as looking out for a friend to arrive at an airport terminal. According to Watson and Humphreys (1997), visual search can be facilitated in this type of situation by actively ignoring unwanted or irrelevant information that is already present in the field via a process they termed visual marking. Thus visual marking is a mechanism for prioritizing and controlling the selection of visual information over time. It operates by actively inhibiting old unwanted (previewed) information, which allows a selection advantage for new objects when they appear (termed the preview benefit). Visual marking is a top-down process that requires limited attentional resources. Because of these and other features of visual marking (see Watson, Humphreys, & Olivers, 2003, for a summary), we expected to find age-related deficits.

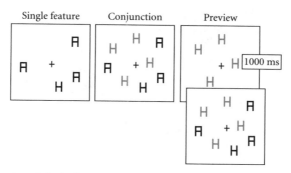

Fig. 3.7 Examples of single feature, conjunction and preview conditions in Watson and Maylor's (2002, experiment 1) visual marking experiment in which participants searched for a red H among red As (single feature) or among red As and green Hs (conjunction and preview). In the preview condition, the green Hs were presented for 1000 ms before the appearance of the red As and red H (if present). (Red and green letters are shown here in black and gray, respectively. The screen background and fixation point are shown with black/white reversed.)

Visual marking can be demonstrated using a modified conjunction search (Treisman & Gelade, 1980) task in which one set of distractors (green Hs) is presented for some time (typically 1000 ms) before a second set (red As and a red H target when present) is added (see right panel of Figure 3.7). Participants are required to indicate the presence or absence of the target among a varying number of distractors and are told that if the target is present, it will be in the second display.

In order to assess whether observers are able to ignore the old previewed distractors, search in the preview condition is compared with two baseline conditions (see middle and left panels of Figure 3.7). In the conjunction (or full element) baseline, all the search elements are presented simultaneously. This condition therefore provides a measure of search performance if all the items have to be searched in the preview condition. Displays in the single feature (or half element) baseline are composed of the same number and type of stimuli presented in the second set of items from the preview condition, thus providing a measure of search performance expected if observers can restrict their search to the new (second set) items only. Accordingly, Watson and Humphreys (1997) argued that if the old unwanted information can be successfully ignored, search in the preview condition should be as efficient as that in the single feature condition. However, if the old unwanted items cannot be ignored, search in the preview condition should be equivalent to that in the conjunction condition.

Watson and Maylor (2002, experiment 1) tested 12 young and 18 old adults (mean ages of 20 and 72 years, respectively) in these three conditions. The RT

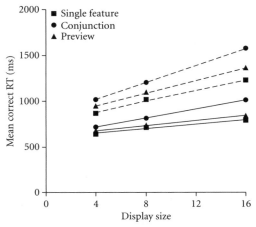

Fig. 3.8 Mean correct reaction times (RTs) to determine target presence for young (solid lines) and old (dashed lines) adults from Watson and Maylor (2002, experiment 1). See Figure 3.7 for summary of experimental conditions. Search rates for the single feature, preview, and conjunction conditions were 12, 14, and 24 ms/item, respectively, for young adults, and 29, 35, and 46 ms/item, respectively, for old adults. For both age groups, the single feature and preview search rates did not differ but each was faster than the conjunction search rate, indicating that participants were able to ignore the previewed items while searching for the target. Data taken from figure 1 of Watson and Maylor (2002), *Psychology and Aging, 17*, 321–339. Copyright © 2002 by the American Psychological Association. Adapted with permission.

data for target present trials[3] are shown in Figure 3.8.[4] First, as expected from the results of Rabbitt (1965), the old adults were slower overall than the young adults and their search slopes were approximately twice as steep. Second, for both young and old, the slope for the preview condition was not significantly steeper than that of the single feature condition but was significantly flatter than that of the conjunction condition (see Figure 3.8 caption for search

---

[3] Greater emphasis is usually placed on target-present trials than on target-absent trials because when the target is absent, people tend to rely on a number of different strategies and are often more cautious (particularly old adults) in responding absent than present (e.g. Humphreys and Müller, 1993; Plude and Doussard-Roosevelt, 1989). In fact, for both experiments reported here from Watson and Maylor (2002), it can be noted that the data patterns were qualitatively similar for target-present and target-absent trials.

[4] Following Watson and Humphreys (1997), the data for the single feature condition are plotted as if there were twice as many items in the display. Thus, if search rate in the preview condition matches that of the single feature condition, then we can conclude that the previewed items have been excluded from subsequent search.

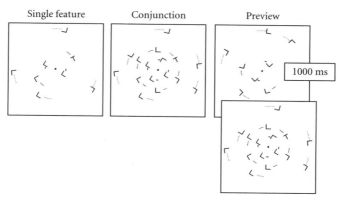

Fig. 3.9 Examples of single feature, conjunction and preview conditions in experiment 3 of Watson and Maylor (2002), with stimuli rotating clockwise around virtual concentric rings at a rate of 38°/s. The screen background and stimuli are shown with black/white reversed. Participants searched for a target letter T among distractor letters L, oriented randomly at 0°, 90°, 180°, and 270°.

rates). That is, both age groups could successfully exclude the first set of items from further search, thus demonstrating age-related sparing of visual marking. Similar results were observed in an earlier study by Kramer and Atchley (2000) who used different stimuli and much larger display sizes to show that both young and old adults can ignore at least 15 irrelevant (previewed) items.

However, objects in the world are not always static—people in the airport terminal are usually moving—and so in two further experiments, Watson and Maylor (2002) compared visual marking in young and old adults with moving stimuli. The procedure for one of these (experiment 3) is illustrated in Figure 3.9. All the stimuli rotated smoothly and continuously clockwise around the fixation point. In this case, the target was the letter T and the distractors were letter Ls. The single feature and conjunction conditions therefore differed only in terms of the numbers of stimuli (2, 4, and 8 vs. 4, 8, and 16) but we have retained the descriptions for comparability with the previous experiment. In the preview condition, the Ls appeared for 1000 ms and rotated clockwise before the remaining stimuli (including a T if present), also rotating, were added.

The data for 18 young and 18 old adults (mean ages of 20 and 73 years, respectively) are shown in Figure 3.10. For the young adults, the preview search slope matched that of the single feature baseline but was significantly flatter than that of the conjunction baseline, thereby displaying a full preview benefit (see also Watson, 2001). In contrast, there was no evidence of visual marking for the old adults for whom the preview search slope matched that of

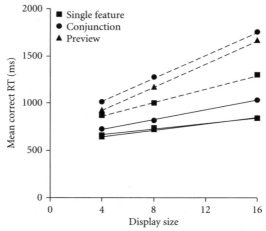

Fig. 3.10 Mean correct reaction times (RTs) to determine target presence for young (solid lines) and old (dashed lines) adults from Watson and Maylor (2002, experiment 3). Search rates for the single feature, preview and conjunction conditions were 14, 17, and 26 ms/item, respectively, for young adults, and 36, 62, and 61 ms/item, respectively, for older adults. For young adults, the single feature and preview search rates did not differ but each was faster than the conjunction search rate. For old adults, the preview and conjunction search rates did not differ but each was slower than the single feature search rate. Data taken from figure 3 of Watson and Maylor (2002), *Psychology and Aging, 17*, 321–339. Copyright © 2002 by the American Psychological Association. Adapted with permission.

the conjunction baseline and was significantly steeper than that of the single feature baseline.[5]

In summary, new items can be prioritized for selection by visual marking, that is, the top-down attentional inhibition of old items already in the field (see Watson & Humphreys, 1997). At least for the conditions explored by Kramer and Atchley (2000) and by Watson and Maylor (2002, experiment 1), there appears to be no age-related impairment in visual marking for static stimuli. This therefore provides a further qualification to Rabbitt's (1965) proposal of an age decrement in the ability to ignore irrelevant information. However, it is consistent with the relative sparing in old age of some other

---

[5] Similar results were found in experiment 2 of Watson and Maylor (2002) in which the task was identical to experiment 1 as illustrated in Figure 3.7 except that all the stimuli moved smoothly and continuously down the screen (i.e. linear rather than circular motion). As in experiment 3 (see Figure 3.10), visual marking was apparent for young but not for old adults.

location-based inhibitory functions such as the passive inhibition of items that have already been processed (i.e. inhibition-of-return, IOR; see Faust & Balota, 1997; Hartley & Kieley, 1995; Langley, Fuentes, Hochhalter, Brandt, & Overmier, 2001).

Visual marking of moving stimuli, in contrast, can be either feature-based (Watson & Humphreys, 1998) or object-based (Watson, 2001), and here there is a clear age-related decrement (Watson & Maylor, 2002, experiments 2 and 3). Moreover, it cannot be explained by any simple account of generalized slowing because there is no linear transformation that can change the preview condition slope so that it matches the single feature condition in the young but the conjunction condition in the old (see Figure 3.10). However, there is another possibility. Generalized slowing could still account for the data if there is age-related slowing in the time course of visual marking. Thus, for static stimuli, 1000 ms between the previewed and new items may be sufficient for visual marking to be fully applied by both young and old adults even if it takes the latter twice as long (say 800 ms rather than 400). It is conceivable that visual marking of moving stimuli may take longer so that 1000 ms is still sufficient for young adults but not for old adults. To check this possibility, Watson and Maylor (2002) tested additional participants in their third experiment (see Figure 3.9) but with a preview duration of 2000 ms rather than 1000 ms. The old adults' data were exactly as before with mean search slopes of 30, 65, and 56 ms/item for the single feature, preview and conjunction conditions, respectively (cf. Figure 3.10), thereby discounting a slower time course of visual marking as an explanation for the age deficit with moving stimuli.

This apparent age-related reduction in the ability to ignore irrelevant moving objects is perhaps of some general concern. As noted earlier, objects in the real world are rarely stationary for long and it is perhaps in such complex scenes that successful time-based selection may provide the greatest utility. However, the practical impact of this particular form of inhibitory deficit on real world performance of course awaits future research.

Visual search vs. enumeration

The final set of studies compares age decrements in the ability to ignore irrelevant information in visual search tasks (cf. Rabbitt, 1965) and in enumeration tasks, which require the processing and keeping track of multiple targets in a display in order to determine as quickly as possible how many targets are present. Typically, RTs to enumerate items in the absence of distractors do not increase linearly as the number of items increases. Instead, RTs remain relatively flat (<100 ms/item) up to about 3–4 items after which they increase linearly with each additional item (>300 ms/item). This results in a bilinear enumeration function with a flex point at around 3 or 4 items. The fast and accurate enumeration for small numbers of items has been termed subitization and the slower and less accurate enumeration of larger numbers has been termed counting (e.g. Kaufman, Lord, Reese, & Volkman, 1949; Mandler & Shebo, 1982; Sagi & Julesz, 1985; Trick & Pylyshyn, 1993, 1994b). A number of mechanisms have been proposed to account for subitization. These range from the involvement of a preverbal counting system that is accurate and reliable only for small numbers of items (Gallistel & Gelman, 1992), to the use of pattern information as a cue to numerosity (Mandler & Shebo, 1982).

A relatively recent model (Trick & Pylyshyn, 1993, 1994a, 1994b) proposed that subitization occurs as a result of the visual system being able to simultaneously tag up to about four items that are individuated at a preattentive level of processing (Pylyshyn, 1989). These tags are called FINSTs (from FINgers of INSTantiation) and, according to FINST theory, subitization arises because small numbers of items can be enumerated by assigning FINSTs to them in parallel and then associating the number of bound FINSTs directly with number names. When the number of objects exceeds the number of FINSTs (about 4), enumeration has to proceed via a serial process of disengaging and reassigning FINSTs (and/or a single focus of attention) to the remaining items. This set of additional relatively complex operations results in a substantial and linear increase in RT as numerosity increases. In addition to accounting for subitization (and other findings), there are several reasons why an efficient visual system requires the ability to tag multiple items simultaneously. Some examples include the efficient relocation of attention around multiple relevant stimuli, the computation of spatial relationships and the integration of information across saccades (e.g. see Pylyshyn, 1989; for recent summaries see Pylyshyn, 1998, 2001). Therefore, if aging reduced the number of FINSTs or impaired the ability to assign or use FINSTs efficiently, this would have an impact on the efficiency of visual functioning in everyday tasks over and above those related to enumeration.

Trick and Pylyshyn (1993) examined enumeration of easy- and difficult-to-find targets (single-feature and conjunction defined, respectively) and found that subitization occurred only with easy-to-find targets. When target items required focused attention for their detection, subitization did not occur and enumeration slopes were substantial and linear even for small numbers of items. This is consistent with the proposal that the FINST mechanism is located between a preattentive and serial attentive level of processing (Pylyshyn, 1989). Thus FINSTs can only be assigned in parallel to items that are represented and individuated preattentively.

Since Rabbitt (1965), a number of studies have examined aging and visual search for a single target (e.g. Foster, Behrmann, & Stuss, 1995; Gilmore, Tobias, & Royer, 1985; Hommel, Li, & Li, 2004; Humphrey & Kramer, 1997; Kramer, Martin-Emerson, Larish, & Andersen, 1996; Plude & Doussard-Roosevelt, 1989; Scialfa & Joffe, 1997; see Kline & Scialfa, 1996, for a summary) and have shown that easy search is relatively unaffected by old age but difficult search is less efficient. In contrast, relatively few studies have assessed the effects of old age on enumeration and these have produced inconsistent results, possibly because (among other differences) some have included distractors (Kotary & Hoyer, 1995; Sliwinski, 1997) whereas others have not (Basak & Verhaeghen, 2003; Geary & Lin, 1998; Nebes, Brady, & Reynolds, 1992; Trick, Enns, & Brodeur, 1996).

Therefore, in our first study (Watson et al., 2002) we assessed the effects of age on the enumeration of 1–9 targets both with and without the presence of distractors. In the former case, there were 19–11 distractors accompanying the 1–9 targets, respectively, so that the total number of stimuli was always 20. In addition, there was a standard visual search task using the same target and distractors. Figure 3.11 includes illustrations of the three conditions. Participants enumerated Os (top panel), enumerated Os while ignoring Xs (middle left), and searched for the presence of a single O among variable numbers of X distractors (bottom left).[6] The third condition was included to check that there was no age deficit in single feature search. Indeed, for the 30 young and 35 old participants (mean ages of 21 and 72, respectively), RTs plotted against display size revealed search functions that were virtually flat in both age groups, indicating parallel detection of the single feature target across the visual field, as expected (e.g. see Plude & Doussard-Roosevelt, 1989).

Enumeration RTs are shown in Figure 3.12. Without distractors, the old were slower overall than the young but both age groups showed the classic bilinear pattern of faster subitizing (small numerosities) than counting (large numerosities). Moreover, the subitizing and counting rates were equivalent for young and old. When distractors were added, the old were slowed considerably more by their presence overall than were the young, showing again a marked deficit in their ability to ignore irrelevant information. In addition,

---

[6] Participants responded by pressing the space bar of the computer keyboard and then entering the response (i.e. numerosity, or target present/absent) when prompted. RT was measured from the onset of the display to the press of the space bar. See Watson, Maylor, and Manson (2002) for a summary of some of the advantages of this technique over other methods.

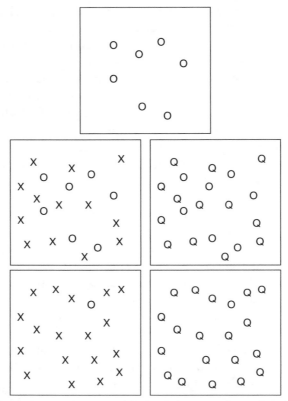

Fig. 3.11 Top panel: Example stimulus display for enumeration task without distractors (how many Os?). Middle panel: Example stimulus displays for enumeration task with X (left) and Q (right) distractors. Bottom panel: Example stimulus displays for search tasks (O present/absent?) with X (left) and Q (right) distractors. Watson, Maylor, and Manson (2002) used X distractors; Watson, Maylor, and Bruce (in press a, experiment 1) used Q distractors. In all cases, luminance inverted (not drawn to scale).

whereas young adults continued to show evidence of subitization, old adults were unable to subitize in the presence of distractors despite evidence of parallel search for a single target among distractors. Finally, enumeration rates for large numbers of targets remained similar in young and old.

These are surprising results for at least two reasons. First, they are contrary to generalized slowing, which predicts that relatively fast and efficient processes (subitization) should be less affected by aging than slower more serial processes (counting beyond four items)—*cf.* single feature vs. conjunction search. This was not the case and (without distractors) enumeration was

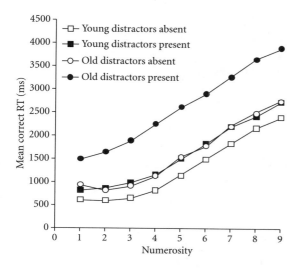

Fig. 3.12 Mean correct response times (RTs) as a function of numerosity and distractor absence/presence for young and old adults in the enumeration tasks from Watson, Maylor, and Manson (2002). Distractors were Xs. From figure 1 of Watson, Maylor, and Manson (2002), *Psychology and Aging, 17*, 496–504.

age equivalent across the whole range of numerosities. Second, when distractors were present, old adults were unable to subitize targets that they were nevertheless able to detect efficiently.

Watson et al. (2002) argued that the age selective deficit for subitization is, however, consistent with a modified FINST account in which they proposed that the assignment of a FINST results in a general reduction in the salience of other items in the field. When there are no distractors present, both young and old adults can assign remaining FINSTs efficiently, resulting in age equivalent subitization. In contrast, when distractors are present, assigning additional FINSTs onto targets is more difficult because of (a) the reduction in salience of the remaining items as a result of earlier FINST assignment, and (b) attentional competition from distractors. For young adults, the saliency of the targets remains sufficiently high to allow efficient FINST assignment even when distractors are present. However, for old adults, an age-related reduction in attentional resources, coupled with the reduced salience of the stimuli and competition from distractors, is sufficient to prevent the efficient assignment of multiple FINSTs; enumeration therefore proceeds serially at small numerosities (see Watson & Humphreys, 1999, for related arguments).

In a subsequent study, Watson et al. (in press a, experiment 1) examined enumeration of Os without distractors (Figure 3.11, top panel), enumeration of Os while ignoring Qs (i.e. difficult-to-find targets; middle right of Figure 3.11), and visual search for the presence of a single O among variable numbers of Q distractors (bottom right of Figure 3.11). Note that

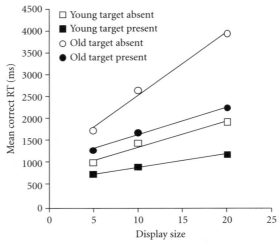

Fig. 3.13 Mean correct response times (RTs) as a function of age, target absence/presence and display size for the visual search task from experiment 1 of Watson, Maylor, and Bruce (in press a). Distractors were Qs. Reworked from the original figure 2 to appear in the *Quarterly Journal of Experimental Psychology (Section A)*, published for The Experimental Psychology Society (see journal website at http://www.psypress.co.uk/journals.asp).

search for targets defined by the absence of a feature relative to the distractors is known to produce relatively inefficient search (Treisman & Souther, 1985). The results from 34 young and 34 old adults (mean ages of 19 and 69 years, respectively) for the visual search task are shown in Figure 3.13, where it can be seen that, as expected, search slopes were no longer either flat or age invariant. Old adults' search rates were approximately twice as slow as those of young adults. Note also that slopes for target absent trials were approximately twice those of target present trials, consistent with a serial and self-terminating search (Treisman & Gelade, 1980; but see Humphreys & Müller, 1993; Townsend, 1972, for alternative limited capacity parallel accounts).

Figure 3.14 shows the enumeration data. In the absence of distractors, we replicated our previous finding of age-equivalent subitizing and counting and, further, showed formally that the span of subitization (i.e. the flex point of the bilinear function) was also age equivalent at 3.3 items for both groups. With distractors present, neither age group was able to subitize, consistent with the results of Trick and Pylyshyn (1993) with difficult-to-find targets. Importantly, because the old adults were less efficient at detecting a difficult-to-find target (Figure 3.13), we expected that their enumeration of such targets would be

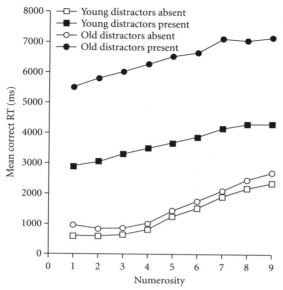

Fig. 3.14 Mean correct response times (RTs) as a function of numerosity and distractor absence/presence for young and old adults in the enumeration tasks from experiment 1 of Watson, Maylor, and Bruce (in press a). Distractors were Qs. Reworked from the original figure 3 to appear in the *Quarterly Journal of Experimental Psychology (Section A)*, published for The Experimental Psychology Society (see journal website at http://www.psypress.co.uk/journals.asp).

particularly inefficient. However, although the old adults' RTs were again much slower overall with distractors present, their enumeration rates were age equivalent.

One reason why counting beyond four items might be spared in old age is because it may require the involvement of a relatively slow but age equivalent process that is not needed either in difficult search or in subitizing single feature targets (which both show age deficits). If this process is sufficiently slow and age equivalent, it may become the rate-limiting process on performance, resulting in the same counting rates for young and old adults. Watson et al. (in press a, experiment 2) tested whether numerical subvocalization (most likely necessary beyond four items) could be this rate-limiting process. Participants were presented with a digit from 1–9 and were asked to count subvocally from one up to the value of the presented digit and then press the space bar. Subvocalizing rates were found to be equivalent in young and old adults but at around 170 ms/number they were much too fast to be the slowest rate-limiting factor in enumeration beyond the subitizing range.

Eye movements

An alternative rate-limiting process to numerical subvocalization is that enumerating beyond four items may require eye movements whereas subitization or visual search may not. In support of this, preventing saccades can make difficult search more efficient (Klein & Farell, 1989; Zelinsky & Sheinberg, 1997) whereas enumeration beyond four items can become less accurate (Atkinson, Campbell, & Francis, 1976; Simon & Vaishnavi, 1996). Methodological issues with the original work on eye movements in enumeration led us to re-examine the role of eye movements in enumeration (Watson, Maylor, & Bruce, 2004). We measured enumeration rates (young adults only) when saccades were or were not allowed and found that preventing eye movements had no effect on subitization rates but counting rates were slowed. We also found that fixation durations were longer before saccades to previously examined locations, which demonstrates for the first time that IOR is involved in visual enumeration. Thus, preventing eye movements does not reduce the accuracy of enumeration but does make it less efficient, which is the opposite of what happens in visual search.

Why should saccades be particularly important in enumeration but not in visual search tasks? For accurate enumeration, it is crucial that each item is processed only once. One way in which old items could be prevented from being reprocessed is via IOR in which attention and eye movements are biased against returning to previously examined locations (Hooge & Frens, 2000; Klein, 2000; Klein & MacInnes, 1999). IOR may thus play a role in ensuring that items are enumerated only once (Simon & Vaishnavi, 1996) and as saccade generated IOR appears to be stronger than IOR generated from covert shifts of attention (Hooge & Frens, 2000) we would expect overt shifts to be more frequent in tasks in which it is particularly important to exclude previously examined items (e.g. enumeration). In contrast, visual search accuracy does not require that items are only processed once, and indeed there may be little memory for what has already been searched (e.g. Horowitz & Wolfe, 1998; but see also Peterson, Kramer, Wang, Irwin, & McCarley, 2001). This might be because visual search is more efficient overall if the cost involved in ensuring that old items are not reprocessed is removed.

If the above account is correct, we would expect the following: (i) subitization should produce relatively few eye movements per item, (ii) enumerating beyond four items should produce more fixations per item than difficult visual search, and (iii) fixation frequency should be age equivalent for enumeration beyond four items. We confirmed these predictions in an experiment that monitored eye movements in easy and difficult visual search and enumeration without distractors in young and old adults (Watson, Maylor, & Bruce, in press b,

Table 3.1 Summary of conclusions from (a) Watson, Maylor, and Bruce (in press b) and (b) Rabbitt (1965)

	Young	Old
(a) Fixation rate (n/item)		
Difficult visual search[a]	0.09	0.18
Enumeration (>4 items)	~1	~1
(b) Size of search set		
Condition 1 (2 targets)	Large	Small
Condition 2 (8 targets)	Small	Small

[a] Target present trials.

experiment 1). Both easy search and subitization resulted in low rates of eye movements that were equivalent for young and old. Old adults made twice as many fixations per item in difficult search than did young adults (see Table 3.1(a)). This is consistent with an age-related reduction in visual or attentional capacity (e.g. reduced useful-field-of-view; Ball, Beard, Roenker, Miller, & Griggs, 1988; Scialfa, Kline, & Lyman, 1987; Sekuler, Bennett, & Mamelak, 2000), which is compensated for by an increase in fixation frequency (rather than duration). In contrast, counting produced much slower and age equivalent fixation rates (Table 3.1(a)). Thus the experiment provides direct evidence that the counterintuitive age equivalence in counting rate beyond four items arises because of the need for both young and old adults to make eye movements. Because the process of programming and executing saccades is relatively slow and can be age invariant (Abrams, Pratt, & Chasteen, 1998), this then becomes the rate-limiting factor on enumeration.

Watson et al. (in press b, experiment 2) also examined fixation frequency for enumeration of difficult-to-find targets (*cf.* Figure 3.14). This revealed that the overall RT difference was associated with many more fixations by the old than the young. In addition, their fixation enumeration slopes were slightly shallower. This shows that under conditions of high attentional competition, the old were processing the displays less efficiently (more exhaustively) than were the young adults. In addition to fixation frequency, we also examined how often locations were refixated. This indicates the extent to which observers needed to recheck locations or restart their enumeration of a display as a result of a failure to keep track of what had already been enumerated. When distractors were absent, refixations increased as a function of numerosity only beyond four items and there were no age differences. This finding is consistent with the memory for what has been processed being based on IOR, which has been shown to be unaffected by old age (see earlier). However, the addition of distractors did cause an increase both in fixation and refixation frequency and the increase in both was greater for the old adults. This is consistent with our account as IOR has been shown to be limited to about five or six locations (Danziger, Kingstone, & Snyder, 1998; Snyder & Kingstone, 2000) and so we would expect IOR-based memory failures to increase as a function of the total fixation frequency.

In summary, the main findings from this series of experiments were that: (i) eye movements are particularly important in enumeration but not in search tasks, (ii) eye movement-based IOR is the likely basis by which old items are prevented from being enumerated more than once, (iii) the reliance of enumeration on eye movements is the reason for the counterintuitive age equivalent enumeration performance, and (iv) age equivalent subitization only holds when distractors do not also compete for attention with the target items.

Rabbitt (1965) revisited

Briefly returning to Rabbitt (1965), there was in fact a second condition in the experiment that has received far less attention in which participants were required to sort the packs of visiting cards into eight rather than only two piles according to which of the letters from A–H appeared among the different numbers of distractors. Sorting times were obviously longer for both young and old adults in this more difficult condition but, more importantly, there was less sign of the interaction between age and the number of irrelevant items that was found in the first condition (Figure 3.1). Rabbitt (1965) suggested that "when young Ss search for two relevant letters they ignore irrelevant symbols more quickly because they process them in larger groups than when they search for eight relevant letters . . . old Ss cannot sample letters in a display in large groups in either condition" (p. 236). This is summarized in Table 3.1(b). Interestingly, the argument is qualitatively similar to our own in relation to the comparison between search and enumeration. That is, the slower or more difficult condition in each case forces the young to adopt the same slow strategy as the old, which of course leads in both cases to violations of generalized slowing.

In summary, our aim has been to convey something of Patrick Rabbitt's influence by taking just one article and showing how it has influenced recent theories of cognitive aging and also inspired many subsequent studies. As Scialfa and Joffe (1997) commented, "Rabbitt's hypotheses motivated many of the attempts to find specific age-sensitive mechanisms to explain the deficits exhibited by older adults in visual search tasks" (p. 228). Madden and Whiting (2004) even describe a recent PET study of a variant of Rabbitt (1965). In the work presented here (on perceptual load, visual marking, and the comparison between search and enumeration), there was some evidence in each case of an age decrement in the ability to ignore irrelevant information. Like the Rabbitt (1965) study, the data were only partially consistent with generalized slowing. A closer look at Rabbitt's (1965) original conclusions reveals an interesting parallel with our current interpretation of enumeration data that suggests we should always be careful to consider the involvement of task-specific factors (such as the need to make eye movements) that may become the rate-limiting process on performance. More generally, if increasing task difficulty results in the involvement of additional processes that are both relatively slow and age equivalent, then age-related differences can disappear. Thus, predictions based on a generalized slowing account will fail whenever a task requires multiple processes and one of the processes is both rate limiting and age equivalent. Determining in which situations and tasks this issue arises will be an important goal for future research.

References

Abrams, R. A., Pratt, J., & Chasteen, A. L. (1998). Aging and movement: Variability of force pulses for saccadic eye movements. *Psychology and Aging, 13*, 387–395.

Atkinson, J., Campbell, F. W., & Francis, M. R. (1976). The magic number 4 ± 0: A new look at visual numerosity judgments. *Perception, 5*, 327–334.

Ball, K. K., Beard, B. L., Roenker, D. L., Miller, R. L., & Griggs, D. S. (1988). Age and visual search: Expanding the useful field of view. *Journal of the Optical Society of America A, 5*, 2210–2219.

Basak, C., & Verhaeghen, P. (2003). Subitizing speed, subitizing range, counting speed, the Stroop effect, and aging: Capacity differences and speed equivalence. *Psychology and Aging, 18*, 240–249.

Birren, J. E. (1965). Age changes in speed of behavior: Its central nature and physiological correlates. In A. T. Welford & J. E. Birren (Eds.), *Behavior, aging and the nervous system* (pp. 191–216). Springfield, IL: Charles C Thomas.

Brinley, J. F. (1965). Cognitive sets, speed and accuracy of performance in the elderly. In A. T. Welford & J. E. Birren (Eds.), *Behavior, aging and the nervous system* (pp. 114–149). Springfield, IL: Charles C Thomas.

Cerella, J. (1985). Information processing rates in the elderly. *Psychological Bulletin, 98*, 67–83.

Cerella, J. (1990). Aging and information processing rate. In J. E. Birren & K. W. Schaie (Eds.), *Handbook of the psychology of aging* (3rd ed., pp. 201–221). San Diego, CA: Academic Press.

Cerella, J., & Hale, S. (1994). The rise and fall in information-processing rates over the life span. *Acta Psychologia, 86*, 109–197.

Danziger, S., Kingstone, A., & Snyder, J. J. (1998). Inhibition of return to successively stimulated locations in a sequential visual search paradigm. *Journal of Experimental Psychology: Human Perception and Performance, 24*, 1467–1475.

Eriksen, B. A., & Eriksen, C. W. (1974). Effects of noise letters upon the identification of a target letter in a nonsearch task. *Perception and Psychophysics, 16*, 143–149.

Faust, M. E., & Balota, D. A. (1997). Inhibition of return and visuospatial attention in healthy older adults and individuals with dementia of the Alzheimer type. *Neuropsychology,* 11, 13–29.

Foster, J. K., Behrmann, M., & Stuss, D. T. (1995). Aging and visual search: Generalized cognitive slowing or selective deficit in attention. *Aging and Cognition,* 2, 279–299.

Gallistel, C. R., & Gelman, R. (1992). Preverbal and verbal counting and computation. *Cognition,* 44, 43–74.

Geary, D. C., & Lin, J. (1998). Numerical cognition: Age-related differences in the speed of executing biologically primary and biologically secondary processes. *Experimental Aging Research,* 24, 101–137.

Gilmore, G. C., Tobias, T. R., & Royer, F. L. (1985). Aging and similarity grouping in visual search. *Journal of Gerontology,* 40, 586–592.

Hartley, A. A., & Kieley, J. M. (1995). Adult age differences in the inhibition of return of visual attention. *Psychology and Aging,* 10, 670–683.

Hasher, L., & Zacks, R. T. (1988). Working memory, comprehension, and aging: A review and a new view. In G. H. Bower (Ed.), *The psychology of learning and motivation* (Vol. 22, pp. 193–225). New York: Academic Press.

Hasher, L., Zacks, R. T., & May, C. P. (1999). Inhibitory control, circadian arousal, and age. In D. Gopher & A. Koriat (Eds.), *Attention and performance XVII. Cognitive regulation and performance: Interaction of theory and application* (pp. 653–675). Cambridge, MA: MIT Press.

Hommel, B., Li, K. Z. H., & Li, S.-C. (2004). Visual search across the life span. *Developmental Psychology,* 40, 545–558.

Hooge, I. Th. C., & Frens, M. A. (2000). Inhibition of saccade return (ISR): Spatio-temporal properties of saccade programming. *Vision Research,* 40, 3415–3426.

Horowitz, T. S., & Wolfe, J. M. (1998). Visual search has no memory. *Nature,* 394, 575–577.

Huang-Pollock, C. L., Carr, T. H., & Nigg, J. T. (2002). Development of selective attention: Perceptual load influences early versus late attentional selection in children and adults. *Developmental Psychology,* 38, 363–375.

Humphrey, D. G., & Kramer, A. F. (1997). Age differences in visual search for feature, conjunction, and triple-conjunction targets. *Psychology and Aging,* 12, 704–717.

Humphreys, G. W., & Müller, H. J. (1993). Search via recursive rejection (SERR): A connectionist model of visual search. *Cognitive Psychology,* 25, 43–110.

Kaufman, E. L., Lord, M. W., Reese, T. W., & Volkman, J. (1949). The discrimination of visual number. *American Journal of Psychology,* 62, 498–525.

Klein, R., & Farrell, M. (1989). Search performance without eye movements. *Perception and Psychophysics,* 46, 476–482.

Klein, R. M. (2000). Inhibition of return. *Trends in Cognitive Sciences,* 4, 138–146.

Klein, R. M., & MacInnes, W. J. (1999). Inhibition of return is a foraging facilitator in visual search. *Psychological Science,* 10, 346–352.

Kline, D. W., & Scialfa, C. T. (1996). Visual and auditory aging. In J. E. Birren & K. W. Schaie (Eds.), *Handbook of the psychology of aging* (pp. 181–203). London: Academic Press.

Kotory, L., & Hoyer, W. J. (1995). Age and the ability to inhibit distractor information in visual selective attention. *Experimental Aging Research,* 21, 159–171.

Kramer, A. F., & Atchley, P. (2000). Age-related effects in the marking of old objects in visual search. *Psychology and Aging, 15*, 286–296.

Kramer, A. F., Martin-Emerson, R., Larish, J. F., & Andersen, G. J. (1996). Aging and filtering by movement in visual search. *Journal of Gerontology: Psychological Sciences, 51B*, 201–216.

Langley, L. K., Fuentes, L. J., Hochhalter, A. K., Brandt, J., & Overmier, J. B. (2001). Inhibition of return in aging and Alzheimer's disease: Performance as a function of task demands and stimulus timing. *Journal of Clinical and Experimental Neuropsychology, 23*, 431–446.

Lavie, N. (1995). Perceptual load as a necessary condition for selective attention. *Journal of Experimental Psychology: Human Perception and Performance, 21*, 451–468.

Lavie, N., & Cox, S. (1997). On the efficiency of visual selective attention: Efficient visual search leads to inefficient distractor rejection. *Psychological Science, 8*, 395–398.

Lavie, N., Hirst, A., de Fockert, J. W., & Viding, E. (2004). Load theory of selective attention and cognitive control. *Journal of Experimental Psychology: General, 133*, 339–354.

Lavie, N., & Tsal, Y. (1994). Perceptual load as a major determinant of the locus of selection in visual attention. *Perception and Psychophysics, 56*, 183–197.

Madden, D. J., & Langley, L. K. (2003). Age-related changes in selective attention and perceptual load during visual search. *Psychology and Aging, 18*, 54–67.

Madden, D. J., & Plude, D. J. (1993). Selective preservation of selective attention. In J. Cerella, J. Rybash, W. Hoyer, & M. L. Commons (Eds.), *Adult information processing: Limits on loss* (pp. 273–300). San Diego, CA: Academic Press.

Madden, D. J., & Whiting, W. L. (2004). Age-related changes in visual attention. In P. T. Costa & I. C. Siegler (Eds.), *Recent advances in psychology and aging* (pp. 41–84). Amsterdam: Elsevier.

Mandler, G., & Shebo, B. J. (1982). Subitizing: An analysis of its component processes. *Journal of Experimental Psychology: General, 111*, 1–22.

Maylor, E. A., & Lavie, N. (1998). The influence of perceptual load on age differences in selective attention. *Psychology and Aging, 13*, 563–574.

Maylor, E. A., & Rabbitt, P. M. A. (1993). Alcohol, reaction time and memory: A meta-analysis. *British Journal of Psychology, 84*, 301–317.

Maylor, E. A., Schlaghecken, F., & Watson, D. G. (in press). Aging and inhibitory processes in memory, attentional and motor tasks. In R. Engle, G. Sedek, U. von Hecker, & D. McIntosh (Eds.), *Cognitive limitations in aging and psychopathology.* Cambridge, England: Cambridge University Press.

Nebes, R. D., Brady, C. B., & Reynolds, C. F., III. (1992). Cognitive slowing in Alzheimer's disease and geriatric depression. *Journal of Gerontology: Psychological Sciences, 47*, 331–336.

Park, D. C. (2000). The basic mechanisms accounting for age-related decline in cognitive function. In D. C. Park & N. Schwarz (Eds.), *Cognitive aging: A primer* (pp. 3–21). Hove, East Sussex: Psychology Press.

Peterson, M. S., Kramer, A. F., Wang, R. X. F., Irwin, D. E., & McCarley, J. S. (2001). Visual search has memory. *Psychological Science, 12*, 287–292.

Plude, D. J., & Doussard-Roosevelt, J. A. (1989). Aging, selective attention, and feature integration. *Psychology and Aging, 4*, 98–105.

Plude, D. J., Enns, J. T., & Brodeur, D. (1994). The development of selective attention: A life-span overview. *Acta Psychologica, 86,* 227–272.

Pylyshyn, Z. W. (1989). The role of location indexes in spatial perception: A sketch of the FINST spatial-index model. *Cognition, 32,* 65–97.

Pylyshyn, Z. W. (1998). Visual indexes in spatial vision and imagery. In R. D. Wright (Ed.), *Visual attention* (pp. 215–231). Oxford, England: Oxford University Press.

Pylyshyn, Z. W. (2001). Visual indexes, preconceptual objects, and situated vision. *Cognition, 80,* 127–158.

Rabbitt, P. M. A. (1965). An age-decrement in the ability to ignore irrelevant information. *Journal of Gerontology, 20,* 233–237.

Rogers, W. A. (2000). Attention and aging. In D. C. Park & N. Schwarz (Eds.), *Cognitive aging: A primer* (pp. 57–73). Hove, East Sussex: Psychology Press.

Sagi, D., & Julesz, B. (1985). Detection versus discrimination of visual orientation. *Perception, 14,* 619–628.

Salthouse, T. A. (1985). *A theory of cognitive aging.* Amsterdam: North-Holland.

Salthouse, T. A. (1991). *Theoretical perspectives on cognitive aging.* Hillsdale, NJ: Erlbaum.

Salthouse, T. A. (1996a). Constraints on theories of cognitive aging. *Psychonomic Bulletin and Review, 3,* 287–299.

Salthouse, T. A. (1996b). The processing-speed theory of adult age differences in cognition. *Psychological Review, 103,* 403–428.

Salthouse, T. A. (2000). Steps toward the explanation of adult age differences in cognition. In T. J. Perfect & E. A. Maylor (Eds.), *Models of cognitive aging* (pp. 19–49). Oxford, England: Oxford University Press.

Scialfa, C. T., & Joffe, K. M. (1997). Age differences in feature and conjunction search: Implications for theories of visual search and generalized slowing. *Aging, Neuropsychology, and Cognition, 4,* 227–247.

Scialfa, C. T., Kline, D. W., & Lyman, B. J. (1987). Age differences in target identification as a function of retinal location and noise level: An examination of the useful field of view. *Psychology and Aging, 2,* 14–19.

Sekuler, A. B., Bennett, P. J., & Mamelak, M. (2000). Effects of aging on the useful field of view. *Experimental Aging Research, 26,* 103–120.

Simon, T. J., & Vaishnavi, S. (1996). Subitizing and counting depend on different attentional mechanisms: Evidence from visual enumeration in afterimages. *Perception and Psychophysics, 58,* 915–926.

Sliwinski, M. (1997). Aging and counting speed: Evidence for process-specific slowing. *Psychology and Aging, 12,* 38–49.

Snyder, J. J., & Kingstone, A. (2000). Inhibition of return and visual search: How many separate loci are inhibited? *Perception and Psychophysics, 62,* 452–458.

Townsend, J. T. (1972). Some results on the identifiability of parallel and serial processes. *British Journal of Mathematical and Statistical Psychology, 25,* 168–199.

Treisman, A., & Souther, J. (1985). Search asymmetry: A diagnostic for preattentive processing of separable features. *Journal of Experimental Psychology: General, 114,* 285–310.

Treisman, A. M., & Gelade, G. (1980). A feature-integration theory of attention. *Cognitive Psychology, 12,* 97–136.

Trick, L. M., Enns, J. T., & Brodeur, D. A. (1996). Life span changes in visual enumeration: The number discrimination task. *Developmental Psychology, 32*, 925–932.

Trick, L. M., & Pylyshyn, Z. W. (1993). What enumeration studies can show us about spatial attention: Evidence for limited capacity preattentive processing. *Journal of Experimental Psychology: Human Perception and Performance, 19*, 331–351.

Trick, L. M., & Pylyshyn, Z. W. (1994a). Cueing and counting: Does the position of the attentional focus affect enumeration? *Visual Cognition, 1*, 67–100.

Trick, L. M., & Pylyshyn, Z. W. (1994b). Why are small and large numbers enumerated differently? A limited-capacity preattentive stage in vision. *Psychological Review, 101*, 80–102.

Watson, D. G. (2001). Visual marking in moving displays: Feature-based inhibition is not necessary. *Perception and Psychophysics, 63*, 74–84.

Watson, D. G., & Humphreys, G. W. (1997). Visual marking: Prioritizing selection for new objects by top-down attentional inhibition. *Psychological Review, 104*, 90–122.

Watson, D. G., & Humphreys, G. W. (1998). Visual marking of moving objects: A role for top-down feature based inhibition in selection. *Journal of Experimental Psychology: Human Perception and Performance, 24*, 946–962.

Watson, D. G., & Humphreys, G. W. (1999). The magic number four and temporo-parietal damage: Neurological impairments in counting targets amongst distractors. *Cognitive Neuropsychology, 16*, 609–629.

Watson, D. G., Humphreys, G. W., & Olivers, C. N. L. (2003). Visual marking: Using time in visual selection. *Trends in Cognitive Sciences, 7*, 180–186.

Watson, D. G., & Maylor, E. A. (2002). Aging and visual marking: Selective deficits for moving stimuli. *Psychology and Aging, 17*, 321–339.

Watson, D. G., Maylor, E. A., & Bruce, L. A. M. (2004). *The role of eye movements in subitizing and counting.* Manuscript submitted for publication.

Watson, D. G., Maylor, E. A., & Bruce, L. A. M. (in press a). Effects of age on searching for and enumerating targets that cannot be detected efficiently. *Quarterly Journal of Experimental Psychology (Section A).*

Watson, D. G., Maylor, E. A., & Bruce, L. A. M. (in press b). Search, enumeration and aging: Eye movement requirements cause age-equivalent performance in enumeration but not search tasks. *Psychology and Aging.*

Watson, D. G., Maylor, E. A., & Manson, N. J. (2002). Aging and enumeration: A selective deficit for the subitization of targets among distractors. *Psychology and Aging, 17*, 496–504.

Zelinsky, G. J., & Sheinberg, D. L. (1997). Eye movements during parallel-serial visual search. *Journal of Experimental Psychology: Human Perception and Performance, 23*, 244–262.

Chapter 4

Individual differences and cognitive models of the mind: using the differentiation hypothesis to distinguish general and specific cognitive processes

Mike Anderson and Jeff Nelson

Abstract

This chapter uses a particular hypothesis from research on individual differences in cognitive ability—the differentiation hypothesis—to show that individual differences can be informative for cognitive models of the mind. The differentiation hypothesis comes in two forms. The developmental differentiation hypothesis argues that as children develop their abilities become more differentiated and that as adults age their abilities become de-differentiated. The individual differences differentiation hypothesis states that abilities are more differentiated at higher IQ. Differentiation is usually inferred from either a smaller g-factor or a lower average inter-test correlation. Simulations of alternative models that specify different functional relationships between processes underlying the g-factor and specific abilities are presented. They reveal that empirical outcomes are likely to be sensitive to nontrivial assumptions about the precise relationships between the hypothetical processes. In particular, a common but simple interpretation of the apparent de-differentiation of abilities with advancing age, and increasing differentiation with development in children, is that a single common factor underlies both g and developmental change (e.g. speed of processing). The simulations reveal that this simple interpretation is unwarranted. Evidence from the analysis of two datasets (elderly adults and young children) confirms this conclusion.

Introduction

In 1957 the then president of the American Psychological Association, Lee Cronbach, used his annual address to the Association to argue for the greater integration of what he called the "Two Psychologies" (Cronbach, 1957). One of these was individual differences psychology and the other experimental psychology. The individual differences approach was characterized mainly by what he called the method of correlations and the experimental approach by the method of means. Essentially the former's research agenda was to explore the observed relationships amongst a set of individual differences variables and the latter's was to use manipulations of independent variables to test hypotheses by comparing differences in means between experimental conditions. In 1957 Cronbach included social and abnormal psychology as part of the individual differences approach, while the experimental approach was best characterized by perception and learning theory, with the latter about to be superseded by the cognitive revolution. An over-arching concern of this chapter is to show how these two approaches to studying a common topic—intelligence—might inform each other.

There has been a burgeoning of work using measures derived from cognitive psychology that, on the surface at least, seems to bring these two traditions together (see, for example, Hunt (1980), Sternberg (1983)). However, I have argued elsewhere that this drawing together is more apparent than real (Anderson, in press). Part of the reason for this is what it is that individual differences researchers of intelligence have taken from the cognitive approach. Rather than take the ideas or theories of cognitive psychology, it is the potential to derive new measures of cognitive ability that has been seized upon. Individual differences researchers are in the main indifferent to theories from cognitive psychology about the cognitive structure of the mind. In turn the major discovery of individual differences research on cognitive abilities—Spearman's g, or the fact that cognitive abilities covary (Spearman, 1904)—has been almost totally ignored by cognitive psychology. In my view this indicates a shallow relationship between the two disciplines. In this chapter I would like to pick up the advocacy of a rapprochement between the two psychologies—specifically in the domain of intelligence. I hope to "lead by example" by using a cognitive theory of the structure of mind, that was itself designed to explain individual differences in cognitive ability, to show how these two research traditions can be mutually informative.

My central thesis is that the constructs of a cognitive theory can be used to sharpen up predictions about individual differences and developmental changes that no amount of methodological developments in the individual differences field (e.g. structural equation modeling) can sidestep. To do this I will use a particular set of theoretical constructs that predicts the "differentiation" of abilities under certain conditions. Within correlational psychology the study of the differentiation of abilities has waxed and waned at various times over the last 50 years, and has had little input from or little impact on general concerns about the structure of the cognition. Consequently I want to demonstrate how taking cognitive theories of mental structure and mechanisms seriously illuminates unsettled questions in the study of individual differences in intelligence. In turn I hope that by so doing I can illuminate the great question of cognitive psychology—how do general intelligence and specific abilities work together in the cognitive mind?

The first wave of investigation: the developmental differentiation hypothesis

The differentiation of abilities is an idea whose roots are in developmental psychology, and the early differentiation studies should really be labeled the *developmental-differentiation* hypothesis to distinguish it from the *individual-differences* differentiation hypothesis of the late 1980s. One of the earliest formulations of the idea of differentiation was given by Garrett (1946). Garrett postulated that as children develop their intelligence changes from being characterized largely by individual differences in some general intellectual capacity to being characterized by differences in more specific abilities. Thus, the "ability structure" of intelligence becomes more differentiated with development. Garrett proposed only a tentative theoretical basis for this idea. He argued that in the young child general intelligence involved the comprehension and use of symbols in the service of problem solving and that differentiation occurs because symbols become more *domain specific* with growing maturity in children (indeed such a view is not so far away from a current theory of cognitive development, the modularization theory of Karmiloff-Smith (1992)). The evidence on which Garrett's conjecture rested came from two principal sources. The first was the determination of how much of the variance in ability was explained by general intelligence and this method is the basis of most modern studies of differentiation. The amount of variance accounted for was determined either by reference to the size of the first principal component in a factor analysis of tests of heterogeneous cognitive abilities, or by the average intercorrelation amongst the tests. The larger the first principal component or the larger the average correlation, the greater the influence of general intelligence and the less abilities are differentiated. Decreases in both the size of the first principal component and the average intercorrelation with children's age were taken as indications of increased differentiation. The second supporting line of evidence came from the number of factors that could be extracted from the correlation between tests or from factor structures that differ between age groups. The more factors that could reliably be extracted the more differentiated the structure of abilities was taken to be. Both kinds of evidence were found in the early studies (Atkin et al. 1977; Kahn, 1970; Very & Iacono, 1970).

It is important to note that there was no strong commitment in the early studies as to whether differentiation was maturationally or experientially driven, nor was their any strong theoretical commitment to the mechanisms that might underpin it. But the early studies recognized many of the methodological pitfalls associated with testing the differentiation hypothesis. One of the most basic is that the strength of the g-factor can be so great that it tends to mask much smaller group factors. One of the most serious consequences of this for studying the developmental differentiation hypothesis is the requirement to appropriately sample cohorts of children of different ages to ensure that sample variability in the general factor does not swamp any changes in specific factors that might really be there (Atkin et al. 1977)—conditions that are difficult to secure. If the "effect size" of changes in specific abilities is smaller than the sampling error of g within any age group then there is no chance of detecting the predicted changes.

The second wave of investigation: the fluid-crystallized g distinction

At the tail-end of the 1970s a number of studies appeared that took a slightly different tack from examining either the proportion of variance accounted for by general intelligence or the number of factors reliably appeared in a factor analysis of an array of cognitive abilities. The distinction between fluid and crystallized g as formulated by Cattell (Cattell & Cattell, 1960) afforded a different formulation of the differentiation hypothesis—one that echoes up to the present time.

Briefly, fluid intelligence is regarded as the ability to solve abstract problems and is relatively independent of processes of acculturation or instruction. Crystallized intelligence (Gc) is the knowledge base built up through the joint action of fluid intelligence across domains of knowledge and motivational, experiential and instructional processes. Cattell proposed that fluid intelligence (Gf) was subserved by different brain structures and processes to crystallized intelligence, and that they showed different developmental functions across the lifespan. In particular fluid intelligence improves during childhood and declines with aging, leaving crystallized intelligence as a kind of high tide mark of the interaction between previous fluid abilities and experiential variables. Of course, the development of fluid and crystallized g would correlate strongly because the development of Gf would necessarily drive the development of Gc. But Cattell conjectured that the "differentiation" of the two might be driven by heterogeneity in factors that might affect motivation and acculturation—factors particularly associated with schooling. For example, some aspects of formal schooling might drive increased differentiation if it led children into different areas of speciality, while others (common learning goals, for example) might hold differentiation in check. But because secondary schooling is more likely to promote the former and primary schooling the latter there would be a general trend to differentiation.

Despite this promising framework for investigating differentiation there are few empirical studies. Probably the better of these have not been studies of the development of Gf and Gc in children but in the elderly—of which more later. For children, Undheim (1976, 1978) did provide tentative support for the prediction that unlike younger children 10–13 year-olds should show adult-like levels of differentiation of Gf and Gc. However, Undheim (1978, p. 442) put the problem with all the research into differentiation up to that point rather well: "The present study points to the need for specific hypotheses rather than sweeping generalizations regarding the question of ability differentiation." Some more specific hypotheses were just around the corner (as we shall see) but two new approaches that offered promise for investigating the differentiation hypothesis appeared in the 1980s. The first was the application of information processing models to understanding individual differences, and in particular the hypothesis that a single global factor (usually speed of processing) was the basis of developmental and individual differences in g. The second was the claim that there was increasing differentiation with increasing IQ.

Single global models of intelligence

In the 1980s cognitive psychologists finally turned their attention to individual differences in intelligence and showed some interest in g (Hunt, 1980; Sternberg, 1983). The application of information processing psychology to the study of individual differences in intelligence, led to a specific hypothesis that g might be based on individual differences in speed of information processing. This hypothesis appeared in three distinct forms. The first is the hypothesis that speed of processing is related to IQ differences in adults (Jensen, 1980, 1982). The second is that increasing speed of processing is the motor of developmental change in intellectual abilities in children (Kail, 1988, 1991a, 1991b; Kail & Salthouse, 1994). The third is that decreasing speed of processing with age is the cause of cognitive decline in the elderly (Salthouse, 1985, 1991, 1996). The main line of evidence in each domain comes from the association between performance on tasks thought to reflect speed of processing and cognitive performance measured by intelligence tests. Reaction times and inspection times are correlated with IQ differences in adults (Jensen, 1982; Kranzler & Jensen, 1989; Nettelbeck, 1987). Reaction times and inspection times decrease with age during childhood development (Fairweather & Hutt, 1978; Nettelbeck & Wilson, 1985). Finally reaction times and inspection times increase with age in adult samples (Birren et al. 1963; Nettelbeck & Rabbitt, 1992). A more complex analysis involved plotting decision times on a widely varying set of cognitive tasks of old and young participants against each other (Brinley plots). This technique led to amazingly linear functions, with correlations typically greater than 0.95 in the elderly and for childhood development (Cerella, 1985; Hale, 1990; Kail, 1988). Research using Brinley plots to compare groups differing on IQ has been sparse and results have been less impressive (see, for example, Davis & Anderson, 1999). Some have argued that these functions support the idea that developmental change could be explained by positing a single scaling factor on all information processing routines—something that a parameter like speed of processing could accommodate with ease (Kail & Salthouse, 1994).[1] Despite the fact that the single global hypothesis of cognitive ageing has not gone unchallenged for both children (Anderson, 1995; Anderson, Nettelbeck, & Barlow, 1997; Davis & Anderson, 1999, 2001) and elderly adults (Rabbitt, Anderson, Davis, & Shilling, 2003; Rabbitt & Anderson, in press), the focus on the possibility of speed of processing underlying both individual differences in intelligence and developmental change in cognitive abilities provided the theoretical backdrop for developments in the differentiation hypothesis.

The de-differentiation hypothesis

The idea that cognitive ageing may represent a decline in a single global process such as processing speed has been a relatively robust hypothesis in the literature. More recently it has been argued that such a decline predicts the de-differentiation of abilities with advancing age, though others have pointed out that evidence for de-differentiation does not in turn unequivocally support the single global hypothesis (Rabbitt & Anderson, in press). Ghisletta and Lindenberger (2003) used a broad scheme of de-differentiation within the fluid/crystallized intelligence framework. In their scheme de-differentiation

---

[1] It has been pointed out that were such a theory be proven true then this would nullify the usefulness of studying developmental changes in cognition, because if age does not affect some processes more than others then age-effects would be, by definition, uninformative for research that hoped to illuminate the underlying mechanisms of cognition (Rabbitt et al. 2003).

can have three manifestations: (1) increasing correlations between abilities with advancing age; (2) the increasing divergence between fluid and crystallized g with advancing age; (3) the increased correlation between measures of intelligence and measures of "biological" functioning with increasing age. They argue that all are signs of an increasing importance of a biological factor on intellectual performance in the elderly. In our terms this can be thought of as the increased dominance of differences in a single global process, such as speed of processing, as that process goes into decline. Ghisletta and Lindenberger (2003) provide supporting evidence for this general picture using measures of visual processing speed to index the "mechanics" of intelligence (fluid g) and knowledge tests to index the pragmatics of intelligence (crystallized g) in a sample of 513 people aged between 70 and 103 from the Berlin ageing study (Baltes & Mayer, 1999). Using a very complex statistical analysis they found an asymmetry in the causal roles of crystallized knowledge and fluid intelligence/processing speed in their study. Variance in "knowledge" was increasingly predicted by variance in processing speed as age increased in the sample but the complement was not true. Variance in knowledge became increasingly unimportant for the prediction of processing speed as age increased in the sample. Consequently, as ageing advances, cognitive ability becomes increasingly dominated by variance in speed. More simply, Rabbitt and Anderson presented data on correlations between the Alice Heim (AH4) test of intelligence and 11 other tasks involving "fluid abilities" (including various kinds of recall, digit span, visual processing speed, and the Cattell Culture Fair test of g) for samples aged form 49–69 (young) and 70–92 (old). These correlations were higher in the older group on 8 out of the 11 cases.

The study of cognitive ageing represents a contemporary application of the ideas underlying the differentiation hypothesis, but it was the work on its relationship to individual differences in IQ by Detterman and colleagues at the end of the 1980s that gave it a renewed impetus.

The third wave: Detterman's individual differences differentiation hypothesis

Detterman (1987) approached understanding individual differences in intelligence from the perspective of understanding mental retardation. He observed that whatever the specific process some researchers would argue was the fundamental deficit underlying retardation (e.g. stimulus traces in memory (Ellis, 1963), attention (Zeaman & House, 1963) or executive processing (Belmont & Butterfield, 1971)) they were nearly always proven right. In other words the mentally retarded showed deficits on all mental processes where researchers cared to look. Similar to the point raised in the context of studies of aging, this could condemn the study of intelligence to be of little or no interest to students of the mechanisms underlying cognition. If explaining individual differences merely involves applying a single scaling parameter to all underlying processes, then the study of individual differences would be uninformative for those interested in understanding the structure of the cognitive mind. Of course, the finding that all processes are deficient in the mentally retarded is consistent with the single global hypothesis. The claim is that there is no processing specificity to mental retardation and instead mental retardation is caused by a reduction in some single global processing parameter, such as speed of processing, that is also *ipso facto* the fount of *g*. However, Detterman (1987) argued that this conclusion was flawed and based on a measurement confusion. The confusion is that omnibus measures of cognitive abilities from which global IQ scores are derived and mental retardation defined are simply molar measures that themselves are theoretically reducible to more elemental cognitive components. For example, if there were six or so of these elemental components (labeled A, B, C, D, E, and F) then a particular subtest of an intelligence test battery might measure elemental processes A, B, and C and another C, D, E, and F and still another A, D, and F. Molar measures would be correlated not because they share some common processing parameter but because at a lower level of analysis they share common specific processing elements. Because molar measures necessarily consist of different combinations of elemental processes in different relationships to each other, positive correlations between cognitive tests are to be expected and do not unequivocally support the idea that there is a common or global ability that influences all mental tasks. In addition, deficits associated with mental retardation and low IQ are likely to be based on deficits in one or more of several components. So general intelligence is a consequence of molar measurement, and need not imply a single or global process.

Detterman proposed a research strategy of trying to isolate these more elemental processes—making the prediction that if it could be done then the size of the first principal component of the resulting test battery would reduce but with no loss of the predictive power of the linear combinations of the elemental measures for full scale IQs. Detterman et al. (1992) using measures ranging from a wide variety of information processing paradigms claimed to find just this effect. It was but one small step from a reformulation of the differentiation hypothesis.

Returning to his original concern with mental retardation, Detterman argued that if mental retardation was caused by deficits in a small number of different elemental processes, then it was likely that individual differences in molar measures would be more strongly correlated in those groups than in groups of normal or higher IQs. Further he predicted that measures of elemental processes would be more correlated in lower than in higher IQ groups. Both these predictions were confirmed (Detterman & Daniel, 1989) and so the second form of the differentiation hypothesis was given strong currency, namely, that in higher ability groups specific abilities will be more differentiated resulting in lower average test intercorrelations than in lower IQ groups. Replication of Detterman's results has been variable. Perhaps the most methodologically sound study is that of Deary et al. (1996). They analyzed the performance of 10,553 participants on eight tests of mental ability (verbal reasoning, abstract reasoning, numerical ability, mechanical reasoning, space relations, clerical speed and accuracy, spelling, and language usage) from the British–Irish Differential Aptitude Test (Educational Research Centre, 1986). The sample was selected from a population of 272,000 students aged between 14 and 17. The sample was subsequently stratified into a series of categories on the basis of differences in age and ability. The final sample of participants was selected on the basis that (a) complete data sets were available for all participants; (b) each subgroup of age and level of ability had near identical bivariate normal distributions of age and ability, with the standard deviations of each group being half of those in the total sample. As much as can be, this avoids the possibility of sampling artifacts creating or losing the differentiation effect. Their analysis followed the procedure recommended by Dettterman by using a single subtest score to divide the groups on ability (rather than overall IQ) but then omitted that subtest in the subsequent analysis. In a careful analysis of the data Deary et al. found no evidence of age differentiation within their sample but some evidence of differentiation by IQ, although the size of the first principal component only differed by about 2% in the low and high ability groups (49.8% and 47.8%, respectively. The average inter-subtest correlation for the low ability group was 0.342 and for the high ability it was 0.256.

While larger data sets seem to provide the most consistent evidence for differentiation (Lynn, 1992), Carroll (1993) in his majestic survey of factor analytic studies of intelligence argued that there was little or no evidence in its favor. The methodological complications are many (how samples are recruited, what tests are used, deciding whether variances should or should not be equalized with samples, whether correlations should be "corrected" or not for restriction of range, on what tests or indices the groups should be divided into ability ranges, what index of differentiation is the most appropriate—the size of the first principal component or the average inter-subtest correlation, and how that is to be computed; to name but a few), makes the empirical study of differentiation using the factor analysis of large population samples fraught. What is obvious is that if differentiation is a "real" effect it adds little by way of describing or explaining the variance in large data sets. As the Deary et al. data show, to argue that abilities may be more differentiated in higher ability groups is but a small qualification on the overall dominance of g. However, as this study also makes clear a small but significant contribution to the variance can be tremendously important theoretically. After-all the difference between Newton's and Einstein's predictions of planetary motions differed by a mere smidgeon, yet the theoretical consequences of these minor differences turned out to be vast. Current analyses that "test" the differentiation hypothesis pay no attention to possible underlying cognitive mechanisms that could generate the effect and perhaps a better formulation of the theoretical basis of differentiation might lead to clearer predictions and a better understanding of what the data might be telling us.

Anderson's theory of the minimal cognitive architecture

Anderson (1986) had first proposed a theory that like Detterman argued that intelligence as measured by global indices such as IQ obscured the fact that a number of separate components contribute to both individual difference and the development of intelligence. Unlike Detterman, however, he argued that individual differences in speed of processing was the single source of g and that as speed of processing increased so the constraint speed imposes on specific abilities decreased. Consequently, higher IQ groups should show the differentiation effect. However, Anderson also proposed that speed of processing did not change with development, putting a new twist on differentiation—in principle separating it into two hypotheses, one relating to individual differences and one related to developmental change. To see how this works we will have to consider the theory in some more detail.

Like Detterman, Anderson's theory of the Minimal Cognitive architecture underlying intelligence and development argues that IQ tests work because they sample knowledge—both what people can state they know and also how they use knowledge to solve problem. However, the theory argues that there are two routes to acquiring this knowledge. One of those routes (thought) is subject to the large individual differences that are typically measured by IQ-type tests of intelligence. Knowledge is acquired through thought by the implementation of knowledge-acquisition algorithms that are written in a code (a kind of language of thought) that comes in two basic varieties, generated by two alternative specific processors (SP1 and SP2). The theory states that the latent "power" (or ability) of these two processors varies between individuals and moreover is uncorrelated in the population as a whole. This means that if they were the only mechanisms that contribute to individual differences in intelligence then there would be two independent abilities or intelligences. The theory clearly proposes that there are only two such mechanisms and the simulations that follow will make this assumption. The key to the theory is that the knowledge algorithms from each specific processor are implemented on a basic processing mechanism (BPM). The BPM varies in its speed and this constrains the complexity of the algorithms that can be implemented. Simply put, faster speeds allow more complex (powerful) algorithms to be implemented. As a consequence the manifest abilities in each ability domain of the specific processor will become correlated. In this way it is the constraint that speed of processing places on the manifest abilities of the specific processors that is the cause of the g-factor in measured abilities.

The differentiation effect was deliberately built into this architecture, for as speed of processing increases so the constraint on the specific processors decreases. Thus at faster processing speed the latent differences between the specific processors become more manifest and correlations between tasks measuring these abilities should decrease. This makes speed of processing more important for "lower ability" groups and in turn this would make the g-factor stronger in low than in high groups.

Unlike Detterman's model there is also a developmental dimension to the differentiation effect that "falls out of" the basic architecture. A major hypothesis of the theory is that speed of processing does not change with development (contrary to some of the views on the single global hypothesis described above). What might be countenanced, however, is that the power of the specific processors change with development. Nevertheless given that the relationship between speed of processing and the manifest abilities is fully specified in the theory the consequences of a change in either, both or none of these mechanisms can be specified for the developmental dimension to differentiation. For example, the effect of increasing speed of processing with development can be modeled and would make the developmental dimension to differentiation equivalent to the individual differences dimension—in short just as higher ability groups should be more differentiated so too should older children. Rabbitt and Anderson (in press) have already applied the logic of this theory to their data on the de-differentiation of abilities with advancing age and did demonstrate that a higher average correlation between a set of cognitive tests for older elderly compared with younger elderly participants was consistent with the global decline model. However it was clear that there are nontrivial alternative models that might make the same prediction. In the remainder of this chapter I will develop the models further and turn finally to both data on the development of abilities in children and other data on elderly adults to try to determine what version of the differentiation hypothesis might best fit the data.

Testing alternative models of differentiation

The approach to modeling differentiation was first developed by Anderson (1992, 1999) and was based on the theory of the minimal cognitive architecture. Simply put, the basic model states:

$$SA = \log (BPM) \times \log (SP_L).$$

The manifest specific ability (SA) is a function of the natural logarithm of the latent power of the specific processor (SP_L) multiplied by the natural logarithm of the speed of the basic processing mechanism (BPM). This equation captures the requisite property of the theory, namely that the constraint of speed of processing on the manifest power of a specific processor decreases as speed increases. While this equation captures the functional relationship between speed of processing and the manifest specific abilities, we still need to enter the individual differences parameters. This is done by creating a "population" of hypothetical individuals with equivalent means and standard deviations on the fundamental attributes: the speed of the basic processing mechanism (BPM) and the latent power of each of the two specific processors ($SP1_L$ and $SP2_L$). The equivalence of means and standard deviations is a simplifying assumption. It would be a matter of empirical investigation to determine the consequences of those assumptions— something we will leave for the moment. In the simulations reported below 5000 such individuals were "created" with the constraint that each of these attributes are uncorrelated in the population (it is only through the constraint of the BPM that the manifest abilities (SA1 and SA2) become correlated). Because in a later section we want to put a developmental dimension into the models we want the tests scores to be located on a common scale. Consequently the manifest abilities in all models are transformed to z-scores.

To test the consequences of this basic model for psychometric measures of ability we need to model the influence of the manifest abilities of the specific processors on cognitive test performance. This requires a further stage where we construct a "battery" of cognitive tests that "load" on different specific processors. This can be done simply by determining that individual differences on a hypothetical test will have a different contribution from each of the specific processors. In the simulations reported below it is also assumed that the contributions of these processors will only ever account for 50% of the variance on any one test. The rest of this variance is allocated to random normally distributed "noise," though in future simulations part of this variance could be allocated to nonability factors. Because the noise and manifest abilities are in effect distributions of z-scores then the weights of these distributions determine the amount of variance that each variable will make to each test. Table 4.1 presents these weights for the "generic" model from the theory of the Minimal Cogntiive Architecture, hereafter referred to as Model 1.

In this way we create 5000 test scores on 10 tests and we are ready to examine three major variables related to the differentiation hypothesis: (1) the size of the average correlation between the tests; (2) the amount of variance accounted for by the first principle component; (3) the size of the variance accounted for by the second principal component, all of which are compared for lower and higher ability groups. That the second principal component is included is the first product of this approach. This is because the simulations allow us to do something that conventional analyses of real data cannot, and that is to examine the relationship between the original processing attributes that generated the data in the first place and the resulting first and second principal components from the conventional psychometric analysis. And what this will reveal is interesting, as we shall see later.

The modeling will be done in two sections. First, the consequences of different functional relationships between the BPM and the specific processors

Table 4.1 Loadings of the manifest specific processors and amount of variance accounted for in each test in the simulated battery

Test	SA1	Variance (%)	SA2	Variance (%)	Noise	Variance (%)
1	0.693	48	0.141	2	0.707	50
2	0.678	46	0.2	4	0.707	50
3	0.632	40	316	10	0.707	50
4	0.592	35	0.387	15	0.707	50
5	0.548	30	0.447	20	0.707	50
6	0.447	20	0.548	30	0.707	50
7	0.387	15	0.592	35	0.707	50
8	0.316	10	0.632	40	0.707	50
9	0.2	4	0.678	46	0.707	50
10	0.141	2	0.693	48	0.707	50

will be examined. Second, alternative developmental models within the architecture will be developed so that predictions from the theory can be tested.

Four alternative functions relating speed of processing to specific abilities

In the original, generic model, the function that described the constraint that the speed of the BPM imposed on the specific processors was a logarithmic one. So:

$$SA = \log(BPM) \times \log(SP_L) \hspace{2cm} \text{(generic model)}$$

The form of this equation was designed to generate differentiation. As speed increases its influence (determined by the amount of variance in manifest specific abilities it accounts for) decreases. However, other functions relating speed and specific abilities would also yield a g-factor but the question becomes—would they also generate differentiation?. Three alternative functions were tested in the first series of simulation. The first, ADD, simply states that speed adds a processing advantage to the specific processors and that advantage is a linear function of speed. So:

$$SA = BPM + SP_L. \hspace{2cm} \text{(ADD model)}$$

The second, MULT, states that speeds acts like a multiplier. The higher an individual's processing speed the greater the effect on the manifest ability. So:

$$SA = BPM \times SP_L \hspace{2cm} \text{(MULT model)}$$

The third, LGLG, accentuates the nonlinearity of the original model by taking the log of the log of the speed of the basic processor as the constraining function. In effect that should accentuate the desired effect that it is at the slowest speeds that changes make the most difference. So:

$$SA = \log(\log(BPM)) \times \log(SP_L) \hspace{2cm} \text{(LGLG model)}$$

These alternative functions underlying the models are plotted in Figure 4.1.

This figure shows the manifest specific ability as a function of increased speed of the BPM for three "levels" of the power of the relevant specific processor for all four alternative models. Note that they represent the effect of speed going from values that range between 3 standard deviations below the population mean and values 3 standard deviations above. The three "levels" of latent specific processor power are chosen similarly, "low" is three SDs below the population mean, "mid" is the mean, "high" is three SDs above the mean. These functions generated manifest specific abilities for the same 5000

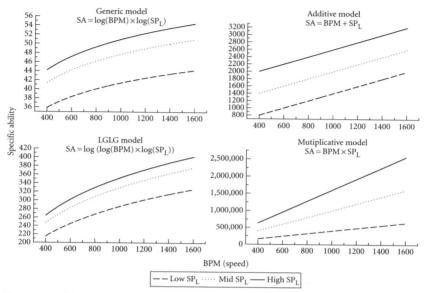

Fig. 4.1 Modeling different functions of the effect of BPM speed and three levels of the latent power of a specific processor specific (SP$_L$) on the manifest specific ability (SA).

individuals (i.e. for the same set of underlying attributes) as used in the generic model. As before those manifest abilities were then transformed to z-scores and then the 10 scores on the "psychometric" test were generated as before (i.e. according to the weights in Table 4.1). It should be borne in mind of course that the majority of the population have speed values that lie in the middle of these ranges and one of the crucial questions becomes does our empirical analysis of these models have sufficient power to detect these effects?

Table 4.2 presents the results of the analyses on the data from all four models for the three major dependent variables—the size of the average correlation in the test battery; the proportion of variance accounted for by the first principal component; and the proportion of the variance accounted for by the second principal component—for the population as a whole and for the population divided into high and low groups (a median split on overall ability, where ability is the sum of the subtest scores). The generic model generates the expected differentiation for high and low groups—the average correlation is much lower in the high group as is the size of PCA1. Note that PCA2 is almost identical for both groups. Even though the average correlation for the additive model is approximately the same size for the population as a whole, the difference between high and low disappears, as

Table 4.2 Average inter-subtest correlations and first and second Principal Components from a factor analysis of the simulated data from the four alternative models

	Average "r"			PCA1 (%)			PCA2 (%)		
	All	**Low**	**High**	**All**	**Low**	**High**	**All**	**Low**	**High**
GENERIC	0.606	0.408	0.276	64.86	47.26	35.57	7.44	11.40	12.73
ADD	0.542	0.277	0.264	58.9	35.10	33.97	7.42	11.09	11.61
MULT	0.538	0.227	0.299	58.50	30.59	37.05	7.38	11.22	11.54
LGLG	0.648	0.463	0.313	68.55	52.18	38.98	5.65	8.45	10.43

Note: The All, Low, and High groups are products of the simulated n = 5000 sample. Performance on the ten tests was assessed and a median split was used to separate the Low and High groups. The All group is the total sample.

does any difference in size of PCA1. In other words the differentiation effect is much smaller for this model. For the multiplicative model (MULT) the difference in average correlation for the high and low groups if anything reverses, as does the difference on PCA1. LGLG has an appreciably higher average correlation for the population as a whole than the generic (single log) model and the difference between low and high is somewhat greater. In other words, increasing the negative acceleration of the curve relating speed of processing to the manifest specific ability increases differentiation—though it also simultaneously increases the strength of the *g*-factor (PCA1) itself. This brings us to a major advantage of simulating models—we can see what it is that the factors in our factor analysis are actually measuring.

Table 4.3 presents the correlations between our major dependent measures from our analyses and the hypothetical cognitive constructs that underpin them. There are two striking features of the data. The first is that we can see while the first principal component (PCA1) is most heavily imbued with the speed of the BPM, for all models the latent power of the specific processors also contribute to the PCA1. This means that while the PCA1 may well be a measure of psychometric *g*, psychometric *g* is not a pure measure of the very process without which there would be no *g*—namely the speed of the BPM. Further, for all the models it is the second principal component (PCA2) that loads exclusively on the specific processors. This means that for all models it is the second principal component that properly reflects the contribution of specific abilities (at least for this theoretical case when there are only two specific processors). The second striking feature of the data is that for both log models (generic and LGLG) the association between speed and the differentiation effect is stronger. In these models the difference between high

Table 4.3 Contribution of original attribute to PCA1 and PCA2 for the population as a whole, for groups divided on ability for each of the four models

	Generic			Mult		
	BPM	SP1$_L$	SP2$_L$	BPM	SP1$_L$	SP2$_L$
PCA1						
All	0.773	0.401	0.440	0.785	0.393	0.398
Low ability	0.630	0.197	0.274	0.629	0.202	0.215
High ability	0.570	0.279	0.320	0.600	0.294	0.208
PCA2						
All	−0.010	−0.632	0.510	0.003	−0.438	0.448
Low ability	−0.028	−0.681	0.596	−0.008	−0.430	0.448
High ability	−0.102	−0.602	0.625	0.026	−0.493	0.507
	Add			**LGLG**		
PCA1						
All	0.795	0.390	0.395	0.893	0.268	0.300
Low ability	0.630	0.259	0.236	0.815	0.109	0.143
High ability	0.620	0.225	0.245	0.749	0.188	0.214
PCA2						
All	0.011	−0.450	0.449	0.026	−0.665	0.395
Low ability	0.026	0.461	0.477	0.022	0.700	0.478
High ability	−0.003	−0.490	0.479	−0.017	−0.609	0.493

Note: The All, Low, and High groups are products of the simulated $n = 5000$ sample. Performance on the ten tests was assessed and a median split was used to separate the Low and High groups. The All group is the total sample.

Table 4.4 Ratio of variance account for by PCA1 to PCA2 for the population and ability groups for the four alternative models

Model	All	Low	High
GENERIC	8.72	4.15	2.79
ADD	7.94	3.17	2.92
MULTI	7.93	2.73	3.21
LGLG	12.13	6.18	3.74

Note: The All, Low, and High groups are products of the simulated $n = 5000$ sample. Performance on the ten tests was assessed and a median split was used to separate the Low and High groups. The All group is the total sample.

and low ability groups in the contribution speed makes to the PCA1 is greater, with speed contributing more to PCA1 in the low than in the high ability groups. Finally Table 4.4 shows the ratio of the variance accounted for by PCA1 and PCA2 for each of the models for the low and high ability groups.

What this table reveals is that for three of the models the ratio of PCA1 to PCA2 is very similar for the population as a whole. PCA1 accounts for about eight times as much of the variance as PCA2. For the LGLG model the respective figure is 12 times. However, when the groups are split on ability we see that the log models (generic and LGLG) stand out from the other two in that the ratio of PCA1 to PCA2 is much larger for the low compared to the high groups. Put this together with the findings shown in Table 4.3 (that PCA2 is exclusively a specific ability factor) and we can conclude that it is only the log models that produce differentiation where the cause of differentiation (in this case speed of processing) is also that which is most related to psychometric g in both high and low ability groups.

In conclusion then, the shape of the function influences not only the extent of differentiation but also influences the causal basis of the g factor in high and low ability groups. It may turn out that it is the second principal component that may be decisive in discriminating alternative models— something not considered before.

Comparing developmental models

We have seen then that the generic model first proposed by Anderson (1992) has the requisite features to generate the differentiation of abilities within same-age populations. The goal of this section is to explore alternative developmental models within this same architecture to determine whether there are detectable patterns of data that will differ between the models. The particular models chosen take the generic model as the base and then shift the distribution of one or more of the underlying attributes that generated the manifest specific abilities two standard deviations above the population mean for the generic model. Note that our own current view (for reasons other than its ability to explain differentiation) is that speed of processing does not change with development in children and therefore our hypothesis is that either model SP1, SP2, or BOTH will turn out to represent the facts of child development. We have no particular position on which of the ageing models is likely to be true.

The models tested are:

- BPM—speed of BPM increases
- SP1—latent power of SP_L1 increases
- SP2—latent power of $SP2_L$ increases
- BOTH—latent power of both SPs increases
- ALL—BPM, $SP1_L$ & $SP2_L$ all increase
- OLD—latent power of one SP_L decreases relative to ALL

The "OLD" model is intended to represent the possible decline in a specific ability with reference to the model that represents the maximum development of all three attributes (ALL) and so while the developmental consequences of the first five models will be compared against the generic model the OLD simulation will be compared against ALL.

Unfortunately while the consequences of the alternative models for the differentiation hypothesis for different levels of ability within the same age population is clear, the same cannot be said for the developmental dimension. The data for all these models are presented in Table 4.5.

The BPM model (increase in speed of processing only) results in a slight decrease in the size of the average correlation and PCA1. More striking is the decrease in the influence of g (measured by the size of PCA1 and the average correlation) within each of the separate ability groups. Both are consistent with increased differentiation with age and of course with the idea that this is caused by a single global factor such as speed of processing.

For the SP1 and SP2 models (where it is the latent power of the specific processors that is developing) there is no change in either the average correlation or size of PCA1. Both of these are consistent with no differentiation with age. This is despite there being considerable developmental change *only* on the specific abilities; emphasizing the different meaning that differentiation can have developmentally. This ambiguity of what differentiation means becomes even more apparent for the BOTH simulation (where both of the specific processors develop). Here there is no change in PCA1 or the average

Table 4.5 Correlation and PCA statistics for the developmental models as a function of ability

	Average "r"			PCA1 (%)			PCA2 (%)		
	All	**Low**	**High**	**All**	**Low**	**High**	**All**	**Low**	**High**
BPM	0.533	0.228	0.083	58.32	31.28	18.15	8.44	16.5	12.65
SP1	0.586	0.363	0.083	62.92	43.17	18.15	6.57	10.08	12.03
SP2	0.591	0.354	0.116	63.36	42.47	20.72	6.58	11.13	11.70
BOTH	0.608	0.397	0.111	64.86	46.05	20.23	5.9	8.87	11.68
ALL	0.572	0.23	0.133	61.74	31.53	22.56	7.06	12.98	12.44
GENERIC	0.606	0.408	0.276	64.86	47.26	35.57	7.44	11.40	12.73
OLD	0.602	0.282	0.171	64.7	36.64	26.69	9.62	18.91	16.05
ALL	0.572	0.23	0.133	61.74	31.53	22.56	7.06	12.98	12.44

Note: The All, Low, and High groups are products of the simulated n 5 5000 sample. Performance on the ten tests was assessed and a median split was used to separate the Low and High groups. The All group is the total sample.

correlation but a decrease in the influence of PCA2, or the unique influence of the specific abilities. For the ALL model there is less of a shift in the major variables compared with the BPM model, but again this global developmental change lessens the influence of the "g-factor" within each ability group. It is *only* for the models that do not incorporate an increase of speed of processing that the importance of the "g-factor" in lower ability groups is maintained for children and adults.

The OLD model (a decline in only one specific ability) sees a slight increase in the average correlation and the size of the PCA1. So this model says a decline in a specific ability might generate data that looks like de-differentiation.[2] In conclusion, it is not the case that increases in PCA1 or the average inter-subtest correlation necessarily reflects the increasing influence of a single global factor such as speed of processing.

Lessons that can be applied to real data?

Finally we will turn to some real data. One dataset on elderly participants from the University of Manchester study has kindly been given to us by Professor Rabbitt, the other is a collection of data from our own study of children (Project KIDS) at the University of Western Australia. The elderly sample is a subsample ($n = 1286$) of a larger study who were selected on the basis that they had scores on all of the following tests: Culture Fair Intelligence Test (Scale 2 Form A): Alice Heim 4, Parts A and B; Mill Hill Vocabulary Parts A and B; Digit Span; Coding—Letter Substitution; Peanuts—Picture Recognition Test; Vocabulary (WAIS); Free Recall; Delayed Recall Memory Drum. The sample of children ($n = 181$) all had scores on the following tests: Culture Fair Intelligence Test (Scale 2 Form A); and WISC 3 tests, Block Design; Object Assembly; Symbol Search; Digit Span (Forward); Mazes; Picture Completion; Similarities; Arithmetic; Coding. Details of both samples are given in Table 4.6.

The elderly groups were divided into subsamples in three different ways. The first was a division into younger and older participants based on chronological age. The second used the AH4 to classify all participants as high or low ability. For the third the participants were divided into young

---

[2] The consequences of a global decline model, such as speed of the BPM decreasing, can be inferred by inverting the logic of comparing the ALL model with BOTH (the latter differs from ALL only by having no change in speed of the BPM)—in this case it predicts a slight increase in the size of the average correlation and PCA1 (de-differentiation) but more of a difference in average correlation between low and high ability groups (individual differences differentiation).

Table 4.6 Sample characteristics of elderly participants and children

Sample	Mean (SD)	Range	n
Manchester sample			
Total sample	64.27(7.05)	49–92	1286
Younger sample	58.82(3.96)	49–64	664
Older sample	70.1(4.51)	65–92	622
Project kids sample			
Total sample	10.04(1.02)	8.11–11.75	181
Younger sample	9.09(0.3)	8.11–9.58	91
Older sample	11(0.39)	9.67–11.75	90

and old as in sample 1, but then the AH4 test score was standardized within age-group to create high and low ability subgroups within each age-group.[3] The children were split into two groups, roughly 7–9.5 and 9.5–11 years. They two were split into different ability groups based on two different WISC3 subtests—either block design or similarities. Arguable Block Design is a more "fluid" test whereas similarities is more crystallized. For both the elderly sample and for the children the test used to split the children into two ability groups was not used in any subsequent correlations for that sample comparison, after the procedure recommended by Deary et al. (1996).

The data from the elderly sample are presented in Table 4.7. The data compaing the older and younger group show that for both the average correlation and the size of the first principal component there is no evidence of differentiation. However, when the elderly are split on a measure of fluid intelligence there is evidence of differentiation on both counts. Interestingly within the younger and older groups when they are further split on fluid intelligence differences within each group there is also consistent evidence for differentiation at higher ability. It seems then that aging obscures rather than reveals ability differentiation, presumably because the amount of age-related variance in ability is actually rather small.

The data from the children are presented in Table 4.8. Consistent with the data from the elderly there is not much evidence of age related differentiation. Again consistent with the elderly sample there is marked differentiation

---

[3] Those groups were 0.5 SD below the mean or lower (low ability group) or 0.5 SD above the mean or higher (high ability group).

Table 4.7 Correlation and PCA statistics for the elderly sample

	Average "r"	PCA1	PCA2
Younger	0.365	44.6	13.4
Older	0.375	45.34	13.2
Low ability	0.284	37.34	14.51
High ability	0.177	30.83	16.87
Young*			
Low	0.298	38.65	12.66
High	0.191	31.33	16.84
Old*			
Low	0.25	34.18	14.01
High	0.149	27.26	18.53

Note: The Low and High Ability Groups were created by a median split on the AH4 test.
* See table 4.6 for age group details.

Table 4.8 Average correlations and size of the principal components for children

	Average "r"	PCA1 (%)	PCA2 (%)
All	0.25	33.7	14.48
Young	0.26	34.82	15.31
Old	0.25	34.79	14.96
Low ability[bd]	0.203	30.38	21.78
High ability[bd]	0.121	22.89	16.81
Low ability[sm]	0.252	34.13	18.36
High ability[sm]	0.202	30.43	15.08
Young			
Low ability[bd]	0.259	37.87	19.79
High ability[bd]	0.151	27.02	17.43
Old			
Low ability[bd]	0.129	31.38	25.15
High ability[bd]	0.117	24.87	17.52

[bd]—WISC3 block design.   [sm]—WISC3 similarities.

between the groups split on ability with a suggestion that that difference might be more marked when the children are split on block design rather than similarities (i.e. fluid rather than crystallized *g*). The analysis of ability differences within the young and old samples reveals if anything a stronger ability differentiation for younger children than older children.

Conclusion

In this paper we have shown how investigating the differentiation hypothesis from the perspective of a cognitive theory establishes a number of important points. First, it makes clear that previous attempts based solely on the factor analysis of ability tests obscures important ambiguities, not least of which is the assumption that what the *g*-factor represents in different age-groups, or different ability levels, is the same thing. If the size of *g* cannot be unambiguously understood as a measure of the relative influence of the fount of *g* (which we have shown it is not) then using this as a measure of differentiation makes little sense, for surely the psychological meaning of differentiation is that abilities other than that which causes *g* become increasingly "important." Second, it is clear that the function relating the process that gives rise to *g* and manifest abilities does itself affect the kind of differentiation expected. It seems clear that the differentiation hypothesis is best tested and the underlying idea advanced by developing measures of these functions rather than by further factor analyses of intelligence test data. Third, there is enough ambiguity in the developmental models to suggest that a simple measure of differentiation does not represent an adequate test of the single global models of developmental change.

References

Anderson, M. (1995). Evidence for a single global factor of developmental change—Too good to be true? *Australian Journal of Psychology, 47*, 18–24.

Anderson, M. (1986). Inspection time and IQ in young children. *Personality and Individual Differences, 7*, 677–686.

Anderson, M. (Ed.) (1992). *Intelligence and development: A cognitive theory.* Oxford, UK: Blackwell Publishers.

Anderson, M. (1999). *The development of intelligence.* Hove, England: Psychology Press/ Taylor & Francis (UK).

Anderson, M. (in press). Marrying intelligence and cognition: A developmental review. In R. J. Sternberg (Ed.), *Cognition and intelligence.* Cambridge University Press.

Anderson, M., Nettelbeck, T., & Barlow, J. (1997). Reaction time measures of speed of processing: Speed of response selection increases with age but speed of stimulus categorisation does not. *British Journal of Developmental Psychology, 15*, 145–157.

Atkin, R., Bray, R., Davison, M., Herzberger, S., Humphreys, L., & Selzer, U. (1977). Ability factor differentiation, grades 5 through 11. *Applied Psychological Measurement, 1*, 65–76.

Baltes, P. B., & Mayer, K. U. (1999). *The Berlin aging study: Aging from 70 to 100.* Cambridge University Press.

Belmont, J. M., & Butterfield, E. C. (1971). Learning strategies as determinants of memory deficiencies. *Cognitive Psychology, 2*, 411–420.

Birren, J. E., Butler, R. N., Greenhouse, S. W., Sokoloff, L., & Yarrow, M. R. (1963). *Human Aging*. Washington, DC: US Government Printing Office Publication. No. 986.

Carroll, J. B. (1993). *Human cognitive abilities: A survey of factor-analytic studies*. New York, NY: Cambridge University Press.

Cattell, R. B., & Cattell, A. K. S. (1960). *The individual or group culture fair intelligence Test*. I.P.A.T. Champaign, IL.

Cerella, J. (1985). Information processing rates in the elderly. *Psychological Bulletin*, **98**, 67–83.

Cronbach, L. J. (1957). The two disciplines of scientific psychology. *American Psychologist*, **12**, 671–684.

Davis, H., & Anderson, M. (1999). Individual differences in development—One dimension or two? In M. Anderson (Ed.), *The development of intelligence* (pp. 161–191). Hove: Psychology Press.

Davis, H., & Anderson, M. (2001). Developmental and individual differences in fluid intelligence: Evidence against the unidimensional hypothesis. *British Journal of Developmental Psychology*, **19**, 181–206.

Deary, I. J., Egan, V., Gibson, G. J., Austin, E. J., Brand, C. R., & Kellerghan, T. (1996). Intelligence and the differentitaion hypothesis. *Intelligence*, **23**, 105–132.

Detterman, D. K. (1987). Theoretical notions of intelligence and mental retardation. *American Journal of Mental Deficiency*, **92**, 2–11.

Detterman, D. K. (Ed.) (1992). *Is mind modular or unitary?* Westport, CT: Ablex Publishing.

Detterman, D. K., & Daniel, M. H. (1989). Correlations of mental tests with each other and with cognitive variables are highest for low IQ groups. *Intelligence*, **13**, 349–359.

Detterman, D. K., Mayer, J. D., Caruso, D. R., & Legree, P. J. (1992). Assessment of basic cognitive abilities in relation to cognitive deficits. *American Journal on Mental Retardation*, **97**, 251–286.

Educational Research Centre. (1986). *Differential aptitude tests. Form T Manual*. Dublin, Ireland: Educational Research Centre.

Ellis, A. (1963). Toward a more precise definition of "emotional" and "intellectual" insight. *Psychological Reports*, **13**, 125–126.

Fairweather, H., & Hutt, S. J. (1978). On the rate of gain of information in children. *Journal of Experimental Child Psychology*, **26**, 216–229.

Garrett, H. E. (1946). A developmental theory of intelligence. *American Journal of Psychology*, **1**, 372–378.

Ghisletta, P., & Lindenberger, U. (2003). Age-based structural dynamics between perceptual speed and knowledge in the Berlin Aging Study: Direct evidence for ability de-differentiation in old age. *Psychology & Aging*, **18**, 696–713.

Hale, S. (1990). A global developmental trend in cognitive processing speed. *Child Development*, **61**, 653–663.

Hunt, E. (1980). Intelligence as an information processing concept. *British Journal of Psychology*, **71**, 449–474.

Jensen, A. R. (1980). Chronometric analysis of mental ability. *Journal of Social and Biological Structures*, **3**, 181–224.

Jensen, A. R. (1982). Reaction time and psychometric g. In H. J. Eysenck, (Ed.), *A model for intelligence*. Berlin, Germany: Springer-Verlag.

Kahn, S. B. (1970). Development of mental abilities: An investigation of the "differentiation hypothesis". *Canadian Journal of Psychology*, **24**, 199–205.

Kail, R. (1988). Developmental functions for speed of cognitive processes. *Journal of Experimental Child Psychology*, **45**, 339–364.

Kail, R. (1991a). Processing time declines exponentially during childhood and adolescence. *Developmental Psychology*, **27**, 259–266.

Kail, R. (1991b). Developmental change in speed of processing during childhood and adolescence. *Psychological Bulletin*, **109**, 490–501.

Kail, R., & Salthouse, T. A. (1994). Processing speed as a mental capacity. *Acta Psychologica*, **86**, 199–225.

Karmiloff-Smith, A. (1992). *Beyond modularity: A developmental perspective on cognitive science*. Cambridge, MA: MIT Press.

Kranzler, J. H., & Jensen, A. R. (1989). Inspection time and intelligence: A meta-analysis. *Intelligence*, **13**, 329–348.

Lynn, R. (1992). Does Spearman's g decline at high IQ levels? Some evidence from Scotland. *Journal of Genetic Psychology*, **153**, 229–230.

Nettelbeck, T. (1987). Inspection time and intelligence. In Vernon, P. A. (Ed). *Speed of information-processing and intelligence*. (pp. 295–346). Westport, CT: Ablex Publishing.

Nettelbeck, T., & Rabbitt, P. M. A. (1992). Aging, cognitive performance, and mental speed. *Intelligence*, **16**, 189–205.

Nettelbeck, T, & Wilson, C. (1985). A cross-sequential analysis of developmental differences in speed of visual information processing. *Journal of Experimental Child Psychology*, **40**, 1–22.

Rabbitt, P. M. A., Anderson, M., Davis, H., & Shilling, V. (2003). Cognitive processes in ageing. In J. Valsiner & K. J. Connolly (Eds.), *Handbook of developmental psychology* (pp. 560–583). London: Sage.

Rabbitt, P. M. A., & Anderson, M. (in press). The lacunae of loss? Aging and the differentiation of cognitive abilities. In F. Craik & E. Bialystok (Eds.), *Lifespan cognition*.

Salthouse, T. A. (1985). *A cognitive theory of aging*. Berlin, Germany: Springer-Verlag.

Salthouse, T. A. (1991). *Theoretical perspectives in cognitive aging*. Hillsdale, NJ: Erlbaum.

Salthouse, T. A. (1996). The processing-speed theory of adult age-differences in cognition. *Psychological Review*, **103**, 403–428.

Spearman, C. (1904). "General Intelligence," objectively determined and measured. *American Journal of Psychology*, **15**, 201–293.

Sternberg, R. J. (1983). Components of human intelligence. *Cognition*, **15**, 1–48.

Undheim, J. O. (1976). Ability structure in 10–11-year-old children and the theory of fluid and crystallized intelligence. *Journal of Educational Psychology*, **68**, 411–423.

Undheim, J. O. (1978). Broad ability factors in 12- to 13-year-old children, the theory of fluid and crystallized intelligence, and the differentiation hypothesis. *Journal of Educational Psychology*, **70**, 433–443.

Very, P. S., & Iacono, C. H. (1970). Differential factor structure of seventh grade students. *Journal of Genetic Psychology*, **117**, 239–251.

Zeaman, D., & House, B. J. (1963). The role of attention in retardate discrimination learning. In, N. R. Ellis (Ed.), *Handbook of mental deficiency*, (pp. 159–223). New York: McGraw-Hill.

Chapter 5

Reaction time parameters, intelligence, ageing, and death: the West of Scotland Twenty-07 study

Ian J. Deary and Geoff Der

Abstract

The West of Scotland Twenty-07 study—a large, population-based, longitudinal study—is used to describe the relationships between reaction times, psychometric intelligence, ageing, and mortality. Being a representative sample, the IQ scores cover the full range and give higher estimates of the correlation with reaction times than are typical of samples with restricted ranges: -0.49 for four choice reaction time and -0.31 for simple reaction time. The Pearson correlation assumes linearity and with a large sample it is possible to examine this assumption. For four choice reaction time the relationship is approximately linear, but for simple reaction time it is complex and nonlinear. The study comprises three age cohorts assessed longitudinally and together spans the ages 16–63. Patterns of ageing and sex differences are described and eight year stability is reported. A novel finding is that women show greater intraindividual variability in choice reaction time across most of the adult age range. The survival of the cohort who were initially aged 56 to age 70 is positively associated with IQ with an effect size similar to those reported elsewhere (hazard ratio 1.41 per standard deviation). In addition, the study was able to show that the association can be accounted for by reaction times.

Introduction

The sciences of individual differences (differential psychology, psychometrics) and epidemiology are natural allies. The former attempts scientifically to characterize and reliably and validly measure psychological aspects of individuals, notably mental states and traits. The latter concerns itself with populations, especially with appropriate sampling techniques and the extent to which findings in samples may be generalized to populations. To the extent that differential psychologists wish to apply their findings to populations, they should be applying epidemiological considerations to their sampling procedures. But this is rare. For example, in the study of intelligence differences, the samples are often heavily biased toward younger and brighter subjects, typically college and university students. And epidemiologists, though they often employ measures such as social class based on, for example, an individual's occupation, they relatively rarely take into account major human traits, especially cognition that is known to be highly correlated with such social factors (Hart, Deary et al. 2003). A number of differential psychologists have recommended a change in research practice by both camps. Lubinski and Humphries (1997) stated that, "The scientific significance of general intelligence is underappreciated in epidemiology and the social sciences." Krueger, Caspi and Moffitt (2000) recommended an "epidemiological personology" approach, in which "individual differences is paired with a population-based sampling frame to yield insights about the role of personality in consequential social outcomes." Bouchard and Loehlin (2001) urged that individual differences researchers address " 'epidemiological questions' . . . we would like to focus the reader on the need for population representative samples for accurate portrayal of the effect size of the causal mechanisms."

The present chapter describes applications of this advice by describing a number of studies in which individual differences variables (psychometric intelligence, reaction times) are applied to population-representative samples. The topics addressed are of interest both to differential psychologists and epidemiologists: the correlates of psychometric intelligence, the ageing of reaction time parameters, and the determinants of mortality. The topics (reaction time, ageing, intelligence differences) and tools (reaction time procedures, Alice Heim 4 test) were specifically chosen for illustration because they related closely to those addressed and employed by Rabbitt for many years.

The Twenty-07 study

Participants

The West of Scotland Twenty-07 study is a longitudinal, population-based cohort study. As we shall see below, it is, in fact, three related studies targeted at different adult ages. Its principal aim is to investigate the processes that generate and maintain sociodemographic differences in health by major axes of social stratification, such as occupational social class, education, gender and area of residence. The study began in 1987 and its target population was the

Central Clydeside Conurbation (CCC), a mainly urban area that includes Glasgow city and its immediate surrounds. In the 1981 census, the total population of this area was 1.7 million people, roughly one-third of the population of Scotland. In terms of health, the area mirrors the generally poor record of the west of Scotland as a whole, with an overall standardized mortality ratio of 109 relative to Scotland, but also with a range of 74–115 for the 11 local authority districts contained within the area (MacIver, 1988).

The study consists of three very narrow age cohorts who were aged 15, 35, and 55 in 1987. They are to be followed up until 2007 when the youngest cohort will be the same age as the middle cohort was at the outset, and the middle cohort will be the same age as the oldest cohort was. To date, four main waves of data collection have taken place: in 1987/8, 1990/1, 1995/6, and 2000/3. Macintyre (1987) gave the rationale for the design and choice of age cohorts.

The sample has two parts: a regional sample, selected to be representative of the CCC; and a locality sample, which comprises two contrasting areas chosen for more intensive study of area characteristics. It is the more population-representative regional sample that we have used for this work on reaction times, intelligence, ageing, and mortality. This sample was selected as a clustered, stratified random sample. The primary sampling units were postcode sectors. Whilst the UK postcodes were originally designed by the Post Office for the delivery of mail, in Scotland they have been adopted for many administrative and research purposes. In particular, output from the Census is available at postcode sector level. Postcode sectors with populations of less than 3,000 were combined with similar sectors. From the resulting 175 areas 52 were chosen as a stratified random sample, with probability of selection proportional to their population.

The sampling frame chosen for the selection of individuals within postcode sectors was the Voluntary Population Survey, an enhanced electoral register (Black, 1985), which had the advantage of containing the age and sex of each household member. Individuals were chosen randomly with probability proportional to the overall population of the same age within the postcode sector. Full details of the selection procedure are given in Ecob (1987).

The achieved sample sizes were 1009, 985, and 1042 for the age 15, 35, and 55 cohorts, respectively. A comparison of these samples with equivalent samples drawn from the 1991 UK Census revealed few differences in terms of sex, social class, household tenure, or car ownership (Der, 1998). The only significant differences were for the youngest cohort, but even these did not conform to the usual pattern of over-representation among women and those of higher socioeconomic position. There was an excess of car-owning households, but not of home owners. Nor did the social class differences clearly favor the nonmanual social classes. In short, the comparison shows little evidence of bias in the samples.

Measures

Data collection is by face-to-face interviews with trained nurse interviewers and these are usually conducted in the respondent's home. The interview covers a broad range of topics. There are questions on paid and unpaid work, housing conditions, income, family composition, social support, stress, life events, physical activity, diet, alcohol and tobacco consumption, beliefs and values, and many other material, cultural, and psychological factors, along with measures of physical and mental health and well-being. Other measures include height, weight, girth, blood pressure, respiratory function, and (in 1995/6 only), cardiovascular reactivity and secretory immunoglobulin-A.

Study participants are flagged at the NHS central registry and the study is notified of any deaths.

Cognitive measures include simple and four choice reaction times, measured at waves 1, 3, and 4. Part 1 (65 verbal and numerical reasoning items) of the Alice Heim 4 (AH4) Group Test of General Intelligence (Heim, 1970) was administered to the oldest cohort at wave 1, and to all three cohorts at wave 4. The Paced Auditory Serial Addition Task (PASAT; Crawford, Obonsawin, & Allan, 1998) was measured for all three cohorts at wave 3.

Reaction time was measured using a portable device originally designed for the UK Health and Lifestyle Survey (Cox et al. 1987). A photograph of the device is shown in Figure 5.1. For simple reaction time, the respondent rests the second finger of their preferred hand on the central "0" key and is instructed to press it as quickly as possible after a zero appears in the display window above. There are eight practice trials and twenty test trials. The mean and standard deviation of the test trials are recorded in milliseconds. For choice reaction time, the respondent rests the second and third finger of each

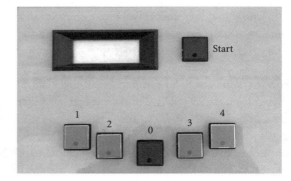

Fig. 5.1 The reaction time apparatus used in the Twenty-07 study. For description see text in Method section.

hand on the keys labeled 1, 2, 3, 4, and presses the corresponding key when one of the four digits appears in the display. There are eight practice trials and forty test trials. In the test trials the digits 1 to 4 each appear ten times in a randomised order. Means and standard deviations of reaction times are recorded separately for correct and incorrect responses as well as the number of errors. The time interval between a response and the display of the next digit varies randomly between one and three seconds for both simple and choice RT. The amount of practice involved is relatively little, though it is similar to the practice involved in most studies that relate reaction times to intelligence differences (Deary, 2000, chapter 6).

We report correlations in this chapter that are based upon the means and standard deviations of the simple and choice reaction times. However, these are attenuated by the period-free reliability of these reaction time variables (and the reliability of the variables with which they are being correlated). We are not aware of any reports of the period-free reliability for the variables obtained by this device. Therefore, for the present chapter, we administered the reaction time procedure to 49 people. They were men (18) and women (31) from our workplaces, and family and friends. Their mean (SD) age was 37.1 years (11.4). The maximum retest period was one day. The test–retest correlations (Spearman's ρ) were: simple reaction time mean = 0.67; simple reaction time standard deviation = 0.20; 4-choice reaction time mean = 0.92; 4-choice reaction time standard deviation = 0.73. Note the low test–retest correlation for simple reaction time standard deviation in this small sample. Of course, a few outliers can influence small samples, but this low value should be kept in mind when this variable, especially, is correlated with others.

More information on the Twenty-07 study

The study is funded by the UK Medical Research Council. More information and a full list of publications are available on the study website at: http://www.msoc-mrc.gla.ac.uk/Twenty-07/Twenty-07_MAIN.html

Reaction time and intelligence

The effect size in a general population sample

It is over 100 years since psychologists first used reaction time variables to try to understand the origins of individual differences in human psychometric intelligence, that is, cognitive ability differences as are now measured by IQ-type tests. Deary (2000) reviews the historical and recent research in this area. Various parameters are used, such as reaction time means, standard deviations, and the differences in times between different stimulus-response contingencies. The reasoning behind this is that reaction times are relatively simple and might reveal fundamental limits to processing efficiency in the nervous system that are related to intelligence differences. It was suggested many years ago that people with higher intelligence scores probably had faster reaction times (Beck, 1933). After the coming of cognitive psychology the main procedure used to study intelligence differences was the Hick reaction time procedure (Jensen, 1987). In this task the main variable used to index processing efficiency was the slope of reaction time as plotted against different levels of stimulus uncertainty. The slope function was hypothesized to assess people's "rate of gain of information" (Hick, 1952). The idea behind correlating the Hick slope with psychometric intelligence was that the more intelligent person had a smaller increment in reaction time as the uncertainty increased. Initial results seemed to support the idea (Roth, 1964). However, what became clear from a large amount of research in this area was that more straightforward aspects of the Hick reaction time procedure, such as the mean and the standard deviation, correlated just as well if not more highly than the Hick slope measure (Jensen, 1987). Deary (2000) suggested that the concentration on the Hick slope was largely an unproductive digression. But a further problem with this area is that the samples were dominated by student participants and the effect sizes (typically about, or sometimes below, $r = 0.2$) were small unless some adjustment was made for attenuation of range in the samples. In the field of reaction time and intelligence Nettelbeck (1987) had called for large-scale testing of normal samples of the population. None had been done until the Twenty-07 data were analyzed.

Deary, Der, and Ford (2001) analysed data on reaction times and AH4 intelligence test scores from 900 participants (487 women, 413 men) with full data from wave 1 of the Twenty-07 study. Their mean age was 56.3 years (SD = 0.6), with a range of 54.5–58.5 years. The sample did not differ in social class distribution from the relevant region in the UK's 1991 census.

For the full sample the Pearson correlation between mean simple reaction time and AH4 score was -0.31 ($p < 0.001$), and for mean 4-choice reaction time was -0.49 ($p < 0.001$); people with higher psychometric intelligence tended to have faster mean response times (Table 5.1). All analyses for choice reaction times and their standard deviations are based on correct responses only. The difference between these correlations is significant ($p < 0.001$). The correlation between AH4 scores and intraindividual variability (standard deviation) of simple and 4-choice reaction times was similar, at $r = -0.26$ ($p < 0.001$); more intelligent people tended to be less variable in response times. There was only a very small association between AH4 scores and errors (77% of participants made no errors) in the 4-choice reaction time procedure ($r = 0.07$). Deary et al. (2001)

Table 5.1 Correlations between Alice Heim 4 Part 1 total test scores and simple (SRT) and 4-choice (CRT) reaction times' means and standard deviations, errors on CRT and CRT-SRT difference for the whole group (N = 900) and for subgroups based on (i) CRT error rates, (ii) sex, (iii) social class (1 = professional, 6 = nonskilled manual), and (iv) educational attainments

	SRT mean	SRT SD	CRT mean	CRT SD	Error	CRT-SRT difference
Whole sample (n = 900)	−0.31	−0.26	−0.49	−0.26	0.07	−0.15
No errors (n = 592)	−0.32	−0.30	−0.49	−0.24	—	−0.09
1–5 errors (n = 308)	−0.28	−0.18	−0.50	−0.30	0.08	−0.30
Men (n = 413)	−0.26	−0.26	−0.44	−0.25	0.07	−0.16
Women (n = 487)	−0.34	−0.26	−0.53	−0.26	0.07	−0.14
Social class 1 (n = 62)	−0.32	−0.11	−0.62	−0.32	0.29	−0.13
Social class 2 (n = 194)	−0.22	−0.15	−0.38	−0.26	0.01	−0.15
Social class 3 (n = 129)	−0.19	−0.14	−0.46	−0.29	0.13	−0.26
Social class 4 (n = 305)	−0.28	−0.26	−0.43	−0.21	0.11	−0.09
Social class 5 (n = 139)	−0.30	−0.40	−0.46	−0.30	−0.01	−0.12
Social class 6 (n = 71)	−0.28	−0.27	−0.32	−0.15	−0.07	−0.05
No educational qualification (n = 696)	−0.28	−0.27	−0.46	−0.25	0.08	−0.15
Any educational qualification (n = 204)	−0.23	−0.15	−0.39	−0.19	−0.00	−0.14

used structural equation modeling and found no significant differences in the correlations (effect sizes) of AH4 with reaction time parameters between subgroups compared on the bases of sex, social class, educational attainment, and errors on the four choice reaction time task (Table 5.1).

In summary, these analyses provided a relatively error free estimate of the association between psychometric intelligence (as measured using the AH4 Part 1) and some reaction time parameters in a general population sample. Previous uncorrected correlations between choice reaction time and intelligence suggested a correlation of about or even below −0.3 rather than about −0.5. The effect size is larger than those reported for most smaller, more biased samples. Sex, occupation, education, and reaction time error rates did not influence the effect size of the associations. The population was aged 56, so these effect sizes have still to be established in younger and older samples. The results agree with those who suggested that it was not necessary to apply the considerations of the Hick's reaction time law to explain reaction time-intelligence correlations: means and standard deviations are sufficient (Beauducel & Brocke, 1993). The Twenty-07 results do not offer a mechanism for these associations, including whether they are due to fundamental limitations in efficiency of information processing or to higher-level differences in strategies, learning, attention and motivation (Neubauer, 1997).

The differentiation hypothesis

In a follow-up study to the above analyses, Der and Deary (2003) inquired whether the larger effect size found for the reaction time-intelligence association in the Twenty-07 sample might be due to the "differentiation hypothesis." This originated as Spearman's (1926) "law of diminishing returns," which stated that the influence of general intelligence on mental ability test scores would be greater at lower absolute test scores and at younger and older ages. It has usually been tested by analyzing the pattern of correlations in a matrix of several mental tests. However, the differentiation hypothesis also implies that there might be a nonlinear association between any two different measures of mental ability, with lower-scoring subsamples having higher correlations. Therefore, the correlations between AH4 scores and reaction time parameters in the Twenty-07 sample were examined for departures from linearity. If the differentiation account of the Twenty-07's findings were correct, there would be an especially high correlation between reaction time parameters and AH4 scores among the lower AH4-scoring individuals.

Reaction times were positively skewed, which is a common finding. Simple reaction time means were especially skewed. The scattergrams between AH4 and 4-choice and simple reaction time means are shown in Figures 5.2 and 5.3, respectively. The AH4–4-choice reaction time scattergram shows a clear negative association across the whole range of AH4 scores. This is not so with the AH4–simple reaction time scattergram; there is a floor-type effect at about 200 ms,

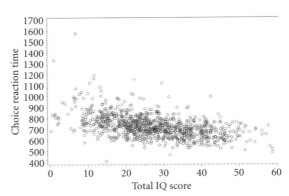

Fig. 5.2 The bivariate association found between 4-choice reaction time and Alice Heim 4 scores in the Twenty-07 study. AH4 scores have been jittered, by adding a random value between zero and one, to improve the representation of point density.

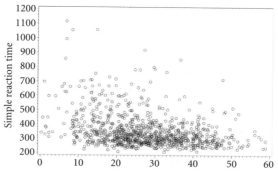

Fig. 5.3 The bivariate association found between simple reaction time and Alice Heim 4 scores in the Twenty-07 study. AH4 scores have been jittered, by adding a random value between zero and one, to improve the representation of point density.

with few mean response times being shorter than that. There are more outliers at lower AH4 scores, and there appears to be decreasing interindividual variation in simple reaction time means as AH4 scores increase. In fact, when AH4 score was divided into deciles, there were large declines in simple and 4-choice reaction time variance as AH4 scores increased (Der & Deary, 2003). In both diagrams the number of outliers is small. The number can appear larger because, in the denser area of the scattergrams, there are many superimposed points.

In the light of these bivariate distributions, especially for simple reaction time, ordinary least squares regression might not be a suitable technique to describe the association between reaction time means and AH4 scores. Reaction times were transformed using a procedure suggested by Box and Cox (1964), which normalizes the distributions and stabilizes the variances. This resulted in homogeneity of variances for simple and 4-choice reaction time means across deciles of AH4 scores. These transformed reaction times were regressed on AH4 scores. There was evidence of significant nonlinear contributions to associations in both simple and 4-choice reaction time means; quadratic, but not cubic. Simple reaction time accounted for 10.8% of the variance in AH4 scores; the quadratic contribution was 0.7%. Four-choice reaction time accounted for 24.7% of the variance in AH4 scores; the quadratic contribution was 0.4%. Predicted values from these models are shown in Figures 5.4 and 5.5. Visualization of the models was assisted by using Kernel Density Estimates of the bivariate distributions of the AH4 scores with simple and 4-choice reaction times. Symbols on the plots also show the mean (circles) and median (solid squares) reaction time for each decile of AH4 score. For simple reaction time the ordinary regression line is clearly less adequate than the regression line using the transformed reaction time: the latter is less influenced by the skewness and heteroscedasticity of the reaction

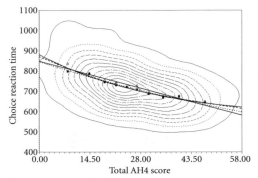

Fig. 5.4 Predicted values from regressions of 4-choice reaction times on AH4 scores, overlaid on contours of the estimated bivariate density, and decile means (circles) and medians (solid squares). To aid the visual assessment of the models, the bivariate distributions of AH4 score with 4-choice reaction means were estimated, using Kernel Density Estimation, and the results displayed as contours here. Also superimposed on the plots are the mean (circles) and median (solid squares) reaction time for each decile of AH4 score. The solid line shows the regression line of the untransformed reaction time on AH4 score. The dotted line represents the regression of transformed reaction times. The solid curve shows the quadratic regression and the dashed curve the locally weighted regression.

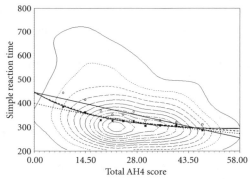

Fig. 5.5 Predicted values from regressions of simple reaction times on AH4 scores, overlaid on contours of the estimated bivariate density, and decile means (circles) and medians (solid squares). To aid the visual assessment of the models, the bivariate distributions of AH4 score with simple reaction time mean were estimated, using Kernel Density Estimation, and the results displayed as contours here. Also superimposed on the plots are the mean (circles) and median (solid squares) reaction time for each decile of AH4 score. The solid line shows the regression line of the untransformed reaction time on AH4 score. The dotted line represents the regression of transformed reaction times. The solid curve shows the quadratic regression and the dashed curve the locally weighted regression.

time data. The quadratic regression line is essentially flat above the mean AH4 score and steeper below it. The ordinary least squares regression line is a much better summary of the 4-choice reaction time data. The transformed data offer only a small improvement, and the curvature in the quadratic curve is small.

In summary, the association between simple reaction time and psychometric intelligence is complex. The relationship is better described by a quadratic than a linear association. Another possibly novel finding is the apparent floor effect in the AH4-simple reaction time association at reaction times at or below 200 ms. This floor effect and the weaker association between AH4 and simple reaction time at higher ability levels could indicate that simple reaction time fails to index cognitive variance at higher ability levels; that is, it might be a qualitatively different task for people of lower and higher ability levels. This would be an alternative to the differentiation hypothesis interpretation, which is also congruent with these findings. The "hard" baseline of 200 ms for mean simple reaction time does occur across the AH4 range. This hard baseline appears to be independent of higher cognitive ability level, and it appears to be that other factors that move response times above this baseline are related to AH4. On the other hand, the Pearson correlation provides an adequate summary of the association between 4-choice reaction time and AH4 scores.

Reaction time and ageing

In the field of cognitive ageing reaction times also feature prominently as tools that might provide parameters of explanatory power in the processes of brain ageing. One reason is that they are thought by some to be indicators of limitations of the brain's information processing efficiency (Madden, 2001). Another is that they account for a moderate to large amount of the age-related variance in higher cognitive functions such as those assessed using psychometric tests (Salthouse, 1991, 1996). Despite this theoretical prominence, and their inclusion in some prominent ageing studies, the reaction time changes that occur with age have not been documented in population-representative samples.

Cross-sectional studies suggest that reaction time means become slower as people grow older (e.g. see summaries by Fozard, Vercruyssen, Reynolds, Hancock, & Quilter, 1994 & Madden, 2001). There are relatively few studies with both cross-sectional and longitudinal data on reaction times and age. For example, the Bonn Longitudinal Study of Ageing (Mathey, 1976) and the Duke Longitudinal Studies (Maddox & Douglas, 1985; Siegler, 1985) provided, on smallish samples and with unusual reaction time procedures, equivocal evidence of reaction times' becoming slower and more variable (intraindividual variability) at older adult ages. The Health and Lifestyle Survey in the United

Kingdom used the same reaction time apparatus and procedure as the Twenty-07 study on a large, broad-based sample of the United Kingdom's adult population. It provided only descriptive data in a nonrefereed report, without statistical analyses (Huppert & Whittington, 1993). The patterns in the summary data suggested some slowing of simple reaction times after about 54–65 years, and quite marked slowing of 4-choice reaction times after about 45–54 years. The Baltimore Longitudinal Study of Aging (Fozard et al. 1994) showed slowing of simple and disjunctive reaction time with age in a well-educated sample.

Therefore, there are no refereed publications which have described reaction time findings on large, representative samples of adults. Moreover, in the four studies described above that have collected cross-sectional and longitudinal data, there are unresolved suggestions that intraindividual variability in reaction time might increase with age, and that there might be sex differences in the ageing of some reaction time variables. The age-related analyses of the Twenty-07 study aimed to add information on all these matters. The notion that intraindividual variability changes with age was explored especially, because changes in this variable have been related to changes in higher cognitive functions and to health (Hultsch & MacDonald, 2004; MacDonald, Hultsch, & Dixon, 2003; Rabbitt, Osman, Moore, & Stollery, 2001). Indeed, there are discussions regarding the possibility that intraindividual variability might have as strong a claim as mean reaction time to be the indicator of some "fundamental" limitation to information processing efficiency: the two are correlated; people with longer mean reaction times tend also to be more variable (Hultsch & MacDonald, 2004).

Deary and Der (in press a) reported the cross-sectional and longitudinal findings on reaction time parameters for the three samples included in the Twenty-07 study; that is, mostly age 16, 36, and 56 at wave 1, and subsequently age 24, 44, and 63, respectively, at the 8-year (wave 3) follow-up.

The basic descriptive findings are shown in Figure 5.6. For simple reaction time mean (panel a) the older cohorts were slower than the younger, and the longitudinal slowing was especially marked with the oldest cohort. For 4-choice reaction time mean, the same cohort pattern appeared, with the older cohorts being slower (panel d). There was longitudinal improvement in the youngest cohort (from age 16 to 24) but slowing in the older two cohorts. For simple reaction time intraindividual variability the older cohorts were more variable, and there was increasing variability in all the cohorts at the 8-year follow up (panel b). This effect was less clear after the intraindividual variability was adjusted for the simple reaction time mean (panel c). The adjustment was done using regression and saving the residuals of intraindividual variability after removing the effects of the mean. For 4-choice reaction

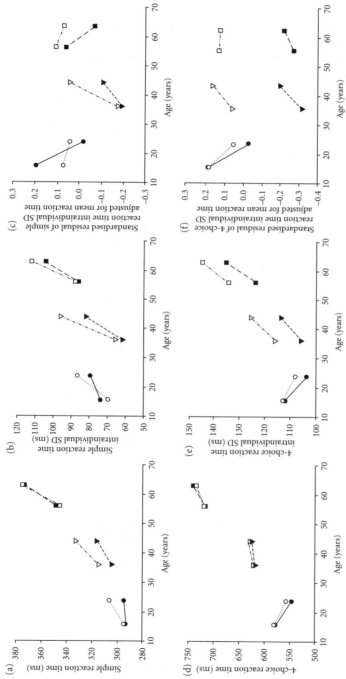

Fig. 5.6 Reaction time findings for three cohorts (age 16, 36, and 56 years) tested at Wave 1 and at 8-year follow-up (Wave 3) of the West of Scotland Twenty-07 study. Closed symbols = men; open symbols = women. Panels are: (a) simple reaction time means (ms); (b) simple reaction time intraindividual standard deviations (ms); (c) simple reaction time intraindividual standard deviations adjusted for simple reaction time mean (standardized scores; mean = 0, SD = 1); (d) four-choice reaction time means (ms); (e) four-choice reaction time intraindividual standard deviations for three cohorts (ms); (f) four-choice reaction time intraindividual standard deviations adjusted for choice reaction time means (standardized scores; mean = 0, SD = 1).

time intraindividual variability, the older cohorts were more variable, but there was longitudinal improvement in the youngest cohort and increased variability in the older two cohorts (panel e). When this was adjusted for 4-choice reaction time mean there was little effect of age among women, who appear consistently more variable then men, especially in the older two cohorts.

The same data were also used to examine age-related changes in interindividual variability, also known as diversity (Hultsch & MacDonald, 2004). This was examined for all reaction time parameters, that is, simple and choice reaction time means and intraindividual variabilities. Generally, diversity was greater in all parameters in the oldest cohort when compared with the two younger cohorts.

The Twenty-07 sample also provided a rare opportunity to examine the 8-year stability of the reaction time parameters (Table 5.2). There were negligible differences in the coefficients between the sexes and the cohorts. The 8-year stability of 4-choice reaction time mean was 0.54, for simple reaction time mean was 0.33, for 4-choice reaction time interindividual variability was 0.34, and for simple reaction time interindividual variability was only 0.15.

With PASAT scores available on the Twenty-07 sample Deary and Der (in press a) found significant effects of age (younger subjects scored better) and sex (men scored better, especially in the younger two cohorts) on this test of information processing and working memory (Table 5.3). However, when adjusted for differences in 4-choice reaction time means and variabilities, the

Table 5.2 Stability coefficients (Pearson's *r*) of reaction time (choice and simple) means and intraindividual standard deviations (SD) for three cohorts (age 16, 36, and 56 years) tested at Wave 1 and at 8-year follow-up (Wave 3) of the West of Scotland Twenty-07 study[a]

	Cohort 1 (age 16)		Cohort 2 (age 36)		Cohort 3 (age 56)	
	Men (*N* = 255)	Women (*N* = 289)	Men (*N* = 310)	Women (*N* = 404)	Men (*N* = 298)	Women (*N* = 374)
Choice RT mean	0.38	0.51	0.57	0.58	0.55	0.63
Simple RT mean	0.34	0.31	0.43	0.38	0.20	0.31
Choice RT intraindividual SD	0.25	0.36	0.39	0.37	0.41	0.27
Simple RT intraindividual SD	0.12	0.10	0.25	0.13	0.04	0.23

[a] Slight differences in subgroup Ns (maximum of three missing subjects in any one cell) reflect occasional instances where some individual variables were unavailable.

Table 5.3 Mean (SD) age and sex effects on paced auditory serial addition test (PASAT) scores before and after controlling for choice reaction time mean and variability

		PASAT score	**Standardized PASAT score**[a]
Women	Cohort 1 (N = 217)	44.8 (8.5)	−0.187 (0.963)
	Cohort 2 (N = 267)	44.1 (9.1)	−0.036 (1.050)
	Cohort 3 (N = 168)	42.0 (8.7)	0.021 (0.987)
Men	Cohort 1 (N = 201)	47.0 (8.0)	0.025 (0.949)
	Cohort 2 (N = 221)	46.5 (8.0)	0.193 (0.961)
	Cohort 3 (N = 177)	41.9 (8.6)	−0.004 (1.040)

[a] Controlling for choice reaction time mean and variability.

influence of age on PASAT scores reduced from an η^2 of 0.036 to 0.005, a reduction of 86%. The sex-related variance remained similar.

In summary, there are probably two main contributions from these analyses of reaction time parameters and age. The first is a formal analysis of the age differences in basic reaction time parameters across a wide range of adult ages in a representative sample of the Scottish population. The second is a clear discovery of the increased 4-choice reaction time variability in women at most adult ages, which remained after adjusting for mean 4-choice reaction time. Deary and Der (in press) considered possible hormonal explanations for these persistent differences. The results' patterns were not consistent with menopausal explanations. A more likely explanation was in terms of persistent sex differences in the effects of estrogens on the brain (McEwen, 2001), especially areas affecting the signal-to-noise ratio in information processing (Li, Lindenberger, & Sikstrom, 2001). Deary and Der (in press) recommended caution in the tendency to adjust reaction time intraindividual variabilities for reaction time means. Because there is debate about which, if either, represents a more "fundamental" indicator of brain ageing, it seems best practice to report the adjusted and unadjusted variabilities.

Reaction time and death

In a relatively new field that has been dubbed cognitive epidemiology, there are replicated findings of associations between cognitive ability level and all-cause mortality: people with higher IQ-type scores tend to live longer. This is found whether the mental ability test scores are available from childhood (Hart et al. 2003; Whalley & Deary, 2001), young adulthood (O'Toole & Stankov, 1990), middle age (Pavlik et al. 2003), or old age (Korten et al. 1999). As the evidence for an ability-mortality association has grown, there have been suggestions about the possible mechanisms (Gottfredson &

Deary, 2004; Whalley & Deary, 2001). Deary and Der (2005) used data from the Twenty-07 study to attempt to replicate the IQ-mortality association, and then tested some extant hypotheses about possible mechanisms of the association.

They examined, using Cox proportional hazards regression, the association between the AH4 scores of the oldest cohort (age 56 when tested) and their survival to age about 70. These participants were flagged at the United Kingdom's National Health Service's Central Register, which records deaths. The analysis included all deaths up to the end of 2002, by which time 185 people had died. Table 5.4 gives hazard ratios between a number of baseline variables and mortality from all causes. These ratios are estimates of the proportionate change in mortality risk for each unit change in the predictor variable. When a ratio, for example that between AH4 score and mortality, is adjusted for another putative mediating/confounding variable, this offers a test of hypotheses about possible mechanisms of the association. Men, smokers, and people with occupations that were more manual than professional were significantly more likely to die between age 56 and 70. AH4 score at wave 1 was significantly related to all-cause mortality: each lowering by a standard deviation was associated with a 41.7% greater chance of dying in the follow-up period. Four-choice reaction time mean had a similar hazard ratio, and that of simple reaction time mean was slightly lower. The intraindividual variabilities of these reaction time measures were also significantly associated with mortality. Overall, slower and more variable reaction times were associated with greater mortality risk. After adjusting for sex, smoking, social class, and education the effects of AH4 and reaction time remained significant, and the hazard ratios were similar to those before adjustment. That is, the associations between mortality and AH4 test scores and reaction times were not accounted for by these factors.

Arguably the most interesting result involved backwards elimination from a fully adjusted model. In Table 5.4 the three rightmost columns show the model of mortality, which is adjusted for sex, smoking, social class, and education, and in which each of the reaction time parameters the AH4 scores are adjusted for all the other variables. Of course, because these are strongly intercorrelated none now remains significant. However, backwards elimination from this model allows the strongest associates of mortality to be identified, and produces hazard ratios that are not shown in Table 5.4. These were 4-choice reaction time mean (hazard ratio = 1.281, 95% CI = 1.102 − 1.488, $p < 0.001$) and simple reaction time standard deviation (hazard ratio = 1.175, 95% CI = 1.026–1.345, $p < 0.020$). After these entered, AH4 score was no longer significantly associated with mortality. That is, reaction time accounts for the AH4-mortality association in this sample.

Table 5.4 Effects on mortality from 1988 to 2002, (N = 898)[a]

	Unadjusted			Adjusted for sex, smoking, social class, and years of education			Fully adjusted		
	Hazard ratio	95% CI	p	Hazard ratio	95% CI	p	Hazard ratio	95% CI	p
Sex (male)	1.428	1.070–1.907	0.016	—	—	—	—	—	—
Smoking (yes)	2.212	1.647–2.976	<0.0001	—	—	—	—	—	—
Social class (more manual)	1.128	1.014–1.255	0.027	—	—	—	—	—	—
Years of education (fewer)	1.059	0.971–1.156	0.20	—	—	—	—	—	—
Alice Heim 4 score (lower)	1.417	1.215–1.654	<0.0001	1.384	1.151–1.665	0.0006	1.197	0.979–1.463	0.080
Choice RT mean (slower)	1.411	1.249–1.595	<0.0001	1.370	1.195–1.571	<0.0001	1.173	0.961–1.433	0.12
Simple RT mean (slower)	1.329	1.186–1.488	<0.0001	1.303	1.158–1.467	<0.0001	1.106	0.931–1.313	0.25
Choice RT SD (more variable)	1.168	1.021–1.335	0.023	1.147	1.001–1.314	0.048	0.995	0.850–1.164	0.95
Simple RT SD (more variable)	1.285	1.146–1.440	<0.0001	1.273	1.129–1.436	<0.0001	1.105	0.941–1.298	0.22

[a] All variables are coded so that higher scores are associated with less favorable outcomes. The direction of each variable associated with higher mortality is shown in parentheses after the variable name.

Note: Sex: male (1) versus female (0). Smoking: nonsmoker (0) versus current smoker (1). Social class: per class, with six classes included; higher numbers represent less professional occupations. Education: per year of education; sign reversed. Alice Heim 4 and reaction time measures: per standard deviation unit, sign reversed for AH4.

Without identifying a single best explanation Deary and Der (2005) discussed a number of possible accounts of the association between reaction time variables and mortality. Given that childhood intelligence is closely correlated with intelligence level in old age (Deary, Whalley, Lemmon, Crawford, & Starr, 2000) and childhood intelligence is associated with survival to old age (Whalley & Deary, 2001), one possible account was that reaction time acts as a trait-like, or life-long indicator of the integrity of the body in terms of information processing efficiency: the better wired-together body lasts longer. On the other hand, reaction time parameters at age 56 might be sensitive indicators of even subclinical illness, a sentinel of terminal decline (Wilson, Beckett, Bienias, Evans, & Bennett, 2003), which would cast reaction time parameters, and also mental ability tests, as sensitive indicators/meters of general bodily states. An association between processing speed and mortality was also found in the Seattle Longitudinal Study (Bosworth, Schaie, & Willis, 1999) and in the Netherlands longitudinal Aging Study (Smits, Deeg, Kriegsman, & Schmand, 1999). In the former study processing speed was still significantly related to mortality after adjusting for sex, age, education, depressive symptoms, and health. However, the follow-up duration was only three years and the subjects ranged in age from 55 to 85, and processing speed was measured using psychometric tests rather than reaction time, limiting the comparisons with the Twenty-07 cohort. In the Netherlands study cognitive decline was a stronger predictor of mortality than cognitive level, indicating that cognitive function does have a function as a bodily state indicator.

In summary, the results from the Twenty-07 study have advanced the new field which studies cognitive associations of mortality. It has ruled out explanations along the lines of intelligence leading to more healthy behaviours (smoking, education) and to safer, professional occupations. On the other hand, it has highlighted the role of reaction time as a powerful predictor of mortality that accounts for the effect of psychometric intelligence.

Discussion

The Twenty-07 study aimed to examine social determinants of health inequalities. None of the novel, recent investigations reported here formed part of the original plans; they were pragmatic uses of an available, high quality dataset. There are new descriptive findings: the changes in reaction time parameters with age. There are new associations: those between reaction time parameters and AH4 scores, and between both and mortality. There are novel examinations of hypotheses and mechanisms: including reaction time-AH4 associations and AH4/reaction time-mortality associations. In all cases there is the unusual benefit of the findings being based on a large, population-representative sample. Perhaps the most interesting and provocative findings are: the greater intraindividual variability of choice reaction time in adult women compared with men; the strong association between reaction time and mortality, and its accounting for the AH4-mortality association; the stronger-than-usually-found reaction time-AH4 association; and the nonlinear AH4-simple reaction time association.

Though differential psychology and epidemiology have different emphases and their strengths have been combined too rarely, they share one aspect by comparison with experimental psychology: the tendency to collect large numbers of subjects at the expense of a detailed phenotype. The reaction time device used here is an example of this. It has proved convenient for population-based studies and has produced novel results, but it has limitations. It does not allow the collection of individual response times. This limits the experimenter's ability to exclude very long or short individual responses, and to extract parameters based on current models of response times (Ratcliff & Smith, 2004). Nevertheless, those parameters that were collected have mostly proved reliable and valid, and related to important human differences. The results from the Twenty-07 study described here provide novel substantive findings and some of the first population estimates of important associations.

References

Beck, L. F. (1933). The role of speed in intelligence. *Psychological Bulletin, 30*, 169–178.

Beauducel, A., & Brocke, B. (1993). Intelligence and speed of information processing: further results and questions on Hick's paradigm and beyond. *Personality and Individual Differences, 15*, 627–636.

Black, R. W. (1985). Instead of the 1986 Census: The potential of enhanced electoral registers. *Journal of the Royal Statistical Society, Series A, 148*, 287–316.

Bosworth, B. H., Schaie, K. W., & Willis, S. L. (1999). Cognitive and sociodemographic risk factors for mortality in the Seattle Longitudinal Study. *Journal of Gerontology: Psychological Sciences, 54B*, P273–P282.

Bouchard, T. J., & Loehlin, J. C. (2001). Genes, evolution and personality. *Behavior Genetics, 31*, 243–273.

Box, G. E. P., & Cox, D. R. (1964). An analysis of transformations. *Journal of the Royal Statistical Society, Series B, 26*, 211–252.

Cox, B. D., Blaxter, M., Buckle, A. L. J., Fenner, N. P., Golding, J. F., Gore, M., et al. (1987). *The health and lifestyle survey*. London: The Health Promotion Research Trust.

Crawford, J. R., Obonsawin, M. C., & Allan, K. M. (1998). PASAT and components of WAIS-R performance: Convergent and discriminant validity. *Neuropsychological Rehabilitation, 8*, 255–272.

Der, G. (1998). *A comparison of the West of Scotland Twenty-07 study sample and the 1991 census SARs* (Working Paper No. 60). Glasgow: MRC Medical Sociology Unit.

Der, G., & Deary, I. J. (2003). IQ, reaction time and the differentiation hypothesis. *Intelligence, 31*, 491–503.

Deary, I. J. (2000). *Looking down on human intelligence: from psychometrics to the brain.* Oxford, U.K.: Oxford University Press.

Deary, I. J., & Der, G. (in press). Reaction time, age, and cognitive ability longitudinal findings from age 16 to 63 years in representative population samples. *Aging, Neuropsychology and Cognition.*

Deary, I. J., & Der, G. (2005). Reaction time explains IQ's association with death. *Psychological Science, 16*, 64–69.

Deary, I. J., Der, G., & Ford, G. (2001). Reaction times and intelligence differences: A population-based cohort study. *Intelligence, 29*, 389–399.

Deary, I. J., Whalley, L. J., Lemmon, H., Crawford, J. R., & Starr, J. M. (2000). The stability of individual differences in mental ability from childhood to old age: follow up of the 1932 Scottish Mental Survey. *Intelligence, 28*, 628–634.

Ecob, R. (1987). *The sampling scheme, frame and procedures for the cohort studies* (Working Paper No. 6). Glasgow: MRC Medical Sociology Unit.

Fozard, J. L., Vercruyssen, M., Reynolds, S. L., Hancock, P. A., & Quilter, R. E. (1994). Age differences and changes in reaction time: The Baltimore longitudinal study of aging. *Journal of Gerontology: Psychological Sciences, 49*, P179–P189.

Gottfredson, L. S., & Deary, I. J. (2004). Intelligence predicts health and longevity, but why? *Current Directions in Psychological Science, 13*, 1–4.

Hart, C. L., Deary, I. J., Taylor, M. D., MacKinnon, P. L., Davey Smith, G., Whalley, L. J., et al. (2003). The Scottish Mental Survey 1932 linked to the midspan studies: a prospective investigation of childhood intelligence and future health. *Public Health, 117*, 187–195.

Hart, C. L., Taylor, M. D., Davey Smith, G., Whalley, L. J., Starr, J. M., Hole, D. J., et al. (2003). Childhood IQ, social class, deprivation and their relationships with mortality and morbidity risk in later life: Prospective observational study linking the Scottish Mental Survey 1932 and the Midspan studies. *Psychosomatic Medicine, 65*, 877–883.

Heim, A. W. (1970). *Manual for the AH4 group test of general intelligence.* Windsor: NFER.

Hick, W. E. (1952). On the rate of gain of information. *Quarterly Journal of Experimental Psychology, 4*, 11–26.

Hultsch, D. F., & MacDonald, S. W. S. (2004). Intraindividual variability in performance as a theoretical window onto cognitive aging. In R. A. Dixon, L. Backman, & L.-G. Nilsson (Eds.), *New frontiers in cognitive aging.* Oxford, U.K.: Oxford University Press.

Huppert, F. A., & Whittington J. E. (1993). Changes in cognitive function in a population sample. In B. D. Cox, F. A. Huppert, & M. J. Whichelow (Eds.), *The health and lifestyle survey: Seven years on.* Aldershot, U.K.: Dartmouth.

Jensen, A. R. (1987). Individual differences in the Hick paradigm. In P. A. Vernon (Ed.), *Speed of information processing and intelligence* (pp. 101–175). Norwood, NJ: Ablex.

Korten, A. E., Jorm, A. F., Jiao, Z., Letenneur, L., Jacomb, P. A., Henderson, A. S., et al. (1999). Health, cognitive, and psychosocial factors as predictors of mortality in an elderly community sample. *Journal of Epidemiology and Community Health, 53*, 83–88.

Krueger, R. F., Caspi, A., & Moffitt, T. E. (2000). Epidemiological personology: The unifying role of personality in population-based research on problem behaviors. *Journal of Personality, 68*, 967–998.

Li, S.-C., Lindenberger, U., & Sikstrom, S. (2001). Aging cognition: from neuromodulation to representation. *Trends in Cognitive Sciences,* **5**, 479–486.

Lubinski, D., & Humphreys, L. G. (1997). Incorporating general intelligence into epidemiology and the social sciences. *Intelligence,* **24**, 159–201.

Mathey, F. J. (1976). Psychomotor performance and reaction speed in old age. In H. Thomae (Ed.), *Contributions to human development, Volume 3: Patterns of aging— Findings from the Bonn longitudinal study of aging* (pp. 36–50). Basel: Karger.

MacDonald, S. W. S., Hultsch, D. F., & Dixon, R. A. (2003). Performance variability is related to change in cognition: Evidence from the Victoria longitudinal study. *Psychology and Aging,* **18**, 510–523.

Macintyre, S. (1987). *West of Scotland Twenty-07: Health in the community. The survey's background and rationale* (Working Paper No. 7). Glasgow: MRC Medical Sociology Unit.

MacIver, S. (1988). *"West of Scotland Twenty-07 Study" Socio-demographic and mortality profiles of the study areas* (Working Paper No. 10). Glasgow: MRC Medical Sociology Unit.

Madden, D. J. (2001). Speed and timing of behavioural processes. In J. E. Birren & K. W. Schaie (Eds.), *Handbook of the psychology of aging* (5th Ed., pp. 288–312). San Diego, CA: Academic Press.

Maddox, G. L., & Douglass, E. B. (1985). Aging and individual differences. In E. Palmore, E. W. Busse, G. L. Maddox, J. B. Nowlin, & I. C. Siegler (Eds.), *Normal aging III: Reports from the Duke longitudinal studies, 1975–1984* (pp. 311–326). Durham, NC: Duke University Press.

McEwen, B. S. (2001). Invited review: Estrogens effects on the brain: Multiple sites and molecular mechanisms. *Journal of Applied Physiology,* **91**, 2785–2801.

Nettelbeck, T. (1987). Inspection time and intelligence. In P. A. Vernon (Ed.), *Speed of information processing and intelligence* (pp. 295–346). Norwood, NJ: Ablex.

Neubauer, A. C. (1997). The mental speed approach to the assessment of intelligence. In J. Kingma & W. Tomic (Eds.), *Advances in cognition and education: Reflections on the concept of intelligence.* Greenwich, CT: JAI press.

O'Toole, B. J., & Stankov, L. (1990). Ultimate validity of psychological tests. *Personality and Individual Differences,* **13**, 699–716.

Pavlik, V. N., de Moraes, S. A., Szklo, M., Knopman, D. S., Mosley, T. H., & Hyman, D. J. (2003). Relation between cognitive function and mortality in middle-aged adults: The Atherosclerosis risk in communities study. *American Journal of Epidemiology,* **157**, 327–334.

Rabbitt, P., Osman, P., Moore, B., & Stollery, B. (2001). There are stable individual differences in performance variability, both from moment to moment and from day to day. *Quarterly Journal of Experimental Psychology,* **54**, 981–1003.

Ratcliff, R., & Smith, P. L. (2004). A comparison of sequential sampling models for two-choice reaction time. *Psychological Review,* **111**, 333–367.

Roth, E. (1964). Die Geschwindigkeit der Verabeitung von Information and ihr Zusammenhang mit Intelligenz. *Zeitschrift fuer Experimentelle und Angewandte Psychologie,* **11**, 616–622.

Salthouse, T. A. (1991). Mediation of adult age differences in cognition by reductions in working memory and speed of processing. *Psychological Science,* **2**, 179–183.

Salthouse, T. A. (1996). The processing-speed theory of adult age differences in cognition. *Psychological Review,* **103**, 403–428.

Siegler, I. C. (1985). Mental performance in the young-old versus the old-old. In E. Palmore, E. W. Busse, G. L. Maddox, J. B. Nowlin, & I. C. Siegler (Eds.), *Normal aging III: Reports from the Duke longitudinal studies, 1975–1984* (pp. 232–237). Durham, NC: Duke University Press.

Smits, C. H., Deeg, D. J., Kriegsman, D. M., & Schmand, B. (1999). Cognitive functioning and health as determinants of mortality in an older population. *American Journal of Epidemiology, 150,* 978–986.

Whalley, L. J., & Deary, I. J. (2001). Longitudinal cohort study of childhood IQ and survival up to age 76. *British Medical Journal, 322,* 819–822.

Wilson, R. S., Beckett, L. A., Bienias, J. L., Evans, D. A., & Bennett, D. A. (2003). Terminal decline in cognitive function. *Neurology, 60,* 1782–1787.

Chapter 6

The wrong tree: time perception and time experience in the elderly

John H. Wearden

Abstract

The chapter discusses age-related differences in timing obtained under *prospective timing* conditions (that is, situations where people are alerted in advance that time is an important dimension of the task), and in particular the question of whether observed changes in timing with increasing age can be related to the idea that humans possess an internal clock, the rate of which "slows down" with ageing. Although there is some evidence for this view, logical and methodological considerations make it difficult to conclusively demonstrate such "slowing down" in the elderly, even if such an effect were really present. Studies of prospective timing also fail to capture many aspects of subjective time experience in the elderly, and such work might be considered to be "barking up the wrong tree". Studies of *retrospective timing*, where people judge the duration of an event retrospectively without being previously alerted that time was important, or *passage of time judgements*, where people make subjective judgements of "how fast or slow" time seems to pass in different situations, are suggested as possible future avenues of research which may help to bridge the gap between laboratory studies of timing and the daily-life changes in time experience which people report as they get older.

Introduction

A prominent psychological feature of ageing is changes in the experience of time. People report that "Christmas comes round quicker every year" as they age, yet "Time lies heavy on their hands," and days may seem to crawl by, in a way they never used to when the person was younger. The two statements together appear at first sight baldly contradictory: the former implies increased rate of the passage of time with ageing, while the latter suggests time seems to drag as we get older.

As will be seen later, modern research in the Psychology of time perception may be able to reconcile these apparent paradoxes, and begin to give us some insight into the ways that time experience might change with increasing age.

The perception of time is a Cinderella who never attended the ball. The number of active workers worldwide remains very small (at the time of writing a few tens of people), and funding for basic research is impossible (in the United Kingdom) or very difficult (elsewhere) to come by. Nevertheless, the few workers that there are in this field show extraordinary productivity, and the last 20 or 30 years have seen a mini-"Golden Age" in the study of time perception in humans, with many fundamental processes being elucidated for the first time, and major discoveries made.

The present chapter is intended to perform a number of different functions. First, it will introduce some basic ideas from contemporary time Psychology, and show how some of these ideas have been applied to the study of some aspects of timing in the elderly. To anticipate slightly, it will become clear that explanations of timing based on some sort of "internal clock" have been recently dominant. Following on from this, a second part will specifically discuss the question of what changes in time experience and behaviour might be occasioned by changes in the "speed" of this internal clock, with a particular focus on any slowing of clock speed that might occur with ageing. The third part of the chapter takes a more radical turn, and essentially argues that most work conducted up until the present time (including work such as Wearden, Wearden, & Rabbitt, 1997), interesting though it may have been, is inappropriate to come to grips in a satisfactory way with important questions about time experience in the elderly, and that new areas, developed from some recent theoretical arguments and developments in time Psychology, need to be explored if a proper understanding of time experience and ageing is ever to be achieved. Much of the work on time perception in the elderly, interesting though it may have been has, according to this view, been "barking up the wrong tree," and some suggestions for a more appropriate location are given.

Prospective timing: a model and some age effects

A distinction central to modern time Psychology is that between *prospective* and *retrospective* timing, although the distinction was introduced only fairly recently in the long history of time perception by Hicks, Miller, and Kinsbourne (1976). Prospective timing involves time judgments made when experimental participants are alerted in advance that duration is an important feature of the procedure. Most common laboratory tasks are of this type (e.g. "hold down this button for one second," "I'm going to present two tones

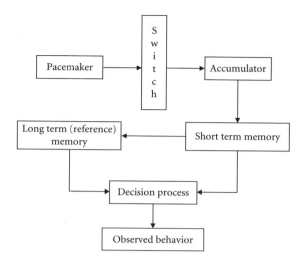

Fig. 6.1 Outline of the timing system proposed by scalar timing theory (or scalar expectancy theory: SET).

and I want you to tell me which lasted longer"). In contrast, retrospective timing involves a time judgment made when the participant is unaware that a question about time is going to be asked (e.g. "how long is it since you started reading this paragraph?").

Contemporary time researchers are (virtually) unanimous that confusing these two is fatal to any proper progress (although they were routinely mixed up until recently, see the work reviewed in Fraisse (1964) for example), and that they are explained by different psychological mechanisms. I will discuss retrospective timing in more detail later (as well as adding a third type of time judgment to the existing list of two), but first I will introduce some ideas and research related to prospective timing.

Figure 6.1 shows the dominant contemporary model of prospective timing (dominant in the sense that all alternative models are either variants of it, or reactions against it), the *scalar timing* model (SET) of Gibbon, Church, and Meck (1984), which is in some ways an elaborated version of an earlier model by Treisman (1963) (for a discussion of the development of this type of approach see Wearden (in press) and for recent reviews of the use of SET as an explanation of human timing see Allan (1998) and Wearden, 2003). SET derives time judgments and timed behaviour from the sequential operation of processes at three levels. "Raw" representations of duration are generated at a clock level by a pacemaker–accumulator clock. This sort of (hypothetical) clock consists of three connected parts: a pacemaker that produces pulses or "ticks," an accumulator that stores the ticks produced during some time period, and a switch that connects the two. So, for example, when a stimulus is timed, the switch closes, allowing pulses to flow from the pacemaker to the accumulator, and when the stimulus goes off, the switch opens, cutting the connection. The accumulator thus contains the number of pulses accrued during the stimulus, and this number is used as the "raw material" for time judgments. Although pacemaker–accumulator clocks are hypothetical in the sense that no brain mechanism corresponding to them has (yet) been found, the operation of the such clocks can be mathematically specified, so very precise predictions about what sort of time representations such clocks can produce can be made (see Gibbon et al. 1984, and Wearden, Edwards, Fakhri & Percival, 1998, for discussions of the mathematics of pacemaker–accumulator clocks).

The next level of the SET system involves two sorts of memory: a working memory for duration (essentially the contents of the accumulator, and in some recent versions of SET the working memory is conflated with the accumulator), and a reference memory storing "important" times, such as standards needed for the particular task used. A final level involves a decision process, and it is only after the operation of all three levels that a time judgment is made.

The task of *temporal generalization* (Wearden, 1992), which has been used with elderly people by Wearden et al. (1997) and by McCormack, Brown, Maylor, Darby, and Green (1999), illustrates the operation of the model. In the normal version of temporal generalization, the participant receives a few pre-sentations of a "standard" duration (e.g. a tone 400 ms long), and must remember this standard. Next, comparison durations (e.g. tones from 100 to 700 ms long) are presented in a random order, and the participant's task is to decide whether each comparison had the same duration as the standard (by making a YES or NO response), with feedback as to performance accuracy usually being given. The resulting behaviour can be presented in the form of a *temporal generalization gradient*, the proportion of YES responses plotted against stimulus duration.

SET explains performance on the task as follows. Presentation of a stimulus causes the switch connecting the pacemaker to the accumulator to close, and "ticks" accumulate until the switch opens again when the stimulus goes off. The accumulator contents are then transferred to working memory, which then contains a raw representation of stimulus duration, coded in terms of the number of ticks stored. At the start of the experiment the identified standards are stored in reference memory, which contains a representation of what the standard (400 ms in our case) "feels like." When a comparison stimulus is presented, the number of ticks in working memory is compared with a sample drawn from reference memory, and if the two are "close enough," according to some decision process, the participant makes the YES response, otherwise he or she responds "NO."

In order to generate behaviour, clock, memory, and decision processes are all involved, so if some intergroup difference (e.g. between elderly participants and younger controls) is found, this could be due to differences at any of the three levels of the SET system. However, SET produces mathematical specifications of the operation of each part of the system, so computer modeling can be used to identify the cause of between-group differences more precisely subject, obviously, to acceptance of the assumptions of the model.

In the case of temporal generalization, the standard treatment (deriving from Wearden, 1992) assumes, in a slightly simplified form, that (a) all the durations are timed on average accurately, (b) the reference memory is represented as a Gaussian distribution of values, with an accurate mean and some variance, which can vary between groups, with a sample being drawn from this distribution on each trial, and (c) the comparison process is based on a threshold (which can also vary between groups, that is, different groups can be more or less conservative about saying that a comparison duration is the standard).

Wearden et al. (1997) used temporal generalization in a wider study of prospective timing in the elderly. In their work, sampling was used to avoid the usual age/IQ confound, so data could be analyzed in terms of either age or IQ. The standard used was a 400 ms tone, and comparison durations ranged from 100 to 700 ms in 100-ms steps. The first interesting finding was how "normal" performance of the elderly groups (60–69 and 70–79 years) was, compared to that of students. In all cases, the temporal generalization gradient peaked at the standard (so on average the 400 ms comparison was identified, correctly, as the standard more than any other comparison value), and was asymmetrical, with durations longer than 400 ms being confused with it more than durations shorter by the same amount. This asymmetry is almost always found, and is explained by the decision processes used (Wearden, 2004).

Wearden et al. (1997) found an age difference between groups, with slightly flatter generalization gradients in the 70–79 year-olds than the 60–69 year-olds. Modeling suggested that the difference was due to greater variability of reference memory in the older subjects. When the same population was divided into three IQ bands, differences between the IQ groups were more marked, but once again the main difference between groups was due to memory variance, with higher variability in the lower IQ groups.

The results of Wearden et al. suggested that prospective timing in the elderly was associated with greater variability of reference memory (or, perhaps, in variability of raw timing processes themselves, see Wearden (in press) and below) than timing in young people, but was essentially very similar in nature, and a similar conclusion from temporal generalization was reached by McCormack et al. (1999). However, differences in timed behaviour between old and younger people are not always found.

A second task used by Wearden et al. (1997), and by McCormack et al. (1999), was *bisection* (see Wearden, 1991, for the original method). Superficially, this task resembles temporal generalization. People are initially presented with two standards, one short (e.g. 200 ms) and one long (e.g. 800 ms), identified as such. They then receive a range of stimulus durations (e.g. from 200 to 800 ms in 100-ms steps), and have to classify each presented duration in terms of similarity to the short or long standards, with a SHORT or LONG response being produced. The resulting behaviour can be plotted as a psychophysical function, the proportion of LONG responses (judgments that a presented duration is more similar to the long than the short standard) plotted against stimulus duration. This produces a monotonically increasing function of ogival shape going from near zero LONG responses when the stimulus with the same duration as the short standard is presented to nearly 100% when the longest stimulus duration occurs. The psychophysical function can be analyzed to yield a number of measures of performance (see Wearden & Ferrara, 1995, 1996), and task performance can be explained by a number of different models (see Wearden, 2004). Among the performance measures that have attracted attention are the *bisection point* (the stimulus duration giving rise to 50% LONG responses), and the *Weber ratio* (essentially a measure of the slope of the psychophysical function, which assesses timing sensitivity).

Wearden et al. (1997) found no age or IQ effects on bisection point (see also McCormack et al. (1999) for a similar result) and, furthermore, the performance of our elderly or low-IQ participants was virtually identical to that of undergraduate students 50 years younger, and (presumably) with higher average IQs. Figure 6.3 of Wearden et al. also suggests that temporal sensitivity did not differ between age and IQ groups either, as the different psychophysical functions superimposed almost perfectly, but Weber ratios were not calculated. It should perhaps be mentioned, however, that bisection is not immune to "developmental" effects, as differences in performance of children of different ages can be consistently found (Droit-Volet & Wearden, 2001, 2002).

The discrepancy between finding consistent age and IQ effects on temporal generalization but not bisection is puzzling, to say the least. A reader might predict that age and IQ effects would be at least as marked on bisection, as people have to remember two standards rather than one (which might be supposed to be more demanding, and is, see Jones & Wearden, 2004), so if the bisection standards in reference memory have increasing variance with increasing age or decreasing IQ, behavioural effects should be obtained, yet are in fact absent. A complete discussion of this result is inappropriate here, but the obvious conclusion is that participants are not using the "standards" in bisection in the same way as the standard in temporal generalization, and there is other evidence for this (e.g. Allan, 2002; Wearden & Ferrara, 1995).

More generally, this generalization/bisection comparison in the elderly may tell us more about how timing tasks are performed (an interesting topic, but not the central focus of the research) than it does about timing processes in the elderly *per se*. In addition, the bisection result shows that age (and IQ) effects on timing are not always obtained. A further complication in timing studies is that a multiprocess theory like SET offers many possibilities for psychological variables, other than "timing ability," which may differ between young and older participants. Attentional effects are well-known in timing (see Lustig, 2003, for a review) although how they should be best understood remains controversial, and age-related differences in memory and decision processes may also play a critical role.

I will discuss some prospective timing studies, which relate to the "speed" of the internal clock later, but before leaving the topic one fairly consistent result needs to be mentioned. Consider the task of temporal generalization described above. When the standard is presented, SET assumes that it is normally stored on average accurately in reference memory (although the storage may involve the introduction of variability to the representation). So, for example, 400 ms is stored as on average 400 ms, and so on. Some data suggest developmental trends not only in the *variability* with which standard durations are represented, but also in the *average* value stored.

McCormack et al. (1999) studied temporal generalization in children of 5, 8, and 10 years (as well as adult groups), and found that the younger groups of children behaved as if they were storing the standard as shorter on average than it really was. This trend disappeared in the older children. Droit-Volet, Clément, and Wearden (2001) found a similar result using children of 3, 5, and 8 years: here, modeling assumed that the youngest children were remembering the standard on average as 83% of its real duration, whereas the oldest children exhibited a much smaller "distortion" of the average, or no distortion at all. The claim that young children remember standard durations are shorter than they really are is controversial, and was not obtained by Droit-Volet (2002), but the bulk of evidence, including new data, seems to support it (see McCormack, Brown, Smith, & Brock, 2004).

The obvious question is this: if children store standards as shorter than they really are, and young adults store them veridically, do older adults store durations as *longer* than they really are? Wearden et al. (1997) and McCormack et al. (1999) effectively assumed in their Modeling that this was not true. However, inspection of their data shows that temporal generalization gradients in the older groups were more skewed to the right than those in younger populations (i.e. older people tended to confuse stimuli *longer* than the standard more with it than younger groups did, although all groups produced asymmetrical gradients), and one obvious suggestion is that the standard is being remembered as (slightly) longer than it is. Other evidence for this comes from a study of absolute identification of duration by McCormack, Brown, Maylor, Richardson, and Darby (2002).

In fact, the suggestion of temporal memory "distortion" in the elderly is supported by earlier work with rats. Meck, Church, and Wenk (1986), and Lejeune, Ferrara, Soffié, Bronchart, and Wearden (1998) both studied aged rats, and younger controls, on a "peak interval" task. To simplify the procedure slightly, lever-presses are reinforced with food but only at some time, *t*, after the onset of a signal. Essentially, the animals should learn that food is available at time *t*, and the procedure enables the measurement of their responding at times both shorter and longer than *t*, on the critical "peak" trials. After considerable training, the response rate of the animals increases from near zero early in the interval to a peak at or near *t*, then declines at longer times, with the overall response versus time curve resembling a Gaussian function. Curve-fitting can be used to determine when the response peak occurs, and this peak location is assumed to be an index of the average value of the animal's reference memory of *t* (see Lejeune et al. (1998) for details). Both studies found that, at least in most cases, the older rats behaved as if they remembered *t* as being longer than it actually was.

Slowing down the clock and the problem of "reference"

The attentive reader will have noted that the possibility that the pacemaker of the internal clock hypothesized by SET slows down with increasing age has not so far loomed large in this chapter. Suppose that the pacemaker does slow down: what are the consequences of this for timing behaviour? SET proposes a pacemaker of a Poisson type, that is, a process which generates ticks at random but at some constant average rate. SET furthermore usually regards the rate of this pacemaker as sufficiently rapid so that the Poisson process makes only a small contribution (which is usually ignored) to the total variance of timing. So, in normal circumstances, the actual speed of the pacemaker (which I will just call "clock speed" from now on), is of no importance in timing.

However, internal-clock based theories like SET have long been interested in the possibility of changing clock speed by various manipulations. Early examples come from attempts to manipulate clock speed in humans by increases or decreases in body temperature (Wearden, 2003, 2004; see also Wearden & Penton-Voak, 1995, for a review). Work with animals has used drugs that increase or decrease dopamine levels (Meck, 1983), and recent work with humans has used a method introduced by Treisman, Faulkner, Naish, and Brogan (1990). With this technique, stimuli or timed responses are preceded by trains of repetitive stimulation (usually in the form of clicks or flashes), and evidence suggests that this stimulation increases clock speed. A complete account of the effects of repetitive stimulation, and other attempts to change clock speed, cannot be given here, but the reader is referred to Penton-Voak, Edwards, Percival, and Wearden (1996), Burle and Casini (2001), Droit-Volet and Wearden (2002: a demonstration of the effect in children), Wearden, Philpott, and Win (1999), and Wearden, Pilkington, and Carter (1999: a rare "slowing down" study).

Almost all the work on changing clock speed, whether by body temperature changes, drugs, or repetitive stimulation, has used a "state change" design, where, for example, timing behaviour with a putatively speeded up or slowed down clock is compared with that obtained with a "normal" clock. In the classic drug experiments by Meck (1983), for example, rats, in some conditions, learned standard durations after saline injections, then were tested with these durations after amphetamine (which speeds up the clock) or haloperidol (which slows it down). The inverse experiments were also conducted by Meck: here, animals were *trained* under haloperidol or amphetamine, then *tested* with saline. In these experiments, rats have a "reference" developed in one state (drug or saline) and use this reference to judge comparisons timed in another state. Logically, if there were no state change, then clock speed differences would not be observed in behaviour, even if present. Meck (1983) showed that this was in fact the case: rats' timing behaviour was identical under amphetamine, haloperidol, or saline, with any differences in clock speed being revealed only when the state was changed (see Meck, 1996, for a discussion and review).

Experiments with humans have employed state change conditions logically similar to those used by Meck (1983): judgments made in one state make reference to standards learned in another one. For example, Droit-Volet and Wearden (2002), in an experimental *tour de force* for which the first author was solely responsible, tested children as young as three in conditions where standards in bisection were learnt with a normal clock, with comparison durations being sometimes presented after flicker, which "sped up" the clock. Wearden, Philpott et al. (1999) show the inverse effect: standards were learned with a speeded up clock, then comparisons were sometimes tested with a "normal" clock. In all cases, the participants behaved as if their clock had sped up or relatively slowed down in the appropriate manner.

To illustrate that some kind of reference is needed to interpret putative clock speed differences, consider the following simple thought experiment. We compare two individuals A and B. For A the internal clock "ticks" at 120/s, for B 80/s (the figures are, of course, imaginary and used only for illustration). Let us suppose that one clock second is represented by 100 ticks. If a stimulus 1 s long is presented, A will overestimate it (1.2 s), and B underestimate it (0.8 s). If, on the other hand, A and B are asked to produce 1 s, and do so by counting ticks, then A will "underproduce" reaching 100 ticks in 0.83 s (100/120), whereas B will "overproduce" 1 s as 1.25 s (100/80). The logic above derives from sketchy and questionable accounts of how verbal estimation and production are performed but, more importantly for present purposes, depends critically on the idea of a "common reference" (100 ticks = 1 s), used by *both* A and B. It assumes that neither A nor B can learn, as a result of everyday experiences, or events presented during the experiment, that 1 s = 120 ticks for A and 80 for B. In experiments where the clock is "speeded up" (e.g. Penton-Voak et al. 1996), participants can establish a "common reference" from state-change conditions, and results are as predicted above: with a faster clock estimations increase but productions decrease. If A and B are a young person and an older one, there can be no state change, so the problem of where the "common reference" comes from remains.

Logically, contemporary internal clock theories appear to forbid the detection of *absolute* clock speed, and allow effects to be manifested only *relatively*, in state change designs, where a "reference" established in one state is used for comparisons in another one. At first sight, this seems to shut the door on timing behaviour in the elderly being explained in terms of changed clock speed compared with younger people, as for example, a person cannot be given the standards on temporal generalization when 18, and tested on the comparisons when 78. In all timing tasks comparing, for example, elderly participants with student controls, comparisons are between-subject so no clock-speed effect can be detected, without some "common reference."

Suppose, for example, that participants are required to hold down a button for 1 s, with accurate performance-related feedback being given after each response. Even if the clock in one group "ticked" at m per second and another group at n per second, the participants could just learn to respond after different numbers of ticks. This suggests that feedback would reduce age, or IQ, effects if these were based on putative clock-speed differences, and it does (see Wearden et al. 1997, figure 6). It may further suggest that "recalibration" of time judgments to take account of clock speed differences may be easy to achieve.

The above discussion suggests that "clock speed" explanations of ageing effects in timing need to be approached with considerable scepticism, as in most cases even if clock speed differences were present they may not affect time judgments. Is there any way out of this quasi-Einsteinian trap, which seems to forbid the detection of absolute clock speed, just as absolute velocity cannot be measured without a "reference?" The conservative answer is "no," but subject to certain assumptions (which may not be correct) progress might be made.

Vanneste, Pouthas, and Wearden (2001), for example, used the idea of "internal tempo," derived from Denner, Wapner, and Werner (1964). This very simple method asks participants to tap at a "speed which is comfortable for them" for a short period of time, and the resulting intertap interval defines that individual's "internal tempo," a measure which is supposed to be related directly to internal clock speed (see Vanneste et al. 2001, and Boltz, 1994, for discussion). Vanneste et al. found that elderly participants (mean age 69) had slower internal tempi than younger ones (mean age 26), a result that can be considered to reflect slower internal clock speed in older people, subject to the assumption that spontaneous tapping reflects internal clock speed directly. Vanneste et al. also tested their participant groups on a "continuation tapping" task introduced by Wing and Kristofferson (1973). Here, people initially receive a periodic signal, and have to tap in synchrony with it. Then the signal stops and the people are required to continue to tap at the same rate.

The synchronization period would be expected to abolish the young/old difference in timing behaviour as even if the internal clock ticked more slowly in the elderly, as the internal tempo result suggests, the participants would compensate for this. This was the result obtained: no differences were found between the young and old group under the continuation tapping phase of the study, even when the "enforced" tap rate was faster than people's spontaneous tapping rates.

The data of Vanneste et al. suggest that some "uncalibrated" conditions, like performance without any kind of feedback or synchronization, might reveal clock speed differences, and this might tempt the reader into thinking that procedures like interval production without feedback might be useful, but this suggestion needs to be treated with the utmost caution. For one thing, we know little about where "references" come from in uncalibrated conditions: when a person is asked to hold down a button for 1 s, we have little or no idea how they do this without feedback (and the role of feedback itself is not understood). For another, some data suggest that the idea in a simple form may not give a coherent account of data

Experiment 4 of Wearden et al. (1997), which asked people to produce 1 s, proceeded in three phases: no feedback, feedback, and post-feedback. No age or IQ effects on mean time produced were found in the feedback or post-feedback conditions, but in the no-feedback conditions, the young participants (60–69) produced longer intervals than the older ones (70–79). Both produced intervals much longer than 1 s without feedback, although the older group's average production (about 1.5 s) was closer to the target. When intervals are produced, faster clock speed leads to *shorter* productions (Penton-Voak et al. 1996), so the conclusion here would be that clock speed is faster in the older participants, which contradicts the general idea of slowing down the clock with increasing age.

However, there are some data consistent with clock speed differences between elderly and younger people, if a common reference is assumed. Craik and Hay (1999), for example, found very large age effects in an experiment where older participants (mean age 72.2) were compared with undergraduates (mean age 22.2). Participants estimated or produced intervals of 30, 60, and 120 s. Both participant groups overproduced real times, but underestimated them. However, very marked age effects were found, with the older groups emitting productions much longer than the younger groups, and productions which were, furthermore, very much longer than the real time. Conversely, estimates produced by the older group were smaller than those produced by the younger one, and sometimes very deviant from real time (e.g. 120 s was estimated as around 40 s in the elderly).

If we assume a clock-speed difference between the groups, the results are consistent with the idea of slower clock speed in the elderly, which will lengthen productions and shorten estimations (as discussed above). However, the logic assumes some common reference for both participant groups, that is, both need to have some standard "clock second" or other unit, which is the same. This may seem at first sight rather implausible as it implies that older people have never, in the course of innumerable experiences with duration in their everyday life, learned to "recalibrate" to compensate for their lower clock speed. One possibility is that Craik and Hay's participants were using the common reference provided by chronometric counting at a subjective rate of 1 count/s. The experiment used long intervals where counting would be expected to be useful, and the procedure did not appear to prevent or discourage it. If, as Vanneste et al. (2001) the results of suggest, older people have slower spontaneous tapping rates than younger ones, then their rate of counting at a subjective rate of 1 count/s might be slower, so counting would produce a common reference, which would produce the effects obtained. When the stimulus finishes, the older people have counted to a smaller number of "seconds" than the younger ones, so report shorter estimates. When they produce some target interval, they count more slowly, so a longer time is needed to get to the "*n* seconds" required, and the interval produced is longer in older people than younger ones. This interpretation is speculative, but does supply a possible "common reference" for judgments in both the old and young people, without which demonstration of a clock speed effect seems impossible.

Obviously, assuming that absolute clock speed can be detected in mean measures of timing behaviour is exceptionally risky, but there may be another way to detect differences. Recall that "classical" SET assumed that pacemaker variance makes a negligible contribution to total timing variance, which is assumed to come from other sources, such as temporal reference memory. Some recent work has questioned this assumption, and some "twenty-first, century" SET tends to the view that the pacemaker of the internal clock itself is an important, or even the principal, source of variance, particularly in human timing. The arguments here are beyond the scope of this chapter, and the reader is referred to Wearden and Bray (2001), and Jones and Wearden (2003, 2004) for (rather technical) discussions.

Suppose that the pacemaker is an important source of timing variance. Virtually any quantitative pacemaker model will produce the mathematical result that *slower* pacemakers produce *greater* relative variance (e.g. variance that is expressed as a fraction of the mean). This is true of standard Poisson pacemakers, but also of variants discussed by Gibbon et al. (1984). In these cases, then, slower clock speed would be expected to result in more variable time judgments in, for example, the elderly compared with younger groups, rather than judgments which differed in mean, as calibration or feedback would eliminate these.

More variable timing performance in the elderly than in younger groups is in fact quite commonly found, consistent with this idea, although the result is not universal. For example, Wearden et al. (1997) found that variability in temporal generalization performance was affected by age and IQ, and was higher even in the high-IQ elderly than student groups (although the differences were small), see their table 1, p. 968. However, no effects were found in bisection. In the interval production study (their experiment 4), although feedback eliminated age and IQ differences in the mean times produced, some variability effects remained. Their figure 7 shows that, in general, the older group produced responses that were relatively more variable than the younger one, although the difference was not significant, but effects of IQ were significant and orderly, with the lowest IQ group producing the highest relative variance, and the highest IQ group the lowest.

In summary, the hypothesis that internal clock speed decreases with age is difficult to directly test, or directly refute, and only has limited usefulness as an explanation of age-related differences in average measures of behaviour. On the other hand, it may explain why relative variability in timing behaviour increases with age.

Retrospective timing and passage of time judgments

The remainder of this chapter does not review any previous empirical work with the elderly, but attempts to indicate what areas of timing research might be useful for the future. Research on prospective timing in the elderly has produced rather small effects, some of which are inconsistent, with even variability differences between groups not always being found. Effects obtained are hard to interpret, and many studies may be more illuminating about issues in time perception *per se* than they are about age-related changes. A further problem is that the issues investigated in prospective timing studies may have little relevance to the time experience of elderly people in their everyday lives. If we wish to come to grips with changes in time experience, we may need to diversify into studies of retrospective timing and what I call "passage of time" judgments.

As mentioned above, retrospective time judgments are those made when an unexpected question about time is asked. Figure 6.2 shows data from a study by Hicks and Kinsbourne (quoted in Hicks, 1992). Ten groups of students examined a tartan pattern presented for from 8 to 54 s, and rated it for complexity and aesthetic value. For people in one condition (retrospective) this was the only task, whereas people in the prospective condition were told that the duration of presentation of the pattern should be estimated without

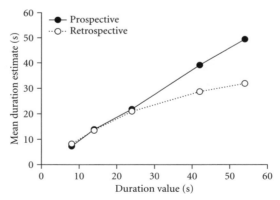

Fig. 6.2 Prospective and retrospective judgments of time from the experiment of Hicks and Kinsbourne. Judgments of the duration of presentation of a tartan pattern are plotted against the real duration of presentation for prospective and retrospective conditions.

counting. After the stimulus presentation, all groups were asked for a judgment of duration. Obviously, people in both the prospective and retrospective conditions showed increased estimates as actual presentation time increased, but the retrospective judgments diverged from the prospective ones at longer durations. However, it might be considered remarkable that retrospective judgments can be performed at all, given that no instructions about timing were given.

Hicks and Kinsbourne's study illustrates an important methodological nuisance in studies of retrospective timing, and that is that once the question about timing has been posed, no further retrospective timing can be measured, as people naturally suspect that time is the focus of the experiment, making the study subsequently prospective. In Hicks and Kinsbourne's experiment, each participant made a single time judgment, essentially participating in only one trial, a methodology that is common in retrospective timing studies (e.g. Block, 1992), but is obviously extremely wasteful of experimental time and effort. However, it is not necessary that each participant gives a single time judgment. Boltz (1994) played participants a short series of distinct auditory stimuli, without any timing instructions, then asked for retrospective time judgments, identifying the stimuli by their content, so did obtain more than one data point from each participant. Overall, retrospective timing studies use much larger participant populations than prospective ones, and collect far fewer data points per subject. Given variability in retrospective time judgments, obtaining statistical significance requires large subject groups, and the arduous nature of the organization and conduct of such studies makes them much rarer than studies of prospective timing and, according to a personal communication from the leading worker in this area (Richard Block of the University of Montana) is a deterrent to carrying them out at all.

How are retrospective time judgments performed? The general idea, deriving from Ornstein (1969), is some sort of "storage size" process. When the participant is asked, unexpectedly, to make a retrospective time judgment, they examine the amount of "memory storage" or "contextual change" during the period in question, and greater amounts of "storage" result in longer time judgments. In other words, retrospective timing is largely based on the amount of "memory-storage" or "information-processing" that has been carried out, and does not depend on internal clock processes in the way that prospective timing does.

Given that elderly people may show poorer memory performance or slower rates of information-processing than younger people, retrospective time judgments would seem to be an area ripe for fruitful investigation, but no study appears to have been done, possibly for the practical reasons outlined above.

Prospective and retrospective timing are commonly distinguished, but I wish to add a third type of time judgment, one that may be particularly useful in studies with elderly people: what I will call "passage of time" judgments. What these are and how they differ from retrospective judgments can be illustrated with reference to a study conducted at Manchester, the grandly-titled "Armageddon" experiment.

The procedure in a slightly simplified form was as follows. A person either watched 9 min of the film "Armageddon" (a virtually violence-free action film), or waited for 9 min in a simulated "waiting room" condition. At the end of this period, the person was asked to judge how quickly time seemed to pass compared with some subjective "normal" condition. The normal result of "time passing quickly when you're enjoying yourself" was found: people rated the passage of time during "Armageddon" as faster than normal, and the "waiting room" time as slower than normal. Note that this implies that the "Armageddon" period was *shorter* than the waiting period (as time passed subjectively quicker in a period that was physically the same), although no judgment of duration was required. Next, both groups read a novel for 10 min, to separate out the two phases of the experiment, then a retrospective time judgment of the previous 9-min period was required. Now, the results were as the storage-size theory predicted: the "Armageddon" period was judged as *longer* than the waiting room period. This result is reminiscent of the paradoxical statements about time experience in the elderly quoted at the start of the chapter, but in reverse: a time period (Armageddon) seems to fly when participants were in it (passage of time judgment), but is judged as relatively long after it has finished (retrospective time judgment).

Studies of passage of time judgments and retrospective timing may enable us to understand changes in time experience with increasing age, changes that are sometimes distressing to elderly people and which greater scientific understanding may help us to alleviate. As mentioned above, such studies are currently completely lacking. What kind of research might it be interesting to do?

The right tree: Toward a new chronogerontology

As mentioned above, the general explanation for our ability to make retrospective time judgments is that we can use the amount of information-processing, or number of items perceived, or remembered, as the basis for judgments of the duration of that period, what from now on I will just call "storage." However, an obvious and persistent difficulty is defining just how much "storage" has occurred. In fact, no study of retrospective timing so far published has done this in a precise way, and most depend on a manipulation as follows: Participants in retrospective conditions are divided into two groups, and receive tasks A or B. An example might be sorting playing cards into red or black (A), or into suits or some more complex arrangement (B). B is putatively more difficult than A, so requires more "information-processing." After tasks A or B have proceeded for some time period, the experiment stops and a retrospective judgment of the duration of A or B is required. In general, more "difficult" tasks produce longer retrospective judgments (see Block, 1992, for discussion).

In the case of the elderly, slowing down of average information-processing rates, and increased intersubject variability in information-processing rates, imply that retrospective timing studies might not only produce large age effects, but also might offer a way of observing more precisely links between "storage" and retrospective time judgments than is possible with younger participants alone. For example, if we have some task A carried out by an elderly group and younger controls for some time period, we might be able to measure (a) the rate of information-processing by individuals during A, (b) subsequent cognitive judgments of events in A, such as the number of items recalled, and (c) link both of these measures to a retrospective time judgment. Experiments such as this, and others employing procedures manipulating information-processing during A, might put possible relations between "storage" and retrospective judgments on a firmer footing than ever before.

However, although experiments of the type outlined above would be very useful, an additional consideration for retrospective time judgments is another problem of "reference." As people age, not only might their internal clock slow down, as discussed earlier, but information-processing rates and memory performance might also decline. However, this decline is gradual in most nonpathological cases, so even in retrospective timing, a person has the opportunity for "recalibration," over a long period of years. We might try to explain the "Christmas comes round quicker every year" effect as follows. Ordinarily, a year contains some amount of "storage" (X). As information-processing rates decrease and memory losses increase with ageing, the amount of storage in a year is less (possibly much less) than X, so the person is surprised that a year has passed, as much less storage has occurred than they expect. The key word here is, of course, "expect," because the obvious question arises of where this expectation comes from: in effect, a "storage" explanation of the "Christmas effect" implies that people are comparing the amount of "storage" in the last year with the amount stored in some other, probably much earlier, year when information-processing rates were higher, and memory losses smaller, effectively employing a "state-change" procedure. This is not impossible, but if people are adjusting to the fact that "less happens" in time periods with increasing age (because people process information more slowly, forget things more, or simply do fewer varied things because of physical limitations) then the "Christmas effect" would be expected to be reduced or even abolished. In general, we need to know much more not only about the cognitive processes on that retrospective time judgments are based, but also on the "reference" used for such judgments. Attributing some real-life timing effects in the elderly to age-related differences in retrospective, rather than prospective, timing may be an essential first step in understanding them, but neither the methodology nor theory of retrospective timing studies currently offer us a completely satisfactory explanation.

Passage of time judgments have been studied quite extensively in the elderly, but usually in a procedure (see Lemlich, 1975), which asks an extraordinary hypothetical question. For example, people are given some standard that represents the passage of time now (a line length or a number), then must rate the passage of time at various ages when they were younger. The usual finding is that people judge time to have passed more slowly when they were young, compared with now.

Even if this procedure yields highly orderly data, it is clearly difficult to know exactly what is being measured here. A more useful line of research, in my view, would be to obtain passage of time judgments from real-life situations (judgments which, ideally, were taken simultaneously with, or just after, the events), and try to understand what influences these. Some work by Zakay (1992) may help to do this. The basic structure of Zakay's approach is illustrated in Figure 6.3. Zakay's model was not initially applied to the study of passage of time judgments, but seems an excellent starting point for it.

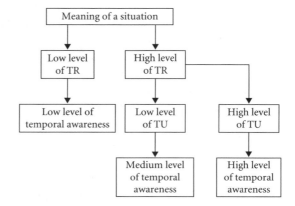

Fig. 6.3 The "temporal awareness" model of Zakay (1992), see text for details. TR = "temporal relevance"; TU = "temporal uncertainty."

According to Zakay, some real-life situation is judged by the participant on the basis of past experience or expectation, in terms of two-dimensions: temporal relevance (how important time is in the task), and temporal uncertainty (how much uncertainty the participant has about the time of event occurrences, or their duration). The outcome variable in Zakay's model is "temporal awareness": if this is high, then the passage of time seems very slow (time seems to "drag"), whereas if it is low, then time can seem to "fly." A situation judged to have very low temporal relevance will induce little temporal awareness, and the passage of time will be subjectively rapid (although a subsequent retrospective time judgment may be long). A high level of temporal relevance can be associated with high or low level levels of temporal uncertainty. Even if the time of some event is critical, then temporal awareness is reduced if uncertainty is reduced (by providing cues as to when the event will occur, for example, or in conditions where things "run like clockwork"). High levels of temporal relevance coupled with high levels of temporal uncertainty produce a high level of temporal awareness, where a person focuses continually on the passage of time, which consequently seems very slow.

Consistent with these ideas, "waiting room" situations produce high temporal awareness, and consequently time seems to drag in them, because (a) time is highly relevant, when waiting for a train or plane, for example, and (b) the exact moment when the train, or plane, arrives can be uncertain, particularly in error-prone transport systems such as the UK-railways at the time of writing.

Zakay's model only gives a starting point, and needs to be elaborated. An important variable might be the amount of attention allocated to temporal and nontemporal aspects of situations (see Brown, 1997, for a review of research). If a person can maintain attention on something other than the passage of time (watching an exciting film, for example), then temporal awareness may be reduced, and time may seem to fly during the time period. To give a personal example, a recently-purchased portable DVD player reduces my temporal awareness during train journeys practically to zero (to the extent of engendering a potential risk of missing the station).

There are many reasons to think that passage of time judgments in the elderly might be a fruitful field of study. For one thing, difficulties in maintaining task attention with increasing age may reduce the capacity for "distraction" away from the passage of time in the elderly. In addition, temporal uncertainty may be higher in the elderly because of increased variability of time representations (caused by slower clock speed or otherwise), or by general memory difficulties such as impairments of prospective memory (Rendell & Craik, 2000). Both reduced ability to focus on nontemporal aspects of situations and increasing temporal uncertainty may increase temporal awareness in older people, thus giving rise to the feeling of "dragging" time sometimes reported.

My general suggestion is that studies of retrospective timing, and passage of time judgments, in the elderly are necessary if we are to gain any proper insight into the subjective distortions of time that accompany old age. Conducting such studies is not, however, easy, and the need for large subject populations may mean that such work can only be performed by research groups which have access to hundreds of elderly participants, and the resources necessary to carry out the studies in any reasonable length of time. Unlike prospective timing research with student participants, which has mostly proceeded using small subject groups, tested easily and at minimal cost, making any serious inroads into understanding the time experience of the elderly will require the allocation of considerable time, effort, and resources. However, the goal of understanding changes in human time experience with ageing may be elusive without such research.

References

Allan, L. G. (1998). The influence of the scalar timing model on human timing research. *Behavioral Processes*, **44**, 101–117.

Allan, L. G. (2002). Are the referents remembered in temporal bisection? *Learning and Motivation*, **33**, 10–31.

Block, R. A. (1992). Prospective and retrospective duration judgement: The role of information processing and memory. In F. Macar, V. Pouth as & W. J. Friedman (Eds.), *Time, action, and cognition: Towards bridging the gap.* (pp. 141–52). Dordrecht: Kluwer Academic Press.

Boltz, M. G. (1994). Changes in internal tempo and effects on the learning and remembering of event durations. *Journal of Experimental Psychology: Learning, Memory, and Cognition*, **20**, 1154–1171.

Brown, S. W. (1997). Attentional resources in timing: Interference effects in concurrent temporal and nontemporal working memory tasks. *Perception and Psychophysics*, **59**, 1118–1140.

Burle, B., & Casini, L. (2001). Dissociation between activation and attention effects in time estimation: Implications for clock models. *Journal of Experimental Psychology: Human Perception and Performance*, **27**, 195–205.

Craik, F. I. M., & Hay, J. F. (1999). Aging and judgments of duration: Effects of task complexity and method of estimation. *Perception and Psychophysics*, **61**, 549–560.

Denner, B., Wapner, S., & Werner, H. (1964). Rhythmic activity and the discrimination of stimuli in time. *Perceptual and Motor Skills*, **19**, 723–729.

Droit-Volet, S. (2002). Scalar timing in temporal generalization in children with short and long stimulus durations. *Quarterly Journal of Experimental Psychology*, **55A**, 1193–1209.

Droit-Volet, S., Clément, A., & Wearden, J. H. (2001). Temporal generalization in 3- to 8-year-old children. *Journal of Experimental Child Psychology*, **80**, 271–288.

Droit-Volet, S., & Wearden, J. H. (2001). Temporal bisection in children. *Journal of Experimental Child Psychology*, **80**, 142–159.

Droit-Volet, S., & Wearden, J. (2002). Speeding up an internal clock in children? Effects of visual flicker on subjective duration. *Quarterly Journal of Experimental Psychology,* **55B**, 193–211.

Fraisse, P. (1964). *The psychology of time.* London: Eyre and Spottiswoode.

Gibbon, J., Church, R. M., & Meck, W. (1984). Scalar timing in memory. In J. Gibbon and L. Allan (Eds.), *Annals of the New York Academy of Sciences,* 423: Timing and time perception (pp. 52–77). New York: New York Academy of Sciences.

Hicks, R. E. (1992). Prospective and retrospective judgments of time: A neurobehavioral analysis. In F. Macar, V. Pouthas, and W. J. Friedman (Eds.), *Time, action, and cognition: Towards bridging the gap.* (pp. 97–108). Dordrecht: Kluwer Academic Press.

Hicks, R. E., Miller, G. W., & Kinsbourne, M. (1976). Prospective and retrospective judgments of time as a function of the amount of information processed. *American Journal of Psychology,* **89**, 719–730.

Jones, L. A., & Wearden, J. H. (2003). More is not necessarily better: Examining the nature of the temporal reference memory component in timing. *Quarterly Journal of Experimental Psychology,* **56**, 321–343.

Jones, L. A., & Wearden, J. H. (2004). Double standards: Memory loading in temporal reference memory. *Quarterly Journal of Experimental Psychology,* **57B**, 55–77.

Lejeune, H., Ferrara, A., Soffié, M., Bronchart, M., & Wearden, J. H. (1998). Peak procedure performance in young adult and aged rats: Acquisition and adaptation to a changing temporal criterion. *Quarterly Journal of Experimental Psychology,* **51B**, 193–217.

Lemlich, R. (1975). Subjective acceleration of time with aging. *Perceptual and Motor skills,* **41**, 235–238.

Lustig, C. (2003). Grandfather's clock: Attention and interval timing in older adults. In W. H. Meck (Ed.), *Functional and neural mechanisms of interval timing* (pp. 261–293). Boca Raton, FL: CRC Press.

McCormack, T., Brown, G. D. A., Maylor, E. A., Darby, A. & Green, D. (1999). Developmental changes in time estimation: Comparing childhood and old age. *Developmental Psychology,* **35**, 1143–1155.

McCormack, T., Brown, G. D. A., Maylor, E. A., Richardson, L. B. N., & Darby, R. J. (2002). Effects of aging on absolute identification of duration. *Psychology and Aging,* **17**, 363–378.

McCormack, T., Brown, G. D. A., Smith, M. C., & Brock, J. (2004). A timing-specific memory distortion effect in young children. *Journal of Experimental Child Psychology,* **87**, 33–56.

Meck, W. H. (1983). Selective adjustment of the speed of internal clock and memory processes. *Journal of Experimental Psychology: Animal Behavior Processes,* **9**, 171–201.

Meck, W. H. (1996). Neuropharmacology of timing and time perception. *Cognitive Brain Research,* **3**, 227–242.

Meck, W. H., Church, R. M., & Wenk, G. L. (1986). Arginine vasopressin innoculates against age-related changes in sodium-dependent high affinity choline uptake and discrepancies in the content of temporal memory. *European Journal of Pharmacology,* **130**, 327–331.

Ornstein, R. E. (1969). *On the experience of time.* Harmondsworth: Penguin.

Penton-Voak, I. S., Edwards, H., Percival, A., & Wearden, J. H. (1996). Speeding up an internal clock in humans? Effects of click trains on subjective duration. *Journal of Experimental Psychology: Animal Behavior Processes,* **22**, 307–320.

Rendell, P. G., & Craik, F. I. M. (2000). Virtual week and actual week: Age-related differences in prospective memory. *Applied Cognitive Psychology,* **14**, S43–S62.

Treisman, M. (1963). Temporal discrimination and the indifference interval: Implications for a model of the "internal clock." *Psychological Monographs, 77*, 1–31.

Treisman, M., Faulkner, A., Naish, P. L. N., & Brogan, D. (1990). The internal clock: Evidence for a temporal oscillator underlying time perception with some estimates of its characteristic frequency. *Perception, 19*, 705–748.

Vanneste, S., Pouthas, V. & Wearden, J. H. (2001). Temporal control of rhythmic performance: A comparison between young and old adults. *Experimental Aging Research, 27*, 83–102.

Wearden, J. H. (1991). Human performance on an analogue of an interval bisection task. *Quarterly Journal of Experimental Psychology, 43B*, 59–81.

Wearden, J. H. (1992). Temporal generalization in humans. *Journal of Experimental Psychology: Animal Behavior Processes, 18*, 134–144.

Wearden, J. H. (2003). Applying the scalar timing model to human time psychology: Progress and challenges. In H. Helfrich (Ed.), *Time and mind II: Information-processing perspectives* (pp. 21–39). Gottingen: Hogrefe & Huber.

Wearden, J. H. (2004). Decision processes in models of timing. *Acta Neurobiologiae Experimentalis, 64*, 303–317.

Wearden, J. H. (in press). Origins and development of internal clock theories of time. *Psychologie Française.*

Wearden, J. H., & Bray, S. (2001). Scalar timing without reference memory: Episodic temporal generalization and bisection in humans. *Quarterly Journal of Experimental Psychology, 54B*, 289–310.

Wearden, J. H., Edwards, H., Fakhri, M., & Percival, A. (1998). Why "sounds are judged longer than lights": Application of a model of the internal clock in humans. *Quarterly Journal of Experimental Psychology, 51B*, 97–120.

Wearden, J. H., & Ferrara, A. (1995). Stimulus spacing effects in temporal bisection by humans. *Quarterly Journal of Experimental Psychology, 48B*, 289–310.

Wearden, J. H., & Ferrara, A. (1996). Stimulus range effects in temporal bisection by humans. *Quarterly Journal of Experimental Psychology, 49B*, 24–44.

Wearden, J. H., & Penton-Voak, I. S. (1995). Feeling the heat: Body temperature and the rate of subjective time, revisited. *Quarterly Journal of Experimental Psychology, 48B*, 129–141.

Wearden, J. H., Philpott, K., & Win, T. (1999). Speeding up and (. . . relatively . . .) slowing down and internal clock in humans. *Behavioral Processes, 46*, 63–73.

Wearden, J. H., Pilkington, R., & E. Carter (1999). "Subjective lengthening" during repeated testing of a simple temporal discrimination. *Behavioral Processes, 46*, 25–38.

Wearden, J. H., Wearden, A. J., & Rabbitt, P. M. A. (1997). Age and IQ effects on stimulus and response timing. *Journal of Experimental Psychology: Human Perception and Performance, 23*, 962–979.

Wing, A. M., & Kristofferson, A. B. (1973). Response delays and the timing of discrete motor responses. *Perception and Psychophysics, 14*, 3–12.

Vanneste, S., Pouthas, V., & Wearden, J. H. (2001). Temporal control of rhythmic performance: A comparison between young and old adults. *Experimental Aging Research, 27*, 83–102.

Zakay, D. (1992). On prospective time estimation, temporal relevance, and temporal uncertainty. In F. Macar, V. Pouthas, & W. J. Friedman (Eds.), *Time, action, and cognition: Towards bridging the gap.* (pp. 109–118). Dordrecht: Kluwer Academic Press.

Section 2

Cognitive control and frontal lobe function

Chapter 7

The chronometrics of task-set control

Stephen Monsell

Abstract

In this chapter I review recent research from reaction-time experiments on the control of task-set, especially experiments in which frequent changes of task are required. The focus is on the reaction-time cost of a task switch, and the reduction in cost usually observed when the subject has time to prepare for a stimulus and foreknowledge of the task to be performed. The latter phenomenon has been interpreted as an index of a control process—task-set reconfiguration (TSR)—being carried out in preparation for the change of task. I defend this interpretation against some recent challenges, and develop a set of recommendations, based on our recent research, on how to conduct a task-cueing experiment in such a way as to allow TSR to reveal itself. I then address the nature of TSR, arguing that a simple associative conception of performance in task-switching experiments is inadequate, although associative binding between stimuli, responses, cues, contexts, and goals undoubtedly contributes to performance. At a minimum, the evidence requires a multi-level associative network in which context selects the task that modulates the lower-level associations by which the stimulus selects the action. The dynamics of such a network must accommodate evidence from RT distributions suggesting discrete rather than incremental changes in task-set readiness. There is also evidence that the fundamental task-set control network we share with infra-human species is supplemented in humans by processes of linguistic self-instruction and perhaps other strategies for getting ready to perform a cognitive task.

Introduction

It was from Pat Rabbitt's lectures to Oxford undergraduates on Human Skill that I first learnt of the mysteries of mental chronometry, as realized through

Research by Monsell & Mizon (submitted a, b) was supported by the Economic and Social Research Council. I am grateful to John Duncan for his helpful comments on the first draft.

the reaction time (RT) experiment pioneered by Donders and others in the nineteenth century. In such an experiment, subjects are asked to respond to each of a series of stimuli from a specified set (e.g. digits, words, objects, etc.) by performing an action (e.g. a key-press, a verbal response, an eye movement), according to a set of task rules (e.g. press the left key if the word names an animal, the right key if not). The subject is instructed with the magic incantation: "Please respond to each stimulus as fast as you can while avoiding errors," and his or her reaction time is measured on a large number of trials. Through manipulating variables such as properties of the stimuli, or the rules, or the responses, or the recent history of the subject, and observing the effect on mean RT (or other properties of the RT distribution) and accuracy you could—or so Pat promised us—make inferences about the hidden mental processes intervening between stimulus input and response output. As things turned out, that is what I have spent much of my research career trying to do.

Although RTs had been measured accurately from the middle of the nineteenth century onwards, even in the late 1960s it remained a laborious process to present visual or auditory stimuli under precise temporal control and record the identity and latency of key-press responses. Much of Pat's pioneering work on sequential effects and error correction in choice reaction time (Rabbitt & Vyas, 1970, 1973, 1974) was done using an electronic beast called SPARTA, which displayed characters on an LED display, absorbed quantities of punched paper tape required to programme its stimulus sequences, and extruded more paper tape recording the reaction times. My own first reaction time experiment involved a bruising encounter with a three-field tachistoscope—quite literally so because to change two stimulus cards on each trial I had to hold each in place with my thumb while slamming a trap-door on it, and precise timing was required to withdraw the thumb at the right moment. Changing the cards and writing down the RTs took so long that I could collect just 60 RTs in an hour, only three or four times more than a well-practiced user of a Hipp chronoscope could record in Wundt's lab in Leipzig in the 1880s. Happily, by the time I was a graduate student, thanks to an MRC equipment grant to Pat and colleagues, the Oxford department had acquired its first lab computer, a Digital Equipment Corporation Linc-8; it occupied a hot and vibrating cabinet the size of a wardrobe, burnt 3 kW an hour, had about 4.5 kB of useable memory, and cost the taxpayer a sizeable sum. This I spent about a year of my time as a research student programming. To a twenty-first century graduate student, who is able to use a PC costing a few hundred pounds, running E-prime or a similar programme with a nice graphic interface, to record RTs to stimuli such as coloured photographs, movies, sound recordings etc. (not to mention the recording of eye or hand movements, ERPs, fMRI BOLD signals etc.), the conduct of RT experiments in the 1960s and early 1970s would seem unbelievably primitive and onerous. But these years nevertheless constituted the transition to an era when we acquired the freedom to choose and manipulate stimuli, conditions, and tasks, while collecting as many hundreds of RTs per session as the subject could bear to produce. We could thus begin to realize the potential of RT as a method for the investigation of a wide range of cognitive skills.

My own research interest at the time was short-term memory. When, in the late 1980s, I began to do experiments on executive control I was pleased to discover that my ex-supervisor was now an authority on this topic, in his case with particular application to ageing research. As I lack any expertise on ageing (other than that derived from personal experience), it seemed appropriate for me to contribute to Pat's Festschrift by addressing the other two elements of the volume title's triad in a review of some recent efforts to investigate control mechanisms—more specifically, control of "task-set"—through the reaction-time experiment.

Task-set

To perform any cognitive task, whether it results in overt action or not, requires some subset of the representations and processes available in our brains, and a particular organization of those processes—a "task-set." To read aloud, for example, I must use processes that represent orthographic patterns (letter identities and their order) in the retinal input, one or more processes that translate orthographic to phonological patterns (including recognition of familiar patterns and retrieval of learned pronunciations) and processes translating phonology into articulatory activity in the vocal tract. I (or some part of my brain) must somehow arrange that information will flow through these stages of processing, that my visual attention is directed appropriately, and that my response criterion and reading rate are adjusted so that I neither initiate speech before an adequate articulatory code is available nor wait too long. (And I can "set" myself to do these things, at least to some extent, before the first word appears on the screen, as has been recognized since the early days of experimental psychology.) When I proof-read, in contrast, I use some of these same processes (such as word recognition) but not others (such as overt articulation); instead I must couple to word-recognition and comprehension processes another set of processes and procedures for detecting and correcting errors. We can speak, therefore, of a reading-aloud "task-set" and a proof-reading "task-set." If I elect to stop reading and start proof-reading, at least some procedures, processes or linkages between processes must be suppressed and others enabled so that I no longer speak aloud the words I look at, but instead begin to detect and correct errors.

Task-set is partly controlled "endogenously"—from within: to some extent we do the tasks we want, or at least intend, to do. Such "top-down" control is most apparent to introspection when dutiful intention must defeat desire, as when I sit down to mark examination scripts. Task-set is also driven "exogenously," or "bottom-up," by the environment: we leap to avoid skateboarders in the street; we answer the phone when it rings (if the context is appropriate); we are prompted to engage in social interaction by chance encounters (if not feeling too grumpy); we "automatically" read text if we happen to fixate it. A novel task-set may be acquired slowly through trial and error, or very rapidly through verbal instruction or demonstration. Practice then develops a procedural representation of the task-set, and it becomes retrievable from memory as a package. As a rule of thumb, the more familiar a task-set, and the more recent its exercise, the easier it is to engage it. Hence at any given moment our task-set "state" reflects the outcome of a complex interaction between internal goals and motivational state, external context and specific stimuli associated with performance of particular tasks, and the frequency and recency with which we have performed particular tasks. A well-adapted brain is one in which endogenous control is neither so strong as to prevent important external events triggering an appropriate change of task-set, nor so weak that unimportant stimuli trigger inappropriate changes (Goschke, 2000).

How can we investigate in the laboratory this complex interaction, so central to our everyday lives, between endogenous control, exogenous influences, and the familiarity and recency of tasks? An increasingly popular method is to incorporate frequent changes of task into the reaction-time experiment. We present a sequence of stimuli, each requiring a rapid response specified by a task-rule, and measure RT. From time to time the task-rule changes. For example, the stimuli might be digits, with one task being to classify the digit as odd/even by pressing a left or right key, and the other being to classify the digit as high/low by pressing one of the same two keys. The phenomenon of interest is the "task switch cost"—the considerable lengthening of RT that is usually observed on trials on which the task changes—*task-switch* trials—relative to the RT on *task-repeat* trials; this is often accompanied by an increase in error rate as well. This "switch cost" suggests that extra mental work of some kind is needed when the task changes; the challenge is to characterize this extra work.

There are several variants of the task-switching experiment, each using a different way of informing the subject which of the several tasks in play to perform (see Monsell, 2003). In this chapter I shall focus on just two. In the *task-cueing* paradigm, each stimulus is preceded or accompanied by a task cue and the task is unpredictable until the cue is presented (Shaffer, 1965). In the *alternating-runs* paradigm, the task is completely predictable: the task changes every *n* trials (Rogers & Monsell, 1995).[1] Although subjects can be required to keep track of the task sequence from memory, external task cues are usually provided to help the subject keep track of where they are in a run of trials (e.g. the task may be specified by location of the stimulus on the screen, the colour or shape of a background, or verbal or pictorial cues).

With both predictable (alternating runs) and unpredictable (cued) changes of task, RT is substantially prolonged on the trial on which the task changes—a "task-switch cost." This is illustrated by the data in Figure 7.1. Note also that when task switches were unpredictable, RT then took two or three more trials to recover fully to an asymptotic level. In contrast, with predictable switches (every four trials in this case) we typically see this abrupt recovery to "baseline" on the trial following the switch (it being understood that this baseline RT is higher than it would be in a block with only one task—the "mixing cost" referred to in Footnote 1). Monsell, Sumner and Waters (2003) suggested that this difference in recovery from a switch with random and predictable switching reflects strategic control of task-set readiness. After the first of a guaranteed run of several more trials on the same task, subjects can fully set themselves for that task (or allow performance of the task so to set them). In the unpredictable case, having just switched tasks, subjects must be prepared to switch back again on the very next trial, and thus resist fully changing their task-set. However, two or three more performances of the task seem to overcome this resistance. One consequence of this difference is that the typical "switch cost" contrast, between RT for task-switch and all task-repeat trials, actually underestimates the true switch cost in the case of unpredictable switching. It should also be mentioned that, after a switch, there may be gradual slowing through a long run of trials following a switch, at least when no time is allowed between each response and the next stimulus (Altmann, 2002). However, from now on

---

[1] If $n = 1$, this is the task-alternation paradigm, often attributed to Jersild (1927)—though Bernstein (1924) cites similar earlier work; performance is compared between alternation blocks and blocks with just one task. However, "alternation cost" includes both long-term "mixing-cost" due to several task-sets being in a state of high availability and the transient "switch-cost" observed following a change of tasks; examining post-switch trials in the alternating-runs paradigm enables us to focus on the latter.

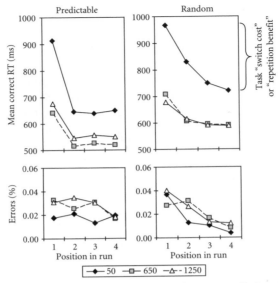

Fig. 7.1 Data from Monsell, Sumner, and Waters (2003, exp 2), in which the stimulus was a digit and the task switched between high/low and odd/even classification. The colour or shape of the background changed on every trial immediately following a response, and either colour (for some subjects) or shape (for others) cued the next task. In predictable switching the task changed every four trials. The data illustrate (a) switch cost, which is (b) limited to the first trial of a run with predictable switching, but (c) shows more gradual recovery with unpredictable switching and (d) reduces in magnitude as the time available for preparation is increased from 50 to 650 ms, but no further as the interval extends to 1250. (Reprinted with permission from Memory and Cognition, Vol. 31 ©2003 The Psychonomic Society.)

I shall ignore these detailed trends in RT over the task-repeat trials following a task switch and focus on the most striking phenomenon—the initial cost of a switch.

I shall begin by addressing the reduction in the switch cost that is observed as the time available to prepare for a task-switch is increased. This effect is often assumed to measure the progress of endogenous task-set reconfiguration. However, this intuitive interpretation has become highly controversial of late. I shall argue that—if the experiment is done right—the intuitive interpretation is correct and provides a means of measuring task-set reconfiguration. I shall then consider in more detail what it is we are measuring, whether this process occurs incrementally or discretely, the role of linguistic coding in aiding this process, and the contribution of associations between stimuli and tasks to performance in task-switching experiments.

Can we measure preparatory task-set reconfiguration with RT?

When you embark on a physical task such as putting up a shelf, the time it will take is generally reduced if you have assembled the tools and materials you need before you start. Intuition suggests that something similar is true of mental tasks: given a warning that you are about to change tasks and a little time to prepare, you can use that time usefully to prepare for the upcoming change of tasks—to "ready" or "set" yourself for the new task. Data from task-switching experiments accord with this intuition—but only partly so. For example, Rogers and Monsell (1995) presented a character pair on each trial. For the letter task, one of the characters was a letter, to be classified as consonant/vowel; for the digit task, one of the characters was a digit, to be classified as high/low; the task changed every two trials. In one experiment the interval between the subject pressing a key and the next stimulus being displayed—the *response-stimulus interval* (RSI)—varied between 150 and 1200 ms, but remained constant during a block of trials. Increasing the RSI up to about 600 ms substantially reduced the switch cost—the difference between mean RT on task-switch and task-repeat trials. I will refer to this interaction (idealized in Figure 7.2) as the "reduction in switch cost" or RISC effect. With further lengthening of the RSI the switch cost reached an asymptote that has come to be called the "residual cost" (Figure 7.2). Experiments with RSIs as long as 5 or 12 s have yielded switch costs (e.g. Kimberg, Aguirre, & D'Esposito, 2000; Sohn, Ursu, Anderson, Stenger, & Carter, 2000). Hence there appears to be a component of the mean switch cost that can be eliminated by voluntary preparation, and a component that cannot.

Rogers and I attributed the RISC effect to an executive process—TSR. If time is available, we argued, this can be done "endogenously" before the stimulus onset, but if there is not, part or all of it must be done after the stimulus to enable task-specific processes such as response selection to proceed

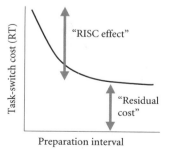

Fig. 7.2 Idealised data showing the reduction in switch cost (RISC) with an increase in time available for preparation and the residual cost.

appropriately; part or all of the duration of TSR will then be included in the RT. At that time we tended to think of TSR as a process that must run to completion before response selection could proceed. But this assumption may be too strong. An alternative possibility is that TSR is an incremental biasing process: enough of a bias must be applied before response selection is complete to ensure that the task-appropriate response is selected, but further opportunity for advance reconfiguration improves the efficiency of response selection by further reducing the influence of the competing task-set. Either way, careful measurement of the RISC effect offers a way to measure the progress of TSR and investigate its properties. It also provides a paradigm for probing the neural correlates of TSR with electrophysiological or haemodynamic methods while at the same time verifying the occurrence of effective TSR behaviourally. However, over the intervening decade, several challenges have been made to the claim that the RISC effect can be used to measure a task-set preparation process in this way. There are (at least) four problematic issues.

Issue 1: Unconfounding active preparation and passive decay
An alternative account of the Rogers and Monsell (1995) result described above was already available when it was published. Allport, Styles and Hsieh (1994) had proposed that the RT switch cost was due to interference with response selection due to a carry-over of task-set state from the previous trial—"task-set inertia" (TSI). If you have just been doing Task A, then persistence of the resulting task-set state (which might include both activation of elements of A and inhibition of elements of B) as you then try to execute Task B somehow prolongs response selection. Thus the switch cost reflected not the duration of a TSR process, but the incompleteness of TSR. On this account, our RISC effect might be due not to active preparation at all, but merely to passive decay or dissipation of TSI: the longer the RSI, the more time available for TSI to "wear off." In the intervening years, evidence that task-set inertia is indeed a contributor to switch costs has accumulated (see Yeung & Monsell, 2003a, 2003b), though its mechanism is still not well understood.

When the task is completely predictable, as in the alternating-runs paradigm, then more opportunity for active preparation is necessarily confounded with more time for dissipation of TSI. But further data on predictable switching indicate that TSI-decay is insufficient to explain the RISC effect. Rogers and Monsell (exp 2) repeated the experiment described above with the single change that the RSI varied randomly from trial to trial. This abolished the RISC effect: the switch cost was about 200 ms at all intervals. Varying the response-stimulus interval from trial to trial rather than between blocks should not stop passive decay of TSI, but inability to predict how long one has to prepare might well deter one from engaging in active reconfiguration.

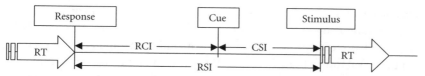

Fig. 7.3 The task-cueing paradigm, which allows one to vary the cue-stimulus interval (CSI) while keeping the response-stimulus interval (RSI) constant, or to vary the response-cue interval (RCI) while keeping the CSI constant (Meiran, 1996).

Goschke (2000) gave subjects two-trial sequences, which they knew in advance would be task-change or task-repeat sequences; the tasks were to identify with a key-press either the colour or the identity of a letter. The RSI was short (14 ms) or long (1500 ms). During the long preparation interval, subjects either named the second task ("colour" or "letter"), said nothing, or said an irrelevant word unrelated to the task ("Monday" or "Tuesday"). In the first two conditions, a long RSI substantially reduced the switch cost, but in the third it did not. Having to say an irrelevant word should surely not prevent decay of TSI; it is entirely plausible that it would interfere with appropriate TSR.

However, if we want to measure TSR uncontaminated by TSI-decay, we need to control the contribution of the latter. Meiran (1996) used the task-cueing paradigm (Figure 7.3) to do this, keeping the response-to-stimulus interval (and hence any decay of TSI) constant, while varying the cue-to-stimulus interval. The assumption is that subjects will not begin active TSR until they perceive a cue indicating that TSR is necessary. And, indeed, Meiran (1996) observed, as have others, a substantial reduction in switch cost with an increase in cue-stimulus interval. In other experiments Meiran, Chorev, and Sapir (2000) showed that increasing the response-to-cue interval while keeping the cue-to-stimulus interval constant also reduced switch costs, suggesting that there was in fact rather rapid decay of TSI over the first second or so. Hence Meiran's constant-RSI version of the cueing paradigm appeared to be the way to measure active TSR while controlling for task-set dissipation.

Issue 2: Failures to observe an interaction of foreknowledge and preparation interval

Several studies have reported failures to observe a reduction in switch cost when subjects are given time to prepare and foreknowledge of the task. In one sense this is not a problem: anticipatory TSR is a voluntary process, and in some circumstances subjects will elect not to prepare in advance of the stimulus onset (*cf.* Braver, Gray, & Burgess, in press, on "proactive: versus reactive" control). The Rogers and Monsell experiment with unpredictable stimulus onsets appears to be one such case. More generally, foreknowledge and opportunity are not sufficient to induce preparation; the subject must be adequately motivated. It is advisable to give explicit instruction on the benefits of preparation and incentives for minimizing RT and errors. Altmann (2004; in press) has recently found that a between-subject manipulation of preparation interval did not yield a RISC effect when an equivalent manipulation within-subjects did so. In predictable switching experiments Nick Yeung and I (Yeung & Monsell, 2003a) also obtained indirect evidence that subjects exposed only to a single long interval did not necessarily take advantage of it. Exposure to a range of preparation intervals may be needed to alert subjects to the benefits of preparation.

More troubling are cases where subjects show a benefit of foreknowledge, but it is the same on switch and nonswitch trials (e.g. Dreisbach, Haider, & Kluwe, 2002; Sohn & Carlson, 2000). One feature of both these experiments was that working out what the upcoming task would be imposed a nontrivial processing load. If interpreting an external cue, or computing the next task from the first, is sufficiently demanding, it may become a task in itself, from which the subject must switch on every trial to perform the specified task, so that every trial becomes a "switch" trial.

Issue 3: Cue interpretation, and the confounding of cue-change and task-change
Even if we use task cues whose meaning is readily apparent, the subject must identify and interpret the task cue to determine what TSR is appropriate, if any. The implicit assumption has been that as cue interpretation is required on both switch and nonswitch trials, its effect on RT, if any, will not interact with the effect of switching task. Most experiments have, moreover, used one cue per task, completely confounding cue change and task change. But it is quite likely that the cue will be processed differently when it is the same as on the previous trial. Logan and Bundesen (2003) controlled for this by using two cues per task. In some of their experiments they used the high/low and odd/even tasks, with a verbal cue—"odd/even," "parity," "high/low," or "magnitude"—preceding each digit by a variable interval. Thus instead of just "switch" and "nonswitch" trials, there were three conditions:

- *both-repeat* (the cue is repeated so the task stays the same)
- *both-change* (a cue for the other task is presented, so the task changes)
- *cue-change* (the other cue for the same task is presented, so the task repeats).

Comparison of the standard switch condition (both-change) and nonswitch condition (both-repeat) showed the usual reduction in "switch cost" with preparation. Their new cue-change condition allowed Logan and Bundesen to separate the contributions to "switch cost" of changing the cue and of changing the task. They found very similar RTs in the cue-change and both-change conditions: i.e. the switch cost was attributable largely to a change in cue, not a change in task.

This is clearly a result that should disturb anyone hoping to use the RISC effect to measure task-set preparation. Logan and Bundesen argued that the switch cost must be a measure of something else: an advantage in processing a repeated cue, that reduces in effect as the preparation interval increases. At about the same time Mayr and Kliegl (2003) also published an experiment in which they used two cues (letters) per task (colour and shape identification), but they obtained a different result. Cue-change accounted for about half the switch cost, and task-change for the rest. So they at least obtained a true cost of changing tasks while controlling for cue change. However, they found no significant reduction in that cost with an increase in preparation time—which is almost as problematic for the standard view. I learned of these results just as I was planning some cueing experiments. The planned experiments were shelved while I embarked with Guy Mizon on a series of experiments using two cues per task to see whether Logan and Bundesen were right (Monsell & Mizon, submitted a).

Our initial findings were perplexing. We sometimes obtained results like Logan and Bundesen's and sometimes did not. In one experiment, for example, we used a pair of tasks with which substantial switch costs have been observed in predictable switching experiments (Aron, Monsell, Sahakian, & Robbins, 2004) and to which we will return later in the chapter. The stimulus is a letter string surrounded by an outline shape (Figure 7.4). For the "arrow task," the outline shape is an arrow pointing left or right, and the subject presses a left or right key accordingly. For the "word" task, the letter string is the word LEFT or RIGHT, and the subject must press the corresponding key. Stimuli were equally often *congruent* (e.g. a left arrow containing the word LEFT), *incongruent* (e.g. a left arrow containing the word RIGHT) or *neutral* (an arrow containing XXXX for the arrow task, an outline rectangle containing the word LEFT or RIGHT for the word task). We used a constant RSI of 2500 ms and the task was cued by one of four easily discriminable sounds presented between 150 and 2000 ms prior to the cue. Subjects were pretrained on a mapping (balanced

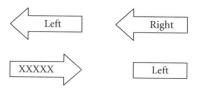

Fig. 7.4 Examples of stimuli used in the word and arrow tasks of Monsell and Mizon (submitted a) and Aron et al. (2004). The top two are congruent and incongruent bivalent stimuli, affording a response in either task; the bottom two are univalent stimuli affording a response in only one task.

over subjects) between each pair of cue sounds and a task. To my chagrin we found that, just as in Logan and Bundesen's experiments, performance on the cue-change and both-change trials was virtually identical: that is, there was no difference in RT between task-switch and task-repeat trials, controlling for a cue change. All the "switch cost" came from the contrast of cue-change and both-repeat conditions: it was significant overall and showed a significant reduction with preparation.

Contrast this outcome to what we found in another experiment (Monsell & Mizon, submitted a, exp 3) with the same basic design. Now the stimuli were object names, and the tasks were to classify them either by the number of syllables (one/two), or by whether the object was big or small (relative to a football). The cues were easy-to-interpret visual icons (e.g. a football or a big and a small double-headed arrow for the size task). The RSI was 1600 ms and a cue appeared above the location of the upcoming word between 150 and 1100 ms prior to the stimulus. Now there was a significant cost of a task-change (with the effect of cue change controlled) and it reduced significantly with preparation. There was also a smaller effect of cue change which did not reduce significantly with preparation.

So, putting together these experiments with two cues per task (ours, Logan & Bundesen's and Mayr & Kliegl's) we had a puzzle. Some of the experiments obtained an effect on RT of task change (controlling for cue change), and in some it reduced with preparation, in a manner appropriate for an index of endogenous TSR. What is the difference between these experiments and those in which no task-change effect (controlling for cue change) was found? We now believe that the critical difference is the probability of a task switch. The experiments in which no true task-switch cost could be detected happened to use a relatively high probability of a task switch (0.5) and an even higher conditional probability of a task switch when the cue changed (0.67). Those in which a task-switch cost was obtained used a lower probability of a task switch (0.33) and a lower conditional probability (0.5). Why might this matter?

Issue 4: Expectation of a task switch
To infer TSR from the interaction between task switch/repeat and preparation time assumes that if subjects have been doing task A, they not only begin to reconfigure for Task B when the cue for B is presented (see Issue 2) but also—just as important—that they do *not* reconfigure themselves for Task B *before* the cue is presented or, indeed, if the cue indicates the same task as before, after the cue is presented. However, we know that people's expectations about random binary sequences are non-normative; they expect alternations more than repetitions, and their expectation of an alternation increases through a run of repetitions. With a 1 in 2 chance of a task switch, subjects may begin to

prepare for the other task, partially and/or probabilistically, even before the cue. Also, in these two-cues-per-task experiments with repeating and nonrepeating cues, if the majority of cue-changes signal a task change, it may seem an optimal strategy to begin to reconfigure for the other task as soon as any cue change is detected, continuing or reversing that preparation when the cue has been fully interpreted.

To test the role of overall expectation of a task-switch we (Monsell & Mizon, submitted a, exp 4) simply manipulated the probability of a task switch. Subjects switched between identifying the shape or colour of the stimulus (four alternatives in each case). To avoid the confound between task- and cue-change, the cue changed on *every* trial between a word cue ("SHAPE" or "COLOUR") and a picture cue (a collage of the four colours or a collage of the four shapes). The RSI was a constant 1650 ms and the CSI was 140 ms or 790 ms. For one group of subjects, there was only a one in four chance of a task switch. For these subjects, there was a switch cost of the order of 200 ms at the short interval, and a substantial reduction in cost at the longer interval. All subjects showed this reduction; for mean RT the percentage reduction in cost was a highly consistent $60 \pm 5\%$. For a second group, the task changed on half the trials. Their switch cost at the short interval was approximately half that of the first group, though still reliable, and although their RISC effect was reliable, it was smaller and less consistent over subjects. For the third group, there was a three in four chance of a switch. The switch cost at the short interval was now of the order of 20 ms, not statistically reliable, and exhibiting no reduction at the longer interval. This seems a clear demonstration that the measured switch cost and RISC effect are sensitive to the expectation of a task switch. To induce an appropriate difference in task-specific preparation between switch and nonswitch trials to measure TSR, it would seem sensible to keep the overall probability of a task switch low enough that subjects tend to reconfigure only after the cue has been interpreted and found to signal a task change.

In a further test of the importance of expectation of a task switch (Monsell & Mizon, submitted a, exp 5), we essentially replicated one of Logan and Bundesen's experiments—high/low and odd/even tasks with digit stimuli, a variable preparation interval, and verbal cues—but altered the sequential probabilities so that p (both repeat) = 0.25, p (cue change, task repeat) = 0.5, and p (both change) = 0.25. The results now looked quite like that of our size/syllable experiment: a substantial effect of task change reducing with preparation, a smaller effect of cue change that did not. When we tested another group of subjects replicating Logan and Bundesen's sequential probabilities (0.25, 0.25, 0.50) the effect of a task change was greatly reduced, supporting the idea that subjects' preparatory strategies are strongly influenced by these probabilities. The effect of a cue change, however, was similar for the two groups, consistent with it reflecting passive priming of cue encoding/interpretation.

Summary: How to measure TSR

If you want to use a particular phenomenon to measure something, other variables have to be appropriately controlled, and critical assumptions have to be satisfied. Our explorations suggest the following recipe for using the task-cueing experiment to measure endogenous task-set reconfiguration:

1 Use a constant response-stimulus interval (to control for decay of task-set inertia).

2 Use easily interpretable cues. (Otherwise interpreting the cue may become a task in itself, and all trials become "task switch" trials).

3 Use two cues per task, changing them on each trial (to unconfound cue change and task change).

4 Keep the probability—and hence expectation—of a task switch low enough so that the subject will not be tempted to reconfigure task set before the cue. (Arguably this also makes the conditions a little more natural: we do not normally oscillate so frequently between tasks.)

5 Use instructions and incentives to motivate subjects to use the cue to prepare appropriately on every trial.

Of course, we cannot promise that even under these conditions subjects will *always* engage in TSR after a cue for the other task or *never* do so before (or after) a cue signalling the same task as before. Nor do we claim that the subject does *nothing* in the preparation interval before the cue, or following a cue indicating a task repeat. In the cueing paradigm we always get a substantial effect of preparation interval on nonswitch trials (albeit smaller than the effect on switch trials). This may in part reflect generic preparation effects such as modulations in phasic alertness, response readiness, etc., which have been known about for decades in the shape of warning signal and foreperiod effects in RT tasks (see Posner, 1978; Sanders, 1998). It may in part reflect the advantage of not having to divide attention between cue and stimulus processing. It may also be that subjects, rather than waiting passively before the cue, actively maintain the task-set that they were in before to prevent its dissipation with the passage of time. And finally, when the cue has been interpreted to indicate a task-repeat, subjects may actively reinforce, or do something to maintain, preparation for the task-set state they were already in. What the reduction in switch cost with preparation measures is the consequence of *extra* processing done to reconfigure task-set in advance when the opportunity permits.

Task-set reconfiguration? Or just associative retrieval?

Being able to measure a process is a necessary preliminary to being able to characterize the process being measured, which is why I have dwelt so long on this troublesome issue. But what are we measuring? In the recent literature authors such as Logan and Bundesen (2003) and Altmann (2003) have argued that—at least for these somewhat impoverished situations with only two or three tasks, relatively few stimuli, a couple of cues per task, and some practice before data are collected—we do not need to invoke a special class of "executive" control processes to explain the data; they can be explained entirely in terms of "standard" processes of associative learning, retrieval and memory dynamics.

Logan and Bundesen, for example, argue that the subject simply retrieves the response associated with the compound of cue + stimulus. The advantage observed for cue-repeat trials in their experiments they attribute to facilitated processing of the cue component of the compound. Evidently their theory was motivated largely by their failure to find a cost of switching task when cue change is controlled, as discussed above. By the same token, our own finding of substantial costs of a task change when cue-changes and expectancies of a switch are suitably controlled undermines this rationale for proposing a compound-cue theory.

Nevertheless, there is an *a priori* case to be made for expecting associative learning to eliminate costs of task-switching when small sets of stimuli (e.g. eight digits) are used, so that each combination of cue, stimulus, and response is repeatedly experienced. Subjects are typically instructed to construe the situation as involving two (or more) tasks, implying perhaps that to process each stimulus they should first select a set of task-rules and then determine which of its rules applies. But surely we would expect them, eventually and automatically, to learn the response for each cue + stimulus compound, thus converting what is presented to them as two tasks (each with two S→R rules) into a single task (with a rather larger set of cue + S→R rules)? In fact, present evidence suggests that, inasmuch as this happens at all, it happens much too slowly to be a major factor in most task-switching experiments.

If learned cue + S→R associations were controlling performance, then introduction of cues or stimuli that have not been seen before should disrupt performance until these new combinations have also been learned. But Rogers and Monsell (1995, exp 1) observed no such increase in switch costs when a new set of consonants not experienced before was introduced after two days of testing. In unpublished experiments on predictable switching, I have observed no increase in switch costs when a new set of external cues is introduced after several hundred trials. In a recent task-cueing experiment we (Monsell & Mizon, submitted b) had subjects classify stimuli from a set of just four digits as odd/even or high/low on the basis of the colour of the background (for some subjects) or its shape (for others). Although RTs reduced substantially over the first 700 trials, there was little sign of switch costs being reduced by learning of the compounds. And when, at that point, a different set of four digits was introduced, performance was only transiently perturbed. It occurred to us that subjects might not use a compound cue strategy because it simply does not occur to them to do so. Hence a second group of subjects was carefully instructed to try to learn the stimulus + cue→response associations. For this group switch costs were reduced by practice, especially for congruent stimuli (which require learning of only the simple association between digit and response) and transfer to a new set of digits was more disruptive. But the performance of this group overall was very much poorer that that of the uninstructed group. Hence, even under conditions that are optimal for the compound-cue strategy, it appears notably inefficient relative to the hierarchical strategy of selecting the task-set, then finding the matching rule within the set.

Hence the idea that the context and stimulus together simply retrieve the associated response seems insufficient to explain the data, and does not licence the conclusion that there is no need to postulate control processes that reconfigure task set.

The nature of task-set reconfiguration

I do not wish to argue that control of task-set is "nonassociative," or that standard processes of memory retrieval and effects of memory trace dynamics (e.g. priming) are not involved in the control of task set. But it does seem appropriate to recognize a distinction between the associative roles of the "stimulus," and the "context." This distinction is recognized in the fundamentally associative framework suggested in Miller and Cohen's (2001) review of the functions of prefrontal cortex (Figure 7.5). They argue, essentially, for two levels of control: relatively direct associative links between stimulus representations and actions habitually associated with those actions, and modulation of the associative strength of those links by a network in prefrontal cortex whose function is to detect at a more abstract level the wider context, both external, and internal (including current goals, desires, and memory-generated cues). The same split is seen, in reduced and schematic form, in Cohen, Dunbar, and McClelland's (1990) well-known connectionist model of the Stroop effect, in which output from "task" nodes modulates the activation of colour name

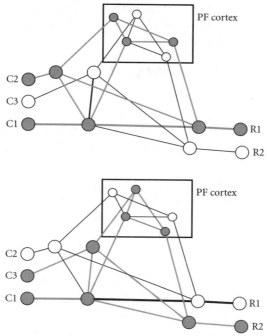

Fig. 7.5 Miller and Cohen's (2001) illustration of the suggested role of prefrontal cortex (PFC) in a multilevel associative-network for task set control. There are processing units representing stimuli and cues such as contextual stimuli, motivational state, memories, etc. (C1, C2, etc.), units representing possible actions (R1, R2), and mediating "hidden" units. PFC is not heavily connected to sensory or response representations, but is richly connected to hidden units in association and premotor cortices. The heavy lines indicate connections well-established by habit; the filled units represent currently active units. "Reward signals foster the formation of a task model, a neural representation that reflects the learned associations between task-relevant information. A subset of the information (e.g. C1 and C2) can then evoke the entire model, including information about the appropriate response (e.g. R1). Excitatory signals from the PF cortex feed back to other brain systems to enable task-relevant neural pathways" (Miller & Cohen, 2001, figure 2 legend). (Reprinted, with permission, from the Annual Review of Neuroscience, Vol. 24 © 2001 by Annual Reviews www.annualreviews.org).

responses by word or colour input via hidden units. This has been elaborated by Braver and Cohen (2000) to deal with a limited form of task switching: a paradigm in which subjects must only respond to a target stimulus if it is preceded by a suitable cue. Gilbert and Shallice (2002) have also developed this family of computational model to account for at least some of the phenomena seen in task switching.

This associative but multi-level conception of task-set control has much to recommend it as a basic template. However, there are several ways in which it may need elaboration. I shall discuss three.

Evidence for the discreteness of task-set reconfiguration

In associative networks like that of Gilbert and Shallice, the effect of top-down input typically varies along a continuum, so that one can be more or less biased toward task-set A relative to task-set B. In such a model, the process of task-set reconfiguration is naturally conceived of as incremental, with top-down input, sustained over an interval, gradually modulating the lower level network from a state that computes task A's associations into one that computes task B's associations. In contrast, some theorists have conceived of task-set reconfiguration as requiring discrete executive control operations such as loading goals (e.g. Rubinstein, Meyer, & Evans, 2001) or retrieving S–R rules (e.g. Mayr & Kliegl, 2000) into a production-system-style procedural working memory—operations that can succeed or fail but, which cannot be half-done. This kind of theory has received some support from additive factor effects on RT (e.g. Rubinstein et al. 2001). However, the most convincing evidence that TSR is accomplished as a discrete process comes from De Jong's (2000) analysis of the effects of preparation on RT distributions. The basic idea is illustrated in Figure 7.6. De Jong proposes that, while trying to prepare for an anticipated change from task A to

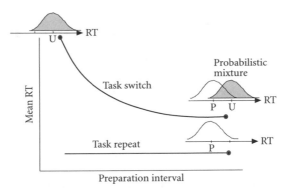

Fig. 7.6 An illustration of De Jong's (2000) model in which RTs on the prepared switch trials are a mixture of RTs from distributions of unprepared trials (estimated by the distribution of RTs on switch trials with no preparation interval) and fully prepared trials (estimated by the distribution of RTs on nonswitch trials with a long preparation interval). P and U mark the means of the distributions of RTs in prepared and unprepared states.

task B, the subject can be in one of only two task-set states: as-yet-unprepared for or fully-prepared for Task-B. The reduction in switch cost with an increase in preparation interval reflects the increasing *probability* of a successful transition to the prepared state as the time available for preparation is increased. The residual cost reflects an upper bound on that probability—the probability that the subject will "fail to engage" effective "intention-activation." The asymptotic switch cost at long RSIs thus reflects a mixture of prepared trials and unprepared trials on the switch trials, compared to the nonswitch trials, on all of which subjects are assumed to be in the prepared state.

The theory can be tested by determining how well individual subjects' RT distributions for long-RSI switch trials can be modeled by mixing some proportion of RTs randomly sampled from their distribution of short-RSI switch RTs (to estimate the unprepared state) and the rest from their distribution of long-RSI task-repeat RTs (used to estimate the prepared state) using the multinomial maximum likelihood method (Yantis, Meyer, & Evans, 1991).[2] De Jong (2000) reports excellent fits, and when Nieuwenhuis and I used the method to fit the data of Rogers and Monsell (1995, exp 3) we also found excellent fits for most subjects, with a mean estimated mixture probability (±s.e.) over subjects of 0.49 ± 0.08 (Nieuwenhuis & Monsell, 2002). A more general model that included an extra duration inserted on all switch trials (to accommodate the hypothesis of a post-stimulus control process or consequence of a switch) did not achieve a significantly better fit, and the fitted duration of the extra process was a trivial and nonsignificant 8 ± 12 ms. Of course the goodness of these fits, though impressive, is hard to assess without contrasting them to the fits of a continuous process model that makes distributional predictions—not currently available—but the fits certainly surprised this author, who had previously assumed that the RISC effect was tracking the average progress of a gradual process.

If we accept these RT distribution data as *prima facie* evidence for the all-or-none character of *achieving* preparatory TSR (though not of the top-down input that *triggers* it) is this incompatible with an associative neural-network theory of the kind developed by, for example, Braver and Cohen (2000)? Apparently not. Recent developments of this approach by Braver and colleagues (personal communication) model proactive control as a process of updating the pattern of activity in PFC context units during the preparation interval (conceived of

---

[2] One constraint on the applicability of this test is that there should be no effect of the preparation interval on nonswitch RT. While this happened to be so for the RSI manipulation in the predictable switching experiments of De Jong (2000) and Nieuwenhuis & Monsell (2002) it is certainly not the case for the effect of cue-stimulus interval in most task-cueing experiments, as already discussed.

as implemented by a phasic burst of dopamine system activity). The updating may or may not "take," with the average behaviour on the prepared switch trials thus being a mixture of two states; the simulations produce RT distributions that are at least qualitatively like those observed by De Jong and ourselves. Those trials on which pro-active control fails to take are compensated for, according to the model, by reactive control triggered by the stimulus and amplified when conflict is detected during post-stimulus processing. Braver and colleagues attribute proactive and reactive control to different brain regions.

Characterizing anticipatory task-set preparation as all-or-none does not explain why it is achieved on only a proportion of trials. One obvious possibility (De Jong, 2000) is that preparation is effortful, and the average subject simply does not try hard enough on all trials. It is also important that subjects understand the benefits of preparation and want to minimize their RT. Nieuwenhuis and I therefore ran an experiment very similar to exp 3 of Rogers and Monsell (1995). We used short blocks to minimize fatigue. We tested bright young subjects, gave them very explicit instruction, monetary rewards for minimizing RT and improving their performance, and ample feedback at the end of each block on mean RT, errors, and earnings. These incentives substantially reduced mean RTs, without increasing error rate, relative to Rogers and Monsell's subjects. But there was still a substantial residual cost. The mixture model again fit well, yielding an estimated mean TSR probability of 0.64. Short of heroic measures that would not pass the scrutiny of an ethics committee, it is hard to imagine getting subjects more motivated. Hence there does seem to be some sort of ceiling on the frequency with which effective proactive preparation can be achieved, at least under laboratory conditions. (De Jong, 2000, suggests that with suitable external cues the residual cost can be eliminated, though I have yet to see evidence for this myself). It remains a mystery, moreover, that extending the preparation interval well beyond 1 s apparently does not enable the subject to crank the cumulative probability of successful preparation closer and closer to unity by repeatedly retrying "intention-activation." Another problem is that the model leaves no room for other contributions to residual cost such as carry-over of task-set activation/inhibition from earlier trials, in spite the accumulation of other evidence for this (Goschke, 2000; Mayr, 2002; Schuch & Koch, 2003; Yeung & Monsell, 2003b).

The role of language and other supplementary processes in TSR

The basically associative but hierarchical view of task-set control expressed in Figure 7.5 arose in part out of observations on the behaviour of monkey prefrontal neurons that appear to maintain a representation of task demands over intervals of a few seconds (e.g. Wallis, Anderson, & Miller, 2001) Macaque monkeys have been trained to task-switch (Stoet & Snyder, 2003a, 2003b), but only with enormous amounts of training. In contrast, humans are able, after brief verbal instructions and experience of only two or three trials, to switch tasks effectively on the basis of arbitrary cues

Obviously language is not available to monkey trainers as a medium for getting task rules into their subjects' heads, whereas humans can be told what to do in a few crisp sentences. And after humans have "got" the task rules, we also have language available to support ongoing control: we can instruct ourselves verbally from trial to trial. Classically, skill acquisition in humans has been seen as a transition from the guidance of actions by external instructions to guidance by a declarative (often linguistic) internal representation of the rules or procedures to, after further practice, control by a procedural representation in memory (Fitts & Posner, 1967). Subjects in task-switching experiments occasionally mutter instructions to themselves, especially at the early stages of an experiment, and it seems likely that covert speech is used to represent task attributes such as the goal ("colour"), the relevant stimulus source ("there") and/or the task-rules ("red . . . left, green . . . right"). Is verbal self-instruction of this kind merely epiphenomenal, or does it play a causal role in reconfiguring task-set?

If verbal self-instruction helps to reconfigure task-set, then interfering with verbal coding by requiring the concurrent articulation of irrelevant material should reduce the benefits of a preparation interval, and increase the difficulty of switching. As already mentioned, Goschke (2000) found that uttering an irrelevant word during the preparation interval eliminated the reduction in switch cost with preparation, but uttering the task name instead did not (though the experiment included no nonverbal interference condition). It has also been shown that concurrent articulation (relative to a tapping control) magnifies switch costs in the Jersild list-alternation paradigm (Baddeley, Chincotta, & Adlam, 2001; Emerson & Miyake, 2003) though evidence from these studies suggests that concurrent articulation had its effect largely by interfering with verbal support for remembering which task was next ("add, subtract, add, subtract") in the absence of external cues. However, Miyake, Emerson, Padilla, and Ahn (2004) have recently demonstrated that continuous articulatory suppression increased switch costs in the task-cueing paradigm, where there is no task sequence to remember. And Mecklinger, von Cramon, Springer & Matthes-von Cramon (1999) has reported a correlation between speech disorder and exaggerated switch costs in patients with left hemisphere damage.

If linguistic self-instruction assists TSR, we might expect an external word (COLOUR) to be a particularly efficient task cue, as it should efficiently evoke the appropriate internal verbal code—or, to put it another way, replace the need to generate an internal verbal code from a prelinguistic representation of the task goal. Direct comparisons of verbal and nonverbal cues are hard to make, as it is hard to match all properties of cues other than their linguistic versus nonlinguistic nature. However, Miyake et al. found that irrelevant speech had less impact in the task-cueing paradigm when a verbal cue was used. In exp 4 of Monsell and Mizon (submitted a), already discussed above, the task cue alternated between word and picture cues. We have subsequently performed a very similar experiment using a dense-electrode EEG recording experiment to examine brain activity during the preparation interval (Monsell, Mizon, & Lavric, in preparation). The contrast of switch versus non-switch trials indicate a slow component of the ERP developing over the second half of the 800 ms preparation interval and more positive, over most electrodes, during preparation for a switch. LORETA source localization indicate that while some of the differential activity associated with preparing for a task change was prefrontal, as one might expect, with a picture cue there was also differential activity in temporal and parietal regions of the left hemisphere, while with a verbal cue there was differential activity in temporal/parietal regions of the right hemisphere. This is explicable if, with an external verbal cue, less linguistic processing is needed to generate a verbal code than with a picture cue. And perhaps the picture cue helps engage task-set in a different way, by perceptually instantiating the relevant visual object attributes. With a verbal cue, the subject may achieve the same effect via endogenous imaging or rehearsal of the target attributes.

In short, while a multi-level associative-network conception of task-set reconfiguration may logically suffice to account for task-switching in monkeys, to account for human performance we need additional mechanisms to account for the rapid acquisition of task-sets and context-task associations. Even when these are established, processes of linguistic self-instruction and, perhaps, nonlinguistic imagery and rehearsal may supplement the bare-bones associative mechanism to facilitate reconfiguration of task-set.

S–R and S-task associations

In suggesting that even a sophisticated multi-level associative network may be insufficient to capture human TSR, I do not want to deny the important contribution of associative learning to performance in task-switching situations. Evidently associative learning is required to establish both the S→R rules of each task (e.g. "if red light press brake pedal") and the context→task rules of an experiment (if the stimulus is in this box, or in this position in the sequence, or preceded by this cue, do task X). In this final section, however, I will focus on the less obvious role of stimulus→task associations, as established by previous experience with particular stimuli and types of stimuli.

Interference from competing S→R associations is a familiar postulate. For example, the Stroop effect is usually attributed to the familiar reading/naming response to a word competing with the required naming of its colour. The Simon effect is similarly attributed to a natural/habitual association between stimulus location and locus of action competing with the less familiar and arbitrary one required by the experimenter (e.g. respond left for red). These are cases where very well-established S–R mappings interfere with less well-established ones. However, when subjects must repeatedly switch between tasks, even relatively novel S–R mappings cause interference: RTs to incongruent stimuli (those associated with competing responses in the currently irrelevant task) are usually longer than those to congruent stimuli (same response in both tasks) or neutral stimuli (response only defined for one task) (e.g. Rogers & Monsell, 1995). Tasks that show very asymmetric interference when just one task is performed (e.g. a conflicting colour word interferes strongly with colour-naming, but there is almost no "reverse-Stroop" interference from a conflicting colour when the task is to name the word) show more symmetrical interference (e.g. there is now a reverse-Stroop effect) when the other task has recently been performed (Allport & Wylie, 2000; Yeung & Monsell, 2003b). Such interference effects indicate that currently irrelevant S–R mappings are not completely disabled if they are habitual or recently active. Presumably this is because well-adapted top-down control is "just-enough" (Goschke, 2000; Gruber & Goschke, 2004; Yeung & Monsell, 2003b); there is no point suppressing the irrelevant mappings more than is necessary because they will then be harder to re-engage when needed.

Stroop-like interference, whether from a pre-experimentally habitual S–R mapping, or from a novel but recently exercised S–R mapping, is typically discussed as if it arises solely from competition between *response* tendencies. However, there is evidence that it arises also at the level of competition between *task-sets*, that is, sets of S–R mappings. For example, Monsell, Taylor & Murphy (2001) investigated the phenomenon first reported by Klein (1964) that even noncolour words interfere with naming of their print colour (relative to XXXX), albeit not as much as colour words. We reasoned as follows. If this interference arises from competition between individual response tendencies associated with the stimulus, it should be greater the higher the associative strength of the irrelevant S–R link. This is easy to manipulate with lexical stimuli: high-frequency words have, by definition, much stronger associations between their spellings and names (and meaning) than low-frequency words, and words have stronger associations than pronounceable pseudo-words (matched for orthographic properties and pronounceability) that have never been pronounced before, as was easily demonstrated by substantial effects of frequency and lexicality on naming latency.

However, when these same stimuli were presented just once for colour naming, the interference (about 40 ms, relative to matched false-font strings) was no greater for words than for pseudowords, nor was it amplified by high frequency for the words. We concluded that, at least when items are unprimed by a prior occurrence in the experiment, the interference observed is due to competition from the irrelevant task-set activated by the stimulus, not from the individual response tendency. Simply put, a pronounceable letter string evokes the tendency to read, and this interferes with the attempt to colour-name. (Under conditions where retrieval of individual responses is primed by stimulus repetition and/or use of colour names then response-level interference undoubtedly augments this task-set-level interference).

In task-switching experiments, competition from stimulus→task associations is revealed by a pattern Rogers & Monsell (1995) observed: RTs substantially shorter for neutral (N) than for congruent (C) stimuli. This ordering would be inexplicable if the effect of the incompletely-suppressed irrelevant S–R associations were solely at the level of individual response tendencies. To the extent that the irrelevant S–R mapping was active, generating a response to a congruent stimulus should be *helped* by the same response being activated by the irrelevant attribute; the neutral stimulus elicits no such irrelevant but helpful response tendency. Hence we argued that observing a positive C–N contrast (i.e. C slower than N) is a marker for competition at the task-set level. That such an effect is not always seen (responses to N stimuli are sometimes slower than responses to C stimuli) does not mean that task-set interference is absent in these cases. The less suppressed the inappropriate task-set is, the more the response tendency it specifies will be activated; the benefit of response facilitation enjoyed by congruent stimuli will eventually outweigh the freedom from interference at the task-set level enjoyed by neutral stimuli. On this account a positive C–N effect is a signature of task-set competition combined with a relatively low level of facilitation or interference at the level of individual responses.

As an illustration, Figure 7.7 shows data replotted from a recent comparison, by Aron et al. (2004), of patients with lesions of left or right pre-frontal cortex (PFC) to age-matched control subjects. Subject had to switch predictably, every three trials, between the right/left arrow and word tasks mentioned above (see Figure 7.4). The task was externally cued with the task-name "WORD" or "ARROW" above the stimulus, and the three-trial runs were

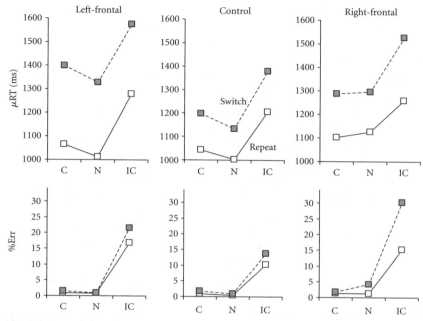

Fig. 7.7 Data plotted from table 2 of Aron et al. (2004) to show the contrast between congruent (C) neutral (N) and incongruent (IC) mean correct RTs and error rates on task-switch and task-repeat trials in patients with left- or right-PFC lesions and matched controls.

indicated by sequentially displaying stimuli round three screen positions. For the data shown, the response-stimulus interval was just 100 ms, so that although the tasks were easy and specified by a external verbal cue, the time pressure was demanding even for an unimpaired young adult. Both left-PFC patients and controls showed the positive C–N effect suggestive of task-set level interference on both switch and nonswitch trials, and the patients also showed a substantially greater switch cost than controls. In the left-PFC patients, the C–N effect, though not significantly larger than that for the controls, was correlated with the extent of damage in medial and inferior frontal gyrus (significantly so in the later case). The right-PFC patients also had larger switch costs than controls, but their data is suggestive of stronger interference at the response level: the C–N difference was negative, the IC–C difference was larger, and there was a substantially elevated probability of making the wrong response to an incongruent stimulus. In addition, the right-PFC patients showed correlations between switch cost, amount of damage to inferior frontal gyrus, and stop-signal latency—a measure of response inhibition.

Aron et al. argue that the left lateral PFC is more involved in establishing and maintaining the appropriate task set, while right inferior PFC is more involved with inhibition of competing response tendencies; see also Aron, Robbins, & Poldrack (2004).

The idea that stimuli retrieve task-sets associated with them, and that the resulting competition is a major determinant of performance in task-switching experiments has been substantially developed by Allport and colleagues (Allport & Wylie, 2000; Waszak, Hommel, & Allport, 2003, in press). They propose that on each encounter a stimulus becomes associatively "bound" not only to the response associated with it, but also to other properties of the episode such as the context and the goal (i.e. the task to be performed). The consequence is that when that stimulus is re-encountered later, the tendency to perform that same task is retrieved, which will facilitate performance if the same task is indeed the one required, but interfere with it if a different task is required. Such bindings are, they suggest, quite long-lasting, so that the associative history of the stimulus over the last few minutes is an important determinant of performance. They argue also that such associative carry-over will have a larger effect on task-switch trials, when task-set is less well-established and more vulnerable to interference. They go so far as to propose that this associatively-evoked task-set competition is the *main* source of the residual task-switch cost. The best evidence for this claim is a series of experiments by Waszak et al. (2003), which elegantly controlled the associative history of particular stimuli. This was accomplished using a large stimulus set of object pictures, each with a word superimposed; the task was to name the object or the word. Using the alternating runs paradigm, they found longer RTs and larger switch costs for reading the word in stimuli which the subjects had previously picture-named than in stimuli they had not picture-named before, even though more than a hundred trials had elapsed. That the enhanced switch cost reflects retrieval of the previously associated task-set rather than the previously associated response is demonstrated by the finding that it occured even for a congruent stimulus—that is, one to which the same response was made on the previous trials (Waszak et al. 2003).

Hence associative retrieval of task-sets can certainly be a powerful determinant of switch costs and of performance in single-task experiments. But is it sufficient to account for the residual switch cost? I doubt this, because in most experiments, a small number of bivalent stimuli occur repeatedly in both task contexts and must become asymptotically associated with both task-sets. It is not obvious why any influence of long-term associations to appropriate and inappropriate task-sets would not just cancel out. If we hypothesize a short-term component of such associations, this predicts that switch costs should be higher the more recently the stimulus has appeared in the other task. Existing data provide no support for this (Monsell et al. 2003; Yeung & Monsell, 2003a) except perhaps with respect to the stimulus on the immediately preceding trial. Hence my current view is that interference due to non-stimulus-specific task-set inertia makes a more universal contribution to the residual cost than stimulus-specific associative retrieval. More data and modeling are needed.

Conclusions

I began by arguing that, in spite of recent scepticism, it is possible to measure the processes that reconfigure task-set in preparation for a task change by using the task-cueing RT paradigm, suitably constrained, to track the reduction in switch cost as more time is allowed for preparation. But what are we measuring: executive control operations or just ordinary old associative retrieval, modulated by familiar memory dynamics? This is a false dichotomy. The aim of research on task-switching is to deconstruct the hitherto mysterious "homuncular" construct of voluntary control of task-set into component processes that can be understood. It would be astonishing indeed if these did not exploit, among others, mechanisms of associative learning and memory retrieval that support all other aspects of cognition. There is certainly evidence, some of which I have summarized, for the critical role of learned associations between stimuli, contexts (including task-goals), responses and task-sets in determining performance in task-switching, as in single-task situations. But to demonstrate this does not solve the problem of control. The brain is undoubtedly a giant associative network, but it is not much of a theory to say that the stimulus plus the context plus goals and motivation somehow retrieve the action; we have to specify the mechanisms. I have argued that any associative-network approach must be sufficiently sophisticated to capture (a) the multi-level hierarchical character of control that naturally parses the realm of action-selection into choice of task and then choice of action within task, (b) evidence for the discreteness of successful task-set reconfiguration, (c) the association of different levels of control with different brain regions (possibly with quite different learning parameters and memory dynamics), and (d) evidence that the basic infra-human multi-level associative network that maps stimulus plus internal and external context to action is augmented in humans by mechanisms such as (but not limited to) linguistic self-instruction.

References

Allport, A., & Wylie, G. (2000). Task-switching, stimulus-response bindings and negative priming. In S. Monsell & J. Driver (Eds.), *Control of cognitive processes: Attention and Performance XVIII* (pp. 35–70). Cambridge, MA: MIT Press.

Allport, D. A., Styles, E. A., & Hsieh, S. (1994). Shifting intentional set: Exploring the dynamic control of tasks. In C. Umiltà & M. Moscovitch (Eds.), *Attention and Performance XV: Conscious and nonconscious information processing* (pp. 421–452). Cambridge, MA: MIT Press.

Altmann, E. M. (2002). Functional decay of memory for tasks. *Psychological Research-Psychologische Forschung, 66,* 287–297.

Altmann, E. M. (2003). Task switching and the pied homunculus: Where are we being led? *Trends in Cognitive Sciences, 7,* 340–341.

Altmann, E. M. (2004). The preparation effect in task switching: Carryover of SOA. *Memory and Cognition, 32,* 153–163.

Altmann, E. M. (2004). Advance preparation in task switching: What work is being done? *Psychological Science, 15,* 616–622.

Aron, A. R., Monsell, S., Sahakian, B. J., & Robbins, T. W. (2004). A componential analysis of task-switching deficits associated with lesions of left and right frontal cortex. *Brain, 127,* 1561–1573.

Aron, A. R., Robbins, T. W., & Poldrack, R. A. (2004). Inhibition and the right inferior frontal cortex. *Trends in Cognitive Sciences, 8,* 170–177.

Baddeley, A., Chincotta, D., & Adlam, A. (2001). Working memory and the control of action: Evidence from task switching. *Journal of Experimental Psychology-General, 130,* 641–657.

Bernstein, E. (1924). Quickness and intelligence. *British Journal of Psychology Monograph Supplements, 7,* VI-55.

Braver, T. S., & Cohen, J. D. (2000). On the control of control: The role of dopamine in regulating prefrontal function and working memory. In S. Monsell & J. Driver (Eds.), *Control of cognitive processes: Attention and Performance XVIII* (pp. 713–737). Cambridge, MA: MIT press.

Braver, T. S., Gray, J. R., & Burgess, G. C. (in press). Explaining the many varieties of working memory variation: Duel mechanisms of cognitive control. In A. Conway, C. Jarrold, M. Kane, A. Miyake, & J. Towse (Eds.), *Variation in working memory:* Oxford University Press.

Cohen, J. D., Dunbar, K., & McClelland, J. L. (1990). On the control of automatic processes: A parallel distributed processing account of the Stroop effect. *Psychological Review, 97,* 332–361.

De Jong, R. (2000). An intention–activation account of residual switch costs. In S. Monsell & J. Driver (Eds.), *Control of cognitive processes: Attention and Performance XVIII* (pp. 357–376). Cambridge, MA: MIT Press.

Dreisbach, G., Haider, H., & Kluwe, R. H. (2002). Preparatory processes in the task-switching paradigm: Evidence from the use of probability cues. *Journal of Experimental Psychology-Learning Memory and Cognition, 28,* 468–483.

Emerson, M. J., & Miyake, A. (2003). The role of inner speech in task switching: A dual-task investigation. *Journal of Memory and Language, 48,* 148–168.

Fitts, P. M., & Posner, M. I. (1967). *Human performance*. Belmont, CA: Brooks-Cole.

Gilbert, S. J., & Shallice, T. (2002). Task switching: A PDP model. *Cognitive Psychology,* **44**, 297–337.

Goschke, T. (2000). Intentional reconfiguration and involuntary persistence in task set switching. In S. Monsell & J. Driver (Eds.), *Control of cognitive processes: Attention and Performance XVIII* (pp. 331–355). Cambridge, MA: MIT Press.

Gruber, O., & Goschke, T. (2004). Executive control emerging from dynamic interactions between brain systems mediating language, working memory and attentional processes. *Acta Psychologica,* **115**, 105–121.

Jersild, A. T. (1927). Mental set and shift. *Archives of psychology,* **89**.

Kimberg, D. Y., Aguirre, G. K., & D'Esposito, M. (2000). Modulation of task-related neural activity in task-switching: An fMRI study. *Cognitive Brain Research,* **10**, 189–196.

Klein, G. S. (1964). Semantic power measured through the interference of words with color-naming. *American Journal of Psychology,* **77**, 576–588.

Logan, G. D., & Bundesen, C. (2003). Clever homunculus: Is there an endogenous act of control in the explicit task-cuing procedure? *Journal of Experimental Psychology-Human Perception and Performance,* **29**, 575–599.

Mayr, U. (2002). Inhibition of action rules. *Psychonomic Bulletin and Review,* **9**, 93–99.

Mayr, U., & Kliegl, R. (2000). Task-set switching and long-term memory retrieval. *Journal of Experimental Psychology-Learning Memory and Cognition,* **26**, 1124–1140.

Mayr, U., & Kliegl, R. (2003). Differential effects of cue changes and task changes on task-set selection costs. *Journal of Experimental Psychology-Learning Memory and Cognition,* **29**, 362–372.

Mecklinger, A., von Cramon, D. Y., Springer, A., & Matthes-von Cramon, G. (1999). Executive control functions in task switching: Evidence from brain injured patients. *Journal of Clinical and Experimental Neuropsychology,* **21**, 606–619.

Meiran, N. (1996). Reconfiguration of processing mode prior to task performance. *Journal of Experimental Psychology-Learning Memory and Cognition,* **22**, 1423–1442.

Meiran, N., Chorev, Z., & Sapir, A. (2000). Component processes in task switching. *Cognitive Psychology,* **41**, 211–253.

Miller, E. K., & Cohen, J. D. (2001). An integrative theory of prefrontal cortex function. *Annual Review of Neuroscience,* **24**, 167–202.

Miyake, A., Emerson, M. J., Padilla, F., & Ahn, J. C. (2004). Inner speech as a retrieval aid for task goals: The effects of cue type and articulatory suppression in the random task cuing paradigm. *Acta Psychologica,* **115**, 123–142.

Monsell, S. (2003). Task switching. *Trends in Cognitive Sciences,* **7**, 134–140.

Monsell, S., & Mizon, G. A. (submitted, a). Can the task-cueing paradigm measure "endogenous" task-set reconfiguration?

Monsell, S., & Mizon, G. A. (submitted, b). Task switching and associative learning.

Monsell, S., Mizon, G. A., & Lavric, A. (in preparation).

Monsell, S., Sumner, P., & Waters, H. (2003). Task-set reconfiguration after a predictable or unpredictable task switch: Is one trial enough? *Memory and Cognition,* **31**, 327–342.

Monsell, S., Taylor, T. J., & Murphy, K. (2001). Naming the color of a word: Is it responses or task sets that compete? *Memory and Cognition,* **29**, 137–151.

Nieuwenhuis, S., & Monsell, S. (2002). Residual costs in task switching: Testing the failure-to-engage hypothesis. *Psychonomic Bulletin and Review, 9*, 86–92.

Posner, M. I. (1978). *Chronometric explorations of mind*. Hillsdale, NJ: Lawrence Erlbaum Associates.

Rabbitt, P. M. A., & Vyas, S. (1970). An elementary preliminary taxonomy for some errors in laboratory tasks. *Acta Psychologica, 33*, 56–76.

Rabbitt, P. M. A., & Vyas, S. (1973). What is repeated in the 'repetition effect'? In S. Kornblum (Ed.), *Attention and Performance* (p. 327). New York: Academic Press.

Rabbitt, P. M. A., & Vyas, S. (1974). Interference between binary classification judgements and some repetition effects in a serial choice reaction time task. *Journal of Experimental Psychology, 103*, 1181–1190.

Rogers, R. D., & Monsell, S. (1995). The costs of a predictable switch between simple cognitive tasks. *Journal of Experimental Psychology-General, 124*, 207–231.

Rubinstein, J. S., Meyer, D. E., & Evans, J. E. (2001). Executive control of cognitive processes in task switching. *Journal of Experimental Psychology-Human Perception and Performance, 27*, 763–797.

Sanders, A. F. (1998). *Elements of human performance: Reaction processes and attention in human skill*. Mahwah, NJ: Lawrence Erlbaum Associates.

Schuch, S., & Koch, I. (2003). The role of response selection for inhibition of task sets in task shifting. *Journal of Experimental Psychology-Human Perception and Performance, 29*, 92–105.

Shaffer, L. H. (1965). Choice reaction with variable S-R mapping. *Journal of Experimental Psychology, 70*, 284–288.

Sohn, M-H., & Carlson, R. A. (2000). Effects of repetition and foreknowledge in task-set reconfiguration. *Journal of Experimental Psychology-Learning Memory and Cognition, 26*, 1445–1460.

Sohn, M-H., Ursu, S., Anderson, J. R., Stenger, V. A., & Carter, C. S. (2000). The role of prefrontal cortex and posterior parietal cortex in task switching. *Proceedings of National Academy of Sciences, 97*, 13448–13453.

Stoet, G., & Snyder, L. H. (2003a). Executive control and task-switching in monkeys. *Neuropsychologia, 41*, 1357–1364.

Stoet, G., & Snyder, L. H. (2003b). Task preparation in macaque monkeys (*Macaca mulatta*). *Animal Cognition, 6*, 121–130.

Wallis, J. D., Anderson, K. C., & Miller, E. K. (2001). Single neurons in the prefrontal cortex encode abstract rules. *Nature, 411*, 953–956.

Waszak, F., Hommel, B., & Allport, A. (2003). Task-switching and long-term priming: Role of episodic stimulus-task bindings in task-shift costs. *Cognitive Psychology, 46*, 361–413.

Waszak, F., Hommel, B., & Allport, A. (in press). Semantic generalization of task-set bindings. *Psychonomic Bulletin and Review*.

Yantis, S., Meyer, D. E., & Evans, J. E. K. (1991). Analyses of multinomial mixture distributions: New tests for stochastic models of cognition and action. *Psychological Bulletin, 110*, 350–374.

Yeung, N., & Monsell, S. (2003a). The effects of recent practice on task switching. *Journal of Experimental Psychology-Human Perception and Performance, 29*, 919–936.

Yeung, N., & Monsell, S. (2003b). Switching between tasks of unequal familiarity: The role of stimulus-attribute and response-set selection. *Journal of Experimental Psychology-Human Perception and Performance, 29*, 455–469.

Chapter 8

An evaluation of the frontal lobe theory of cognitive aging

Louise H. Phillips and Julie D. Henry

Abstract

In the 1990s the predominant theoretical explanation of adult age differences in cognition shifted from general resource theories (e.g. speed or capacity of processing) to neuropsychological theories relating cognitive changes to neural changes in localized brain areas. Most influentially, it has been argued that age-related changes in the frontal lobes predict cognitive changes in older adults. However, evidence for this hypothesis from behavioural and neuroimaging studies has been equivocal at best. Four issues will be reviewed. (1) There is little strong evidence to support the conclusion that executive control is differentially affected by age in comparison to other cognitive functions. (2) There are differences in the pattern of deficits seen following focal frontal lobe damage and those accompanying the aging process, particularly in relation to the distinction between laboratory and real world performance. (3) The effects of age on social and emotional functioning have been largely ignored, despite considerable evidence linking such functions to the frontal lobes of the brain. (4) Functional neuroimaging data do not support a straightforward version of the frontal lobe theory of aging. Future work needs to adopt more sophisticated models of the structural and functional neuroanatomy of frontal lobe regions and their integration with other brain areas, and also to focus more on regulation of social, emotional, and behavioural functioning in naturalistic tasks rather than solely concentrating on complex "frontal lobe" tests.

Aging and cognitive control functions: the influence of Pat Rabbitt

In the 1980s the dominant theory of cognitive aging explained deficits in memory and reasoning in terms of general slowing of information processing in the brain (e.g. Cerella, 1985; Salthouse, 1985). Such theories arose to explain the fact that age differences in tasks such as reaction time paradigms, which apparently measure simple information processing speed often explain age variance in much more complex tasks such as episodic memory or visuo-spatial reasoning. Age differences in such speed measures overlap with age variance in a wide range of other cognitive tasks. This information-processing speed explanation for cognitive aging remains an important influence on aging research, and measures proposed to be proxy indices of processing speed (usually speeded coding tasks such as the Digit Symbol task) are often taken in cognitive aging studies. Pat Rabbitt has been a vociferous critic of simple speed-of-information-processing causal models of aging (for recent summaries of such arguments see Rabbitt, 2000, 2002). For example, the positive manifold of numerous task parameters does not logically indicate that one basic aspect of neural functioning must underlie such relationships (Rabbitt, 2000)—it is also possible that intercorrelations between many tasks may reflect the ability to utilize effective control strategies. Also, there is so far no evidence which shows a clear causal link between particular parameters of brain aging and slowed information processing (Rabbitt, 2002). This does not mean that declines in processing speed cannot underlie age deficits on some tasks—rather the evidence used to support the speed-of-processing model is susceptible to alternate interpretations, and strong causal links have not been shown in the available evidence.

In the past decade, influenced by findings from neuroimaging, the main explanatory variables within cognitive aging research have changed from general resource measures to more specific cognitive control functions. In particular, there has been a focus on the role of frontal-executive processes in explaining cognitive changes with age (e.g. West, 1996). In neurophysiological terms, the frontal lobe theory of aging (outlined in more detail below) proposes that age-related changes in cognition are explained by early, localized changes found in the frontal lobes of the brain. In cognitive terms, dysfunction of the frontal lobes of the brain has long been linked with poor cognitive control or executive functions. Age changes in memory and reasoning are therefore attributed to poorer executive functions, that is, less efficient operation of cognitive control processes such as inhibition, switching, monitoring, and planning. Aging research is not alone in this focus on the role of the frontal lobes in explaining cognitive deficits: the frontal lobes have shifted from being conceptualized as "the silent lobe" of the 1940s that could be partially removed without consequence, to the most fashionable lobe of the 2000s involved in all aspects of cognition, emotion, consciousness, and behaviour.

From the early 1960s onward, long before neuroimaging technology suggested that aging might have localized effects on the frontal lobes,

Pat Rabbitt consistently argued for the importance of studying executive control processes in aging (e.g. Rabbitt, 1963). Pat's ingenious strategy was to take apparently simple tasks such as choice reaction time (RT), and show that such tasks were, in fact, not so simple. Choice RT tasks can tell a canny experimental psychologist more than just "information processing speed." Such tasks are informative about speed-accuracy trade-offs, error monitoring and correction, learning curves, motor control functions, etc. (see, for example, Rabbitt & Vyas, 1970). Even understanding performance on simple RT tasks (responding as quickly as possible to a single stimuli) means considering self-monitoring, error detection, and maintenance of control processes (Rabbitt, 2002). For example, Rabbitt (1963) argued that age differences in the speed of learning associations between simple patterns and arbitrary labels (a process likely to be involved in the Digit Symbol task so commonly used to assess "simple speed of processing" in current aging research) could be explained by a reduced ability to ignore irrelevant information and focus on the critical stimulus dimensions. The methodological logic here is to take a simple task and deconstruct performance to allow the nature of the cognitive deficits that underlie age differences to be identified. Unfortunately most of the literature on aging and frontal-executive functioning has lurched violently in the opposite direction: rather than taking elegant paradigms and manipulating those tasks to understand the action of specific control processes, researchers have tended to steal complex "frontal lobe" tasks from clinical neuropsychology such as the Wisconsin Card Sort task, and have then struggled to identify what cognitive processes (or brain mechanisms) might underlie age differences.

The frontal lobe theory of aging: from brain to behaviour

The frontal lobe theory of aging proposes that early, localized age changes in the frontal lobes of the brain are associated with deficits on executive control processes (Daigneault, Braun, & Whitaker, 1992; Mittenberg, Seidenberg, O'Leary, & DiGiulio, 1989; Moscovitch & Winocur, 1992; Troyer, Graves, & Cullum, 1994; West, 1996). The theory predominantly derives from evidence that there are greater age-related changes in both the neuroanatomy and neurochemistry of the frontal lobes than in other cortical areas (Fuster, 1989; Woodruff-Pak, 1997). These neural changes are thought to cause disturbances in affect, cognition, and behaviour that parallel the dysfunction associated with damage to the frontal cortex (Daigneault et al. 1992; Moscovitch & Winocur, 1992). Thus, it has been explicitly proposed that in order to better understand the process of cognitive aging, we need to look to the functions associated with the frontal lobes (Parkin, 1997; West, 1996) and in particular to try to map the deficits seen in older adults to those shown by patients with focal frontal lobe lesions (Moscovitch & Winocur, 1992). There is a great deal of evidence that the neural substrates of executive processes lie at least partially in the frontal cortex (see Stuss & Benson, 1986). Patients who sustain damage to this cortical region often experience difficulty with tasks that require the integration and synthesis of information, and may exhibit impaired self-regulation and planning, perseveration with cognitive rigidity and stimulus-boundedness, and a lack of spontaneity (Eslinger, Grattan, & Geder, 1995). This deficit profile is consistent with most definitions of executive impairment (Crawford & Henry, 2005; Lezak, 1993; Moscovitch & Melo, 1997; Perret, 1974; Phillips, 1997; Shallice, 1988; Stuss & Benson, 1986).

In the rest of this chapter we will review the frontal lobe theory of aging, describing evidence that challenges the idea that age related declines in cognition can be neatly mapped to localized atrophy in the frontal lobes. We will review some of Pat Rabbitt's work in this area, which emphasizes the importance of detailed investigation of task performance to understand cognitive control functions, and raises some major criticisms of the frontal lobe theory as a causal explanation for cognitive aging. Issues covered include: (1) the lack of evidence for differential age changes in executive functions compared to other aspects of cognition, (2) a double dissociation between the effects of aging and focal frontal lesions on laboratory and realistic tasks, (3) lack of age effects on emotional and social regulation, and (4) the complex pattern of age effects on functional activation in the frontal lobes during cognitive task performance.

Are there differential effects of aging on control as compared to noncontrol cognitive functions?

It is impossible to measure executive aspects of cognition without also tapping other functions such as perception or memory: control functions cannot be measured in isolation (Phillips, 1997). This means that it is difficult to determine why an individual performs poorly on a given executive test without a detailed analysis of test performance. Numerous studies have found evidence of age-related decline on tasks that are considered to tap executive functioning, including planning (Andrés & Van der Linden, 2000; Gilhooly, Phillips, Wynn, Logie, & Della Sala, 1999; Robbins et al. 1998), inhibition (Cohn, Dustman, & Bradford, 1984; Daigneault et al. 1992; Shilling, Chetwynd, & Rabbitt, 2002), and cognitive switching (Hughes & Bryan, 2002; Isingrini & Vazou, 1997; Parkin & Java, 1999). However, attempts to investigate whether age deficits in these complex tasks reflect specific problems with executive functioning or other types of cognitive deficit have not produced a clear pattern of results. Below we review studies, which investigate whether age-related performance declines in three tasks commonly used to tap executive functions (Stroop, fluency, and Tower of London) reflect changes in specific cognitive control functions, or instead might reflect declines in other parameters such as slowed information-processing speed or poorer memory capacity.

One of the tasks most widely used to measure inhibition is the Stroop task, in which the inhibitory condition requires participants to name the colour of ink in which a colour word is printed—requiring the suppression of the tendency to read the colour word. A review of aging studies on the Stroop task make clear how difficult it can be to interpret age differences in performance on even relatively simple tasks aimed to assess executive functioning. There are many studies that indicate greater age-related slowing on the inhibition condition of the Stroop task compared to baseline conditions (naming the colour of patches or rows of Xs). However, the inhibitory condition of this task takes considerably longer than baseline conditions for young adults as well as old, and so the aging effect may simply reflect a scalar factor of slowing (Rabbitt, Lowe, & Shilling, 2001). Verhaegen and De Meersman (1998) show through meta-analysis of mean response times on the Stroop task that a single function can explain age differences in both baseline and interference conditions of the Stroop task, unlike in Alzheimer's Disease where the effects of dementia on baseline and interferences conditions can be explained by separate functions (Amieva, Phillips, Della Sala, & Henry, 2004). Verhaegen and De Meersman argue that their result indicates that Stroop effects can be explained in terms of slowed information processing with age. However, Rabbitt (2002) argues that the conclusions drawn by Verhaegen and De Meersman (1998) from their scalar analysis are inappropriate since only *mean* reaction times for old and young were considered, and the mean does not constitute an adequate summary of the complex effects of age on reaction time distributions.

Other evidence contradicts the theory that age differences in Stroop task performance are due to general slowing. Evoked potential studies of brain activity during Stroop indicate selective age-related attentuation of frontal activation reflecting parameters of inhibition but no evidence that general age-related slowing influenced inhibition (West & Alain, 2000). Despite a considerable number of studies investigating this issue there is still debate in the literature as to whether age related variance in the critical Stroop condition of the task reflects a specific inhibitory deficit or instead is better interpreted within a framework of slowed information processing. Factors such as task-specific practice and the exact type of stimuli used may influence the results obtained (Lowe & Rabbitt, 1997; Rabbitt, 2002; Shilling et al. 2002). Shilling et al. (2002) argue that the lack of correlation between different versions of the Stroop task indicates that individual differences in Stroop performance are due to other factors than a common inhibitory component. Rabbitt (2002) proposes that in order to demonstrate age differences in inhibitory function using the Stroop task it is necessary to look at the proportionate age-related slowing on both inhibitory and noninhibitory task conditions that are matched for complexity or mean time of processing. No published studies have matched this stringent condition.

Another family of tasks commonly used to assess executive functions are measures of verbal fluency. These tasks require time-restricted retrieval of words based on phonemic or semantic criteria. Phonemic fluency tasks in particular are proposed to load cognitive control components because they require novel strategies to retrieve *phonological* information from a *semantic* store. In recent meta-analytic reviews phonemic and semantic fluency were found to be particularly sensitive to the presence of focal frontal cortical injuries (Henry & Crawford, 2004a) and traumatic brain injury (Henry & Crawford, 2004b), disorders for which there is a great deal of evidence that executive dysfunction is particularly prominent (see, for example, Crawford & Henry, in press; Shallice, 1988; Stuss & Benson, 1986). Whilst a number of researchers have documented that fluency performance is negatively related to aging (Capitani, Laiacona, & Barbarotto, 1999; Kempler, Teng, Dick, Taussig & Davis, 1998; Parkin, Yeomans, & Bindschaedler, 1994; Phillips, 1999; Tombaugh, Kozak, & Rees, 1999), in other studies it has been found that there is no age effect (Bolla, Lindgren, Bonaccorsy, & Bleecker, 1990; Crawford, Bryan, Luszcz, Obonsawin, & Stewart, 2000; Miller, 1984), whilst a positive relationship between age and phonemic fluency performance has also been documented (Henry & Phillips, in press; Parkin & Walter, 1991; Yeudall, Fromm, Reddon, & Stefanyk, 1986). Some authors have argued that where age deficits are found on phonemic fluency tasks, these are not due to executive factors such as retrieval strategy selection or strategic switching but may instead be attributable to differences in the speed of responding (Phillips, 1999; Salthouse, 1996; Troyer, Moscovitch, & Winocur, 1997). There is a pattern of greater age decline in semantic compared to phonemic fluency, which more closely resembles the pattern of effects seen in patients with Alzheimer's Disease or temporal lobe damage rather than the pattern of fluency deficits seen in frontal lobe patients (Henry & Crawford, 2004; Henry, Crawford, & Phillips, 2004; Henry & Phillips, submitted). Age deficits in fluency may only reflect distinctive executive dysfunction when alternate indices of fluency performance such as word repetitions are used, or fluency paradigms are investigated that specifically load retrieval switching (Henry & Phillips, submitted).

The Tower of London task (TOL; Shallice, 1982) has also been widely used to assess an aspect of executive functioning: in this case, planning. Coloured disks must be moved one-by-one from an initial state to match a goal state, and instructions are generally given to mentally plan the sequence of moves before executing that plan. Older adults tend to be slower than younger adults on the TOL, and need more moves to solve TOL trials, which suggests less efficient planning (Andrés & Van der Linden, 2000; Gilhooly et al. 1999; Robbins et al. 1998). Patients with frontal lobe injuries tend to have particular problems in their first encounter with goal–subgoal conflict (Morris, Miotto, Feigenbaum, Bullock, & Polkey, 1997) while older adults do not show particular difficulty in dealing with goal conflict (Gilhooly et al. 1999) suggesting that age differences do not reflect difficulties in planning multiple subgoals. Phillips, Gilhooly, Logie, Della Sala, & Wynn (2003) investigated the effects of various secondary tasks on age differences in the TOL task. Articulatory suppression was used to load verbal rehearsal, pattern tapping to load spatial rehearsal, and verbal and spatial random generation tasks were used to load the executive resources in addition to the domain-specific rehearsal systems. Older adults showed generally high levels of interference between the secondary tasks and concurrent TOL, while younger adults showed a more specific interference pattern between TOL and the random generation tasks. These results indicate that for younger adults the TOL task specifically depended upon executive resources, whereas for older adults the task loaded on verbal and spatial maintenance as well as executive resources. These results suggest that for older adults, the TOL task loads many cognitive systems. This finding mirrors the less differentiated neural activation often seen in older adults during cognitive task performance (for a review see the section on functional imaging below), and may be interpreted to reflect the involvement of more widespread cognitive systems to carry out cognitive tasks in old compared to young adults.

As the evidence from the Stroop, fluency and TOL tasks illustrate, there are difficulties in interpreting the nature of age-related differences in performance on tasks intended to measure cognitive control. In fact, replication of basic age performance deficits in many frontal lobe tasks is often unreliable from one study to the next (Rabbitt et al. 2001). Where clear age declines in performance on frontal lobe tasks are found in an individual study, these *may* reflect changes in other parameters such as speed, memory, attention, or motivation, rather than indicating a specific executive deficit (Rabbitt, 2002). In other words assumptions cannot be made about the cognitive nature of age-deficits seen on frontal lobe tasks without detailed task analysis. For example, some studies indicate that age variance in executive test performance is statistically explained by measures of fluid intelligence (e.g. Burgess, 1997; Crawford et al. 2000; Henry & Phillips, submitted; Rabbitt et al. 2001). Rabbitt and Lowe (2000) show that while age changes in fluid intelligence can explain variance in executive tasks, the age variance in memory tasks is independent of fluid intelligence measures. However, fluid intelligence tests depend on many different processes, including cognitive control functions, and so the overlap in variance between these tasks and standard executive measures is unsurprising. There is neuropsychological evidence (e.g. Duncan, Burgess, & Emslie, 1995) that fluid intelligence tests depend upon the functioning of some regions within the frontal lobes, and so in that sense can be considered "frontal lobe tests" themselves.

Do older adults and frontal lobe patients show the same pattern of deficits on laboratory and real-life cognitive tasks?

One critical variable in both the literature on cognitive aging and studies of human frontal lobe function is whether a task is novel and artificial or instead taps skills used in real world situations. The use of standard neuropsychological executive tests to assess frontal lobe deficits has been criticized for not picking up the fundamental deficit associated with frontal lobe dysfunction: inability to deal with the type of open-ended, poorly-structured situations encountered in real life (Channon & Crawford, 1999; Shallice & Burgess, 1991; Stuss & Levine, 2002; Wilson, Alderman, Burgess, Emslie, & Evans, 1996). Most neuropsychological tests have explicit instructions and task demands, relatively short and constrained trials, and explicit prompts by the tester to initiate and terminate performance (Garden, Phillips, & MacPherson, 2001). Shallice & Burgess (1991) point out that it is only when brain-injured patients are required to plan activities over longer time periods, or weigh up priorities in the face of competing demands that their cognitive deficit is exposed. Executive tasks demanding self-initiation set in complex virtual environments have proven to be more sensitive to head injury than standard executive test batteries carried out in the laboratory (e.g. McGeorge et al. 2001).

Shallice and Burgess (1991) show that patients with frontal lobe lesions who performed well on standard executive tasks failed on two tasks designed to mimic the complex multiple goal scheduling demands of real life situations— the Six Elements and Multiple Errands tasks. The behaviour of frontal lobe patients was characterized by poor planning, rule-breaking, and inappropriate social conduct. However, Garden et al. (2001) found no significant age effect on either of these multiple subgoal scheduling tasks, although there was a trend for younger adults to be more likely to break task rules—that is, evidence of an age-related benefit on the real-environment planning task. This coupled with the finding of Garden et al. (2001) that there were significant age deficits on standard executive tasks provide evidence of opposite patterns of frontal lobe and aging effects: whilst aging causes greatest decline in standard laboratory executive tasks, frontal lobe lesions have greatest effect on realistic scheduling tasks. A review of age effects on cognitive planning (Phillips, MacLeod, & Kliegel, 2005) confirms this pattern of relative age sparing or improvement on the most realistic tasks. These findings do not support the frontal lobe theory of aging but instead are more consistent with the disuse hypothesis of aging, which proposes that age declines on cognitive performance are largest on skills that have not been recently practised.

These findings also fit in with a recent meta-analysis of age effects on prospective memory tasks which require participants to remember to carry out an intended action in response to a particular internal or external cue (Henry, Macleod, Phillips, & Crawford, 2004). Henry et al. (2004) report that there are strong age-related *declines* in performance on laboratory-based prospective memory tasks, but equally strong age-related *improvements* in performance on naturalistic prospective memory tasks. Naturalistic studies that found aging to be associated with improvement in prospective memory included tasks in which the participant is required to telephone the experimenter at a specific time over four weeks (Devolder, Brigham, & Pressley, 1990), three weeks (Poon & Schaffer, 1982) two weeks (Moscovitch, 1982) and five days (Maylor, 1990), mail postcards to the experimenter (Patton & Meit, 1993), and periodically log the time on an electronic organiser (Rendell & Thomson, 1993, 1999). In addition, older adults tend to show better prospective memory for attending appointments (Martin, 1986). Thus, these tasks require the ability to organize and plan ahead, often over considerable periods of time, and in the absence of explicit prompts from the experimenter. That is, they are precisely the kinds of tasks that patients with focal frontal lobe injuries typically experience difficulties with (Channon & Crawford, 1999; Shallice & Burgess, 1991). The finding of substantial age-benefits on realistic prospective memory measures is therefore incongruent with the predictions of the frontal theory of aging.

Overall, the clinical picture presented by at least some patients with focal frontal lobe damage does not seem to match the pattern of age related decline in fluid abilities accompanied by preservation of knowledge and life skills

(Phillips, MacPherson, & Della Sala, 2002). For patients with substantial frontal lobe damage there is often a dissociation between impaired wisdom (use of knowledge in the world) and relatively spared intelligence as assessed by standardized intelligence tests (e.g. Brazzelli, Colombo, Della Sala, & Spinnler, 1994; Damasio & Van Hoesen, 1983; Eslinger & Damasio, 1985; Rolls, Hornak, Wade, & McGrath, 1994; Shallice & Burgess, 1991). Reviews often emphasize the intact performance of patients with frontal lobe damage on intelligence and laboratory tests along with impaired social behaviour, poor judgment, and inappropriate decisions taken in real-life (Benton, 1994; Damasio & Anderson, 1993; Milner, 1995; Parker & Crawford, 1992). This pattern suggests that precisely those problem-solving abilities which may be relatively spared following frontal lobe lesions (e.g. laboratory experimenter-controlled tasks) are most affected by aging; while the problem-solving abilities which are often impaired after frontal lobe lesions (e.g. social decision-making, using knowledge wisely) are least affected by aging (Phillips & Della Sala, 1998).

Age effects on tasks of social and emotional processing known to be sensitive to frontal lobe functioning

One of the key functions of the frontal lobes of the brain is the control of emotional and social processing (Ochsner & Gross, 2004). There is considerable evidence that patients with focal frontal lesions often exhibit deficits in socio-emotional processes such as decision-making, emotion regulation and social cue identification (for a review see Stuss & Levine, 2002). However, although older adults have been found to be impaired in particular types of emotional tasks, at least some aspects of socio-emotional control appear to be unaffected or even improve with age.

Patients with frontal lobe lesions often make disastrous financial decisions in real life (Eslinger & Damasio, 1985). To tap the emotional processes involved in making financial decisions Bechara, Damasio, Damasio, and Anderson (1994) designed a laboratory-based gambling task. Compared to patients with lesions in other brain areas, patients with ventromedial frontal damage showed dampened emotional reactions to the gambling tasks, and selected more risky cards, resulting in financial losses (Bechara et al. 1994; Bechara, Damasio, Tranel, & Anderson, 1998; Bechara, Tranel, Damasio, & Damasio, 1996). However, there is no effect of normal aging in performance on the Bechara gambling task, including the likelihood of making risky decisions at any stage of the task (Lamar & Resnick, 2004; MacPherson, Phillips, & Della Sala, 2002).

Neuroimaging studies indicate that the experience and control of negative emotions is associated with the activation of regions within the frontal lobes (Dougherty et al. 1999; Ochsner, Bunge, Gross, & Gabrieli, 2002; Phan, Wager, Taylor, & Liberzon, 2002). Patients with frontal lobe damage often experience problems with mood regulation ranging from apathy to a reduced ability to control anger (Paradiso, Chemerinski, & Yazici, 1999). A number of reviews indicate frontal lobe abnormalities are involved in emotional dysregulation (e.g. Davidson, Putnam, & Larson, 2000). However, normal aging has been found in a number of studies to have positive effects on emotion regulation, resulting in better control of negative emotions (e.g. Gross et al. 1997). Phillips, Henry, Hosie, and Milne (in preparation) found that older adults showed improved ability to regulate anger, and further that the age improvement in anger regulation was unrelated to age-related decline in cognitive control functions. Overall, the evidence suggests an age improvement in emotion regulation, in stark contrast to the poorer emotional control associated with frontal lobe damage.

There have been numerous imaging, patient and aging studies investigating the ability to carry out social cue decoding, using tasks such as perception of facial expressions of emotion or understanding the thoughts or feelings of others' in adult theory of mind tasks. Hornak, Rolls, and Wade (1996) found that patients with lesions in the prefrontal cortex were significantly impaired on emotion identification tests compared to patients with lesions elsewhere in the brain. Many neuroimaging studies of emotion identification tasks have been carried out, and these usually indicate involvement of areas of the frontal lobes in identification of facial expressions of emotion (e.g. Sprengelmeyer, Rausch, Eysel, & Przuntek, 1998). Recent studies suggest that there is age-related decline in the ability to identify some negative facial expressions of emotion, particularly sadness (Calder, Keane, & Manly, 2003; MacPherson et al. 2002; Phillips, MacLean, & Allen, 2002; Sullivan & Ruffman, 2004a). However, this may not reflect a frontal deficit. There is some evidence indicating that age variance in emotion perception can be statistically explained by variance in a battery of medial temporal lobe tasks, but not dorsolateral prefrontal tasks (MacPherson et al. 2002), and we have replicated this finding with recent data (Phillips & Allen, in preparation). Recent neuroimaging studies also suggest that age differences in processing negative emotions may relate to diminished activation of limbic regions within the brain rather than changes in frontal lobe functioning (Gunning-Dixon et al. 2003; Mather et al. 2004).

There is evidence that frontal lobe patients experience difficulty identifying others' mental states, that is, have impaired "theory of mind" (Channon &

Crawford, 2000; Rowe, Bullock, & Polkey, 2001; Stone, Baron-Cohen, & Knight, 1998; Stuss, Gallup, & Alexander, 2001). Also, some neuroimaging studies suggest that areas within the frontal lobes are among a network of brain regions involved in carrying out theory of mind tasks (e.g. Gallagher & Frith, 2003; Gallagher, Happe, & Brunswick, 2000). Studies investigating age differences in theory of mind tasks have produced a very mixed pattern of results: age deficits have been found on tasks requiring identification of social cues from pictures of eyes (Phillips, MacLean, et al. 2002), videos of social interactions (Sullivan & Ruffman, 2004b) or stories describing social interactions (Maylor, Moulson, & Muncer, 2002; Sullivan & Ruffman, 2004b). MacPherson et al. (2002) report no age effect on the ability to identify social faux pas from stories. Also, age-related improvement in identifying others' theory of mind from stories has been reported by one study (Happé, Winner, & Brownell, 1998). However, a network of regions in the medial temporal lobes are reliably found to be involved in decoding others' theory of mind (for a review, see Gallagher & Frith, 2003) and so it may be that age changes in theory of mind ability relate to temporal lobe rather than frontal lobe changes. Indeed, age differences in theory of mind task performance were not explained by parallel variance in executive test performance (Maylor et al. 2002), suggesting a possible dissociation between age differences in social functions and age effects on executive tasks sensitive to frontal lobe functioning.

In sum, there are age effects on some aspects of socio-emotional processing but overall the pattern of age differences does not seem to closely match the deficits shown by patients with frontal lobe lesions. Older adults show maintained or improved ability to regulate emotions, and the age deficits seen in identifying social cues to emotion or others' thought processes might be mediated by changes in medial temporal functioning rather than frontal lobe impairment.

Neuroimaging: changes in frontal lobe activation with age

One of the main forces driving the frontal lobe theory of aging came from structural imaging studies indicating earlier neural changes localized to the frontal lobes of the brain. Curiously, relatively few studies have tested specifically the theory that frontal atrophy with age is correlated with changes in cognitive function. However, recently a number of studies have investigated age-related changes in *functional* activation during cognitive performance. It is interesting to contemplate, before reviewing these studies, what the frontal lobe theory of aging might predict about changes in functional activation in the frontal lobes during cognitive task performance. Structural changes might result in lower frontal activation with age. On the other hand, localized structural changes within the frontal lobes might result in a wider pattern of functional activation due to the need to use extra resources to compensate for age-related tissue loss.

In fact, both of these results have emerged from imaging studies. In some tasks, older adults show lower levels of frontal activation than young. Older adults tend to show lower levels of frontal lobe activation when at rest than young (e.g. Petit Taboué, Landeau, Desson, Desgranges, & Baron, 1998). There is evidence of lower frontal activation in older adults during tasks such as memory encoding (Grady, 2002) and attentional control (Milham et al. 2002) and this may be interpreted as older adults engaging in less effortful processing during complex cognitive tasks (Madden et al. 2002). These findings can easily be interpreted within the frontal lobe theory, whether the neural changes in the frontal lobes or less effective use of effortful strategies are the more important causal factor. Perhaps more common has been the reliable finding that older adults tend to show more widespread and often higher levels of activation in frontal lobe regions than young during cognitive task performance. In a range of tasks, whether memory for faces (Grady, 2002) working memory for verbal and spatial information (Reuter-Lorenz, 2002) or tasks demanding inhibitory processing (Nielson, Garavan, & Langenecker, 2002) younger adults tend to show well replicated patterns of lateralized frontal activation while older adults show more widespread bilateral activation. For example, in younger adults there is a well replicated pattern in memory tasks such that encoding differentially activates left prefrontal cortex while retrieval activates right prefrontal regions (e.g. Nyberg, Cabeza, & Tulving, 1996). This neat asymmetry is not replicated in older adults, where bilateral frontal activation is generally seen at both encoding and retrieval (for a review see Cabeza, 2002). This finding of increased bilateral frontal activation in older adults during cognitive tasks has now been extensively replicated.

A number of different explanations have been put forward to explain this increasing bilateral frontal activation during cognitive performance. One possibility links the changing activation patterns to right hemi-field aging. However, there is little evidence to support this explanation (Dolcos, Rice, & Cabeza, 2002). Another possible explanation is the dedifferentiation hypothesis (Li & Lindenberger, 1999) which suggests that old age results in the unravelling of specialized neural mechanisms for particular cognitive functions, and that older adults instead have increased reliance on more general purpose resources to carry out complex cognitive tasks. The final family of explanations propose that compensatory mechanisms explain the age differences, that is, more brain regions are recruited by older adults to make up for deterioration in information processing. A range of different compensatory mechanisms have been proposed: (i) the prefrontal effort hypothesis suggests that tasks which are relatively easy for young participants are more difficult for old, and thus require more widespread neural recruitment (Tisserand & Jolles, 2003). This hypothesis is supported by evidence that younger adults also show increased bilateral frontal activation when the working memory load of a task is increased (e.g. Jonides et al. 1997); (ii) the strategic recruitment hypothesis suggests that additional neural circuits are recruited as a result of age differences in the cognitive strategies used to carry out tasks, in response to changes in processing fidelity; (iii) the reorganization hypothesis proposes that neural circuitry left intact by the aging process changes in organizational pattern to compensate for lost networks. Cabeza (2002) argues that neural reorganization is a more likely explanation than strategic recruitment because similar patterns of decreased lateralization in the frontal lobes is seen in older adults in simple sensory discrimination tasks as well as more complex tasks.

The research into age differences in functional activation indicates that there is not a simple relationship between frontal lobe atrophy and cognitive decline in aging. Instead, it seems likely that age changes in frontal networks may results in compensatory recruitment of both frontal and other neural circuits to carry out information processing.

Requirements for a revised frontal lobe theory of aging

The frontal lobe theory of aging proposes that localized atrophy of the frontal lobes of the brain causes a specific decline in executive control functions, which then impacts upon a wide range of cognitive and behavioural processes. Despite this logic having been clearly stated for over a decade, relatively few studies have actually aimed to test the causal tenets of this theory. In other words, there is relatively little evidence that neural changes in the frontal lobes correlate with executive decline in old age. Tisserand and Jolles (2003) argue that: "At present, there is no direct evidence for a relationship between regional neuronal number and cognitive performance in non-pathological ageing" (p. 1107). In one of the few direct tests of the theory, Raz, Gunning-Dixon, Head, Dupuis, and Acker (1998) assessed the neuroanatomical substrates of cognitive aging using structural MRI. It was found that age-related increases in perseveration on the Wisconsin Card Sort Test (WCST) were related to atrophy in the prefrontal cortex. However, a limitation of this study is that no other measures were used to assess executive functioning. Although the WCST has been widely used to index perseveration both in the aging literature and neuropsychological research in general, questions have persistently been raised with respect to its validity as a measure of "frontal" functioning, as it has failed to consistently differentiate patients with frontal insult from either healthy controls or patients with lesions elsewhere in the brain (Axelrod, Goldman, Heaton, & Curtiss, 1996; Crawford & Henry, 2005; Mountain & Snow, 1993; Reitan & Wolfson, 1994).

The frontal lobe theory also proposes that the effects of aging on behaviour should parallel the effects of focal frontal damage. As reviewed above, the evidence for this is at best equivocal. Patients with frontal lobe damage tend to show deficits in executive functions, working memory, emotional control, and behavioural self-regulation (Stuss & Levine, 2002). Older adults show deficits in tasks intended to assess executive functions and working memory, although agreement has not yet been reached as to whether those deficits truly represent executive dysfunctions as opposed to more general resource deficits. However, older adults do not show the impaired socio-emotional or behavioural regulation in real-life situations that is a core distinctive feature of frontal lobe pathology.

This leaves the frontal lobe theory of aging in need of some refinement. Below we propose some key changes that need to be made in order to salvage the link between age, the frontal lobes and executive functioning into a more coherent theory.

1. *Reinstating the importance of the medial temporal lobes.* Although many authors have emphasised that age changes in the medial temporal lobes are also likely to impact on cognitive and emotional functions (e.g. Greenwood, 2000; Moscovitch & Winocur, 1992; Rabbitt & Lowe, 2000) this is not reflected in the majority of recent literature on cognitive aging (Tisserand & Jolles, 2003). Age changes in functions such as fluency, memory, and emotion perception may be better interpreted as reflecting changes in medial temporal functioning rather than frontal lobe functioning. All cognitive and behavioural changes with age need to be interpreted in relation to the network of frontal lobe connections to other brain regions rather than just considering the frontal lobes in isolation. Behavioural data can give some insight into this issue through the investigation of differential deficits in, and correlations with, tasks tapping temporal and frontal lobe function (e.g. Glisky, Polster, & Routhieaux, 1995). For example, Rabbitt and Lowe (2000) report that age differences were greater in magnitude on a battery of temporal lobe compared to frontal lobe measures. However, all cognitive tasks, and especially executive tasks, are likely to tap an extended network of brain regions, and so care must be taken in over-interpreting such behavioural results. Functional imaging

may also shed some light on this issue, in particular providing evidence for the use of different aspects of the frontal-temporal networks for carrying out the same task in young and old populations. However, it must be emphasised that in order to test the theory that *structural* changes in the temporal-frontal network underlie age differences in cognition, it is necessary to carry out structural imaging studies. There is a pressing need for more studies that investigate the relationship between regional brain atrophy with age and current cognitive functioning in the same population. This requires multidisciplinary research utilising the most recent technology in measuring regional structures in the brain along with sophisticated behavioural testing which allows investigation of particular executive functions using appropriate task decomposition.

2. *Taking heed of the compelling evidence for fractionation within the frontal lobes.* Clinical and neuroimaging evidence has recently allowed a more sophisticated picture of the different behavioural functions underlain by different subregions of the prefrontal cortex. In particular, there is converging evidence that the dorsolateral regions of the frontal lobes are involved in executive control functions while ventromedial regions underlie the control of emotional and social processing (Bechara et al. 1996; Stuss & Levine, 2002). As outlined above, aging tends to result in poorer performance on executive control tasks but does not tend to result in decline in socio-emotional control processes, and this has been interpreted as evidence that age may affect dorsolateral and ventromedial prefrontal functions differentially (MacPherson et al. 2002; Phillips & Della Sala, 1998; Phillips, MacPherson et al. 2002). MacPherson et al. (2002) propose that age causes differential early decline in the dorsolateral prefrontal cortex, which impacts specifically on executive control functions but spares socioemotional control (although note that the opposite pattern has also been proposed by Lamar & Resnick, 2004). This issue needs to be further explored by the combined use of structural neuroimaging and behavioural measurement. Functional imaging may also have a role to play, although relatively few functional imaging studies currently report effects on the most ventromedial prefrontal regions.

3. *Social and emotional functions.* There has been a growing trend within psychology to regard cognitive functioning as having an important interplay with social and emotional processes, and cognitive aging has come belatedly to consider this. Despite the consistent clinical and neuroimaging evidence of the involvement of temporal frontal networks in socio-emotional processing, age-related changes in these processes have rarely been considered within a neuropsychological framework. In order to achieve a complete

neuropsychological model of aging it is necessary to consider behaviour outside of the traditional domain of cognitive functions. The pattern of relatively preserved aspects of socioemotional functioning with age may reflect relative sparing of some of the specific brain areas involved in emotional functioning (Phillips, MacLean et al. 2002), compensatory experience of social skills throughout a lifetime (Pasupathi, Carstensen, Turk-Charles, & Tsai, 1998), or changes in the prioritization of emotional goals (Carstensen, Fung, & Charles, 2003). There is little consensus on how best to explain consistent age related deficits in some aspects of perception of emotional cues (Calder et al. 2003; Phillips, MacLean et al. 2002; Sullivan & Ruffman, 2004a). There are many aspects of the relationship between age changes in neural, emotional and social processing that have barely been explored to date, despite their importance for life skills and well-being.

4. *Importance of life experience and skills.* Executive functions are often thought of as particularly important in "novel" situations (e.g. Burgess, 1997; Denckla, 1994; Phillips, 1997) and tested using laboratory-based abstract tasks. However, it is clear that executive functions are extremely important in everyday life: behavioural and emotional regulation are essential aspects of social functioning, while even simple everyday memory tasks become considerably more difficult without strategic organization. However, the frontal aging hypothesis has so far concentrated almost exclusively on laboratory-based abstract tasks. This may give a very misleading picture of the impact of frontal lobe changes with age on real world functioning. Patients with frontal lobe lesions have great difficulties in coping with planning and social interaction in real life, even when they can effectively complete lab-based tasks (Shallice & Burgess, 1991). In contrast, older adults tend to show good performance on real life measures of planning (Garden et al. 2001; Phillips et al. 2005) prospective memory (Henry, Macleod et al. 2004) and emotional control (Carstensen et al. 2003). It is imperative that future research investigating frontal lobe changes with age explores not just artificial but also well-practised or socially-relevant executive tasks. This would permit a better understanding of the relationship between age, neural changes and the behavioural functions actually utilized in everyday life.

5. *More careful measurement of executive functions.* Aging research should have a moratorium of the use of "frontal lobe tests" such as the Wisconsin Card Sort Test, fluency, Stroop, and Tower of London without more careful thought going into why these tasks are being used. These tasks are generally poor measures of frontal lobe functioning in the sense that they are not selectively sensitive to frontal lobe functions (Crawford & Henry, in press;

Phillips, 1997; Stuss & Levin, 2002). Such complex tasks are difficult to break down to their cognitive components, providing the same psychometric construct validity problem identified in intelligence tests for many decades—it is not clear what the tests are testing—although at least intelligence tests are reliable and predictive of real world behaviours, unlike most "frontal lobe tests." Individual executive functions need to be more carefully defined. Rabbitt (e.g. Rabbitt, 1997; Rabbitt et al. 2001) argues very succinctly that cognitive constructs such as "inhibition" or indeed "speed" are often used carelessly to describe many different levels of neural and behavioural data, which do not necessarily have any links. Studies using evoked potentials to examine neural correlates of specific cognitive contrasts (e.g. West & Alain, 2000) may help to shed light on this issue.

Conclusions

The frontal lobe theory of cognitive aging proposes that localized age-related changes in the frontal lobes of the brain underlie deficits of cognitive control functions that in turn cause difficulties in memory and reasoning. Our evaluation of the current status of this theory is that (1) there is little direct evidence available to evaluate the causal link between brain and behavioural changes with age, (2) the current evidence of specific age deficits in cognitive control functions is weak partly because the research in this area has concentrated on overall scores of complex frontal lobe tasks rather than using more sophisticated task performance breakdowns on carefully designed experimental paradigms, (3) neuropsychological models of aging need to take seriously important evidence of frontal and temporal lobe involvement in real world skills and socio-emotional functioning, and (4) the theory currently relies on a very crude representation of neuroanatomy and greater consideration needs to be given to subregions within the frontal lobes and cortical and subcortical frontal networks.

References

Amieva, H., Phillips, L. H., Della Sala, S., & Henry, J. D. (2004). Inhibitory functioning in Alzheimer's Disease. *Brain, 127*, 949–964.

Andrés, P., & Van der Linden, M. (2000). Age-related differences in supervisory attentional system functions. *Journal of Gerontology: Psychological Sciences, 55B*, 373–380.

Axelrod, B. N., Goldman, R. S., Heaton, R. K., & Curtiss, G. (1996). Discriminability of the Wisconsin Card Sorting Test using the standardisation sample. *Journal of Clinical and Experimental Neuropsychology, 18*, 338–342.

Bechara, A., Damasio, A. R., Damasio, H., & Anderson, S. W. (1994). Insensitivity to future consequences following damage to human prefrontal cortex. *Cognition, 50*, 7–15.

Bechara, A., Damasio, H., Tranel, D., & Anderson, S. W. (1998). Dissociation of working memory from decision making within the human prefrontal cortex. *Journal of Neuroscience*, 18, 428–437.

Bechara, A., Tranel, D., Damasio H., & Damasio, A. R. (1996). Failure to respond autonomically to anticipated future outcomes following damage to prefrontal cortex. *Cerebral Cortex*, 6, 215–225.

Benton, A. L. (1994). Neuropsychological assessment. *Annual Review of Psychology*, 45, 1–23.

Bolla, K. I., Lindgren, K. N., Bonaccorsy, C., & Bleecker, M. L. (1990). Predictors of verbal fluency (FAS) in the healthy elderly. *Journal of Clinical Psychology*, 46, 623–628.

Brazzelli, M., Colombo, N., Della Sala, S., & Spinnler, H. (1994). Spared and impaired cognitive abilities after bilateral frontal damage. *Cortex*, 30, 27–51.

Burgess, P. W. (1997). Theory and methodology in executive function research. In P. Rabbitt (Ed.), *Methodology of frontal and executive function* (pp. 81–116). Hove, UK: Psychology Press.

Cabeza, R. (2002). Hemispheric asymmetry reduction in older adults: The HAROLD model. *Psychology and Aging*, 17, 85–100.

Calder, A. J., Keane, J., & Manly, T. (2003). Facial expression recognition across the adult life span. *Neuropsychologia*, 41, 195–292.

Capitani, E., Laiacona, M., & Barbarotto, R. (1999). Gender affects word retrieval of certain categories in semantic fluency tasks. *Cortex*, 35, 273–278.

Carstensen, L. L., Fung, H. H., & Charles, S. T. (2003). Socioemotional selectivity theory and the regulation of emotion in the second half of life. *Motivation and Emotion*, 27, 103–123.

Cerella, J. (1985). Information processing rates in the elderly. *Psychological Bulletin*, 98, 67–83.

Channon, S., & Crawford, S. (1999). Problem-solving in real-life-type situations: The effects of anterior and posterior lesions on performance. *Neuropsychologia*, 37, 757–770.

Channon, S., & Crawford, S. (2000). The effects of anterior lesions on performance on a story comprehension test: Left anterior impairment on a theory of mind-type task. *Neuropsychologia*, 38, 1007–1017.

Cohn, N. B., Dustman, R. E., & Bradford, D. C. (1984). Age-related decrements in Stroop Colour Test performance. *Journal of Clinical Psychology*, 40, 1244–1250.

Crawford, J. R., Bryan, J., Luszcz, M. A., Obonsawin, M. C., & Stewart, L. (2000). The executive decline hypothesis of cognitive aging: Do executive deficits qualify as differential deficits and do they mediate age-related memory decline? *Aging, Neuropsychology and Cognition*, 7, 9–31.

Crawford, J. R., & Henry, J. D. (2005). Assessment of executive deficits. In P. W. Halligan & N. Wade (Eds.), *The effectiveness of rehabilitation for cognitive deficits* (pp. 233–246). Oxford: Oxford University Press.

Daigneault, S., Braun, C. M. J., & Whitaker, H. A. (1992). Early effects of normal aging on perseverative and non- perseverative prefrontal measures. *Developmental Neuropsychology*, 8, 99–114.

Damasio, A. R., & Anderson, S. W. (1993). The frontal lobes. In K. M. Heilman & E. Valenstein (Eds.), *Clinical Neuropsychology* (pp. 409–459). New York: Oxford University Press.

Damasio, A. R., & Van Hoesen, G. W. (1983). Emotional disturbances associated with focal lesions of the frontal lobe. In P. Satz (Ed.), *Neuropsychology of human emotion* (pp. 85–110). New York: Guilford Press.

Davidson, R. J., Putnam, K. M., & Larson, C. L. (2000). Dysfunction in the neural circuitry of emotion regulation—a possible prelude to violence. *Science, 289*, 591–594.

Denckla, M. (1994). Measurement of executive function. In G. Reid Lyon (Ed.), *Frames of reference for the assessment of learning disabilities. New views on measurement issues.* (pp. 117–142). Baltimore: Paul H. Brookes.

Devolder, P. A., Brigham, M. C., & Pressley, M. (1990). Memory performance awareness in younger and older adults. *Psychology and Aging, 5*, 291–303.

Dolcos, F., Rice, H. J., & Cabeza, R. (2002). Hemispheric asymmetry and aging: Right hemisphere decline or asymmetry reduction. *Neuroscience and Biobehavioral Reviews, 26*, 819–825.

Dougherty, D. D., Shin, L. M., Alpert, N. M., Pitman, R. K., Orr, S. P., Lasko, M., et al. (1999). Anger in healthy men: A PET study using script-driven imagery. *Biological Psychiatry, 46*, 466–472.

Duncan, J., Burgess, P., & Emslie, H. (1995). Fluid intelligence after frontal lobe lesions. *Neuropsychologia, 33*, 261–268.

Eslinger, P. J., & Damasio, A. R. (1985). Severe disturbance of higher cognition after bilateral frontal-lobe ablation: Patient EVR. *Neurology, 35*, 1731–1741.

Eslinger, P. J., Grattan, L. M., & Geder, L. (1995). Impact of frontal lobe lesions on rehabilitation and recovery from acute brain injury. *Neurorehabilitation, 5*, 161–182.

Fuster, J. M. (1989). *The prefrontal cortex* (2nd ed.). New York: Raven Press.

Gallagher, H. L., & Frith, C. D. (2003). Functional imaging of "theory of mind." *Trends in Cognitive Sciences, 7*, 77–83.

Gallagher, H. L., Happe, F., & Brunswick, N. (2000). Reading the mind in cartoons and stories: An fMRI study of "theory of mind" in verbal and nonverbal tasks. *Neuropsychologia, 38*, 11–21.

Garden, S., Phillips, L. H., & MacPherson, S. E. (2001). Mid-life aging, open-ended planning and laboratory measures of executive function. *Neuropsychology, 15*, 472–482.

Gilhooly, K. J., Phillips, L. H., Wynn, V. E., Logie, R. H., & Della Sala, S. (1999). Planning processes and age in the 5 disc Tower of London task. *Thinking and Reasoning, 5*, 339–361.

Glisky, E. L., Polster, M. R., & Routhieaux, B. C. (1995). Double dissociation between item and source memory. *Neuropsychology, 9*, 229–235.

Grady, C. L. (2002). Age-related differences in face processing: A meta-analysis of three functional neuroimaging experiments. *Canadian Journal of Experimental Psychology, 56*, 208–220.

Greenwood, P. M. (2000). The frontal aging hypothesis evaluated. *Journal of the International Neuropsychological Society, 6*, 705–726.

Gross, J. J., Carstensen, L. L., Pasupathi, M., Tsai, J., Skorpen, C. G., & Hsu, A. Y. C. (1997). Emotion and aging: Experience, expression, and control. *Psychology and Aging, 12*, 590–599.

Gunning-Dixon, F. M., Gur, R. C., Perkins, A. C., Schroeder, L. U., Turner, T., Turetsky, B. I. et al. (2003). Age-related differences in brain activation during emotional face processing. *Neurobiology of Aging, 24*, 285–295.

Happé, F. G. E., Winner, E., & Brownell, H. V. (1998). The getting of wisdom: Theory of mind in old age. *Developmental Psychology, 34*, 358–362.

Henry, J. D., & Crawford, J. R. (2004a). A meta-analytic review of verbal fluency performance following focal cortical lesions. *Neuropsychology, 18*, 284–295.

Henry, J. D., & Crawford, J. R. (2004b). A meta-analytic review of verbal fluency performance in traumatic brain injured patients. *Neuropsychology, 18*, 621–628.

Henry, J. D., Crawford, J. R., & Phillips, L. H. (2004). Verbal fluency performance in dementia of the Alzheimer's type: A meta-analysis. *Neuropsychologia, 42*, 1212–1222.

Henry, J. D., Macleod, M. S., Phillips, L. H., & Crawford, J. R. (2004). A meta-analytic review of prospective memory and aging. *Psychology and Aging, 19*, 27–39.

Henry, J. D., & Phillips, L. H. (in press). Covariates of production and perseveration on tests of phonemic, semantic and alternating fluency in normal aging. *Aging, Neuropsychology and Cognition.*

Hornak, J., Rolls, E. T., & Wade, D. (1996). Face and voice expression identification in patients with emotional and behavioral changes following ventral frontal lobe damage. *Neuropsychologia, 34*, 247–261.

Hughes, D. L., & Bryan, J. (2002). Adult age differences in strategy use during verbal fluency performance. *Journal of Clinical and Experimental Neuropsychology, 24*, 642–654.

Isingrini, M., & Vazou, F. (1997). Relation between fluid intelligence and frontal lobe functioning in older adults. *International Journal of Aging and Human Development, 45*, 99–109.

Jonides, J., Schumacher, E. H., Smith, E. E., Lauber, E. J., Awh, E., Minoshima, S. et al. (1997). Verbal working memory load affects regional brain activation as measured by PET. *Journal of Cognitive Neuroscience, 9*, 462–475.

Kempler, D., Teng, E. L., Dick, M., Taussig, I. M., & Davis, D. S. (1998). The effects of age, education, and ethnicity on verbal fluency. *Journal of the International Neuropsychological Society, 4*, 531–538.

Lamar, M., & Resnick, S.M. (2004). Aging and prefrontal functions: Dissociating orbitofrontal and dorsolateral abilities. *Neurobiology of Aging, 25*, 553–558.

Lezak, M. D. (1993). Newer contributions to the neuropsychological assessment of executive functions. *Journal of Head Trauma Rehabilitation, 8*, 24–31.

Li, S., & Lindenberger, U. (1999). Cross-level unification: A computational exploration of the link between deterioration of neurotransmitter systems and dedifferentiation of cognitive abilities in old age. In L. Nilsson & H. J. Markowitsch (Eds.), *Cognitive neuroscience of memory* (pp. 103–146). Ashland, OH: Hogrefe & Huber.

Lowe, C., & Rabbitt, P. (1997). Cognitive models of aging and frontal lobe deficits. In P. Rabbitt (Ed.), *Methodology of frontal and executive functions* (pp. 39–59). Hove, UK: Psychology Press.

MacPherson, S. E., Phillips, L. H., & Della Sala, S. (2002). Age, executive function, and social decision making: A dorsolateral prefrontal theory of cognitive aging. *Psychology and Aging, 17*, 598–609.

Madden, D. J., Turkington, T. G., Provenzale, J. M., Denny, L. L., Langley, L. K., Hawk, T. C. et al. (2002). Aging and attentional guidance during visual search: Functional neuroanatomy by Positron Emission Tomography. *Psychology and Aging, 17*, 24–43.

Martin, M. (1986). Aging and patterns of change in everyday memory and cognition. *Human Learning, 5*, 63–74.

Mather, M., Canli, T., English, T., Whitfield, S., Wais, P., Ochsner, K. et al. (2004). Amygdala responses to emotionally valenced stimuli in older and younger adults. *Psychological Science, 15*, 259–263.

Maylor, E. A. (1990). Age and prospective memory. *The Quarterly Journal of Experimental Psychology, 42A*, 471–493.

Maylor, E. A., Moulson, J. M., & Muncer, A. (2002). Does performance on theory of mind tasks decline in old age. *British Journal of Psychology, 93*, 465–485.

McGeorge, P., Phillips, L. H., Crawford, J. R., Garden, S. E., Della Sala, S., Milne, A. B. et al. (2001). Using virtual environments in the assessment of executive dysfunction. *Presence: Teleoperators and Virtual Environments, 10*, 375–383.

Milham, M. P., Erickson, K. I., Banich, M. T., Kramer, A. F., Webb, A., Wszalek, T. et al. (2002). Attentional control in the aging brain: Insights from an fMRI study of the Stroop task. *Brain and Cognition, 49*, 277–296.

Miller, E. (1984). Verbal fluency as a function of a measure of verbal intelligence and in relation to different types of cerebral pathology. *British Journal of Clinical Psychology, 23*, 53–57.

Milner, B. (1995). Aspects of human frontal lobe function. *Epilepsia, 36*, 81.

Mittenberg, W., Seidenberg, M., O'leary, D. S., & DiGiulio, D. V. (1989). Changes in cerebral functioning associated with normal aging. *Journal of Clinical and Experimental Neuropsychology, 11*, 918–932.

Morris, R. G., Miotto, E. C., Feigenbaum, J. D., Bullock, P., & Polkey, C. E. (1997). The effect of goal–subgoal conflict on planning ability after frontal- and temporal-lobe lesions in humans. *Neuropsychologia, 35*, 1147–1157.

Moscovitch, M. (1982). A neuropsychological approach to memory and perception in normal and pathological aging. In F. I. M. Craik & S. Trehub (Eds.), *Aging and cognitive processes* (pp. 55–78). New York: Plenum Press.

Moscovitch, M., & Melo, B. (1997). Strategic retrieval and the frontal lobes: Evidence from confabulation and amnesia. *Neuropsychologia, 35*, 1017–1034.

Moscovitch, M., & Winocur, G. (1992). The neuropsychology of memory and aging. In F. I. M. Craik & T. A. Salthouse (Eds.), *The handbook of aging and cognition* (pp. 315–372). Hillsdale, NJ: Erlbaum.

Mountain, M. A., & Snow, W. G. (1993). Wisconsin Card Sorting Test as a measure of frontal pathology: A review. *The Clinical Neuropsychologist, 7*, 108–118.

Nielson, K. A., Garavan, H., & Langenecker, S. A. (2002). Differences in the functional neuroanatomy of inhibitory control across the adult life span. *Psychology and Aging, 17*, 56–71.

Nyberg, L., Cabeza, R., & Tulving, E. (1996). PET studies of encoding and retrieval: The HERA model. *Psychonomic Bulleting and Review, 3*, 135–148.

Ochsner, K. N., Bunge, S. A., Gross, J. J., & Gabrieli, J. D. E. (2002). Rethinking feelings: An fMRI study of the cognitive regulation of emotion. *Journal of Cognitive Neuroscience, 14*, 1215–1229.

Ochsner, K. N., & Gross, J. J. (2004). Thinking makes it so: A social cognitive neuroscience approach to emotion regulation. In R. F. Baumeister & K. D. Vohs (Eds.), *Handbook of self-regulation: Research, theory and applications* (pp. 229–255). New York: Guilford Press.

Paradiso, S., Chemerinski, E., & Yazici, K. M. (1999). Frontal lobe syndrome reassessed: Comparison of patients with lateral or medial frontal brain damage. *Journal of Neurology, Neurosurgery and Psychiatry, 67*, 664–667.

Parker, D. M., & Crawford, J. R. (1992). Assessment of frontal lobe function. In J. R. Crawford, D. M. Parker, & W. W. McKinlay (Eds.), *A handbook of neuropsychological assessment* (pp. 267–291). London: Erlbaum.

Parkin, A. J. (1997). Normal age-related memory loss and its relation to frontal lobe dysfunction. In P. M. A. Rabbitt (Ed.), *Methodology of frontal and executive function* (pp. 177–190). Hove, UK: Psychology Press.

Parkin, A. J., & Java, R. I. (1999). Deterioration of frontal lobe function in normal aging: Influences of fluid intelligence versus perceptual speed. *Neuropsychology, 13*, 539–545.

Parkin, A. J., & Walter, B. M. (1991). Aging, short-term memory, and frontal dysfunction. *Psychobiology, 19*, 175–179.

Parkin, A. J., Yeomans, J., & Bindschaedler, C. (1994). Further characterization of the executive memory impairment following frontal-lobe lesions. *Brain and Cognition, 26*, 23–42.

Pasupathi, M., Carstensen, L. L., Turk-Charles, S., & Tsai, J. (1998). Emotion and aging. In H. Friedman (Ed.), *Encyclopedia of Mental Health* (Vol. 2, pp. 91–101). San Diego, CA: Academic Press.

Patton, G. W., & Meit, M. (1993). Effect of aging on prospective and incidental memory. *Experimental Aging Research, 19*, 165–176.

Perret, E. (1974). The left frontal lobe of man and the suppression of habitual responses in verbal categorical behaviour. *Neuropsychologia, 12*, 323–330.

Petit Taboué, M. C., Landeau, B., Desson, J. F., Desgranges, B., & Baron, J. C. (1998). Effects of healthy aging on the regional cerebral metabolic rate of glucose assessed with statistical parametric mapping. *Neuroimage, 7*, 176–184.

Phan, K. L., Wager, T., Taylor, S. F., & Liberzon, I. (2002). Functional neuroanatomy of emotion: A meta-analysis of emotion activation studies in PET and fMRI. *Neuroimage, 16*, 331–348.

Phillips, L. H. (1997). Do "frontal tests" measure executive function? Issues of assessment and evidence from fluency tests. In P. M. A. Rabbitt (Ed.), *Methodology of frontal and executive function* (pp. 191–213). Hove: UK Psychology Press.

Phillips, L. H. (1999). Age and individual differences in letter fluency. *Developmental Neuropsychology, 15*, 249–267.

Phillips, L. H., & Allen, R. Involvement of the frontal and medial temporal lobes in age differences in emotion identification. Manuscript in preparation.

Phillips, L. H., & Della Sala, S. (1998). Aging, intelligence and anatomical segregation in the frontal lobes. *Learning and Individual Differences, 10*, 217–243.

Phillips, L. H., Gilhooly, K. J., Logie, R. H., Della Sala, S., & Wynn, V. (2003). Age, working memory, and the Tower of London task. *European Journal of Cognitive Psychology, 15*, 291–312.

Phillips, L. H., Henry, J. D., Hosie, J. A., & Milne, A. B. Age, anger regulation and well-being. Manuscript in preparation.

Phillips, L. H., MacLean, R. D. J., & Allen, R. (2002). Age and the understanding of emotions: Neuropsychological and sociocognitive perspectives. *Journals of Gerontology: Series B: Psychological Sciences and Social Sciences, 57B*, 526–530.

Phillips, L. H., MacLeod, M., & Kliegel, M. (2005). Adult aging and cognitive planning. In G. Ward & R. Morris (Eds.), *The cognitive psychology of planning* (pp. 111–134). Hove: Psychology Press.

Phillips, L. H., MacPherson, S., & Della Sala, S. (2002). Age, cognition and emotion: The role of anatomical segregation in the frontal lobes. In J. Grafman (Ed.), *Handbook of neuropsychology* (2nd ed., Vol. 7, *The frontal lobes*, pp. 73–97). Amsterdam: Elsevier.

Poon, L. W., & Schaffer, G. (1982). *Prospective memory in young and elderly adults.* Washington, DC: American Psychological Association.

Rabbitt, P., & Lowe, C. (2000). Patterns of cognitive ageing. *Psychological Research, 63*, 308–316.

Rabbitt, P. M. A. (1963). Grouping of stimuli in pattern recognition as a function of age. *Quarterly Journal of Experimental Psychology, 15*, 172–176.

Rabbitt, P. M. A. (1997). Introduction: Methodologies and models in the study of executive function. In P. M. A. Rabbitt (Ed.), *Methodology of frontal and executive function* (pp. 1–38). Hove, UK: Psychology Press.

Rabbitt, P. M. A. (2000). Measurement indices, functional characteristics and psychometric constructs in cognitive aging. In T. J. Perfect & E. A. Maylor (Eds.), *Models of cognitive aging* (pp. 160–187). London: Oxford University Press.

Rabbitt, P. M. A. (2002). Aging and cognition. In H. Pashler & J. Wixted (Eds.), *Steven's handbook of experimental psychology* (Vol. 4, *Methodology in experimental psychology*, pp. 793–860). New York: John Wiley & Sons.

Rabbitt, P. M. A., Lowe, C., & Shilling, V. (2001). Frontal tests and models for cognitive ageing. *European Journal of Cognitive Psychology, 13*, 5–28.

Rabbitt, P. M. A., & Vyas, S. M. (1970). An elementary preliminary taxonomy for some errors in laboratory choice RT tasks. In A. F. Sanders (Ed.), *Attention and performance. Part III* (pp. 56–76). Amsterdam: North-Holland.

Raz, N., Gunning-Dixon, F. M., Head, D., Dupuis, J. H., & Acker, J. D. (1998). Neuroanatomical correlates of cognitive aging: Evidence from structural magnetic resonance imaging. *Neuropsychology, 12*, 95–114.

Reitan, R. M., & Wolfson, D. (1994). A selective and critical review of neuropsychological deficits and the frontal lobes. *Neuropsychology Review, 4*, 161–195.

Rendell, P. G., & Thomson, D. M. (1993). The effect of ageing on remembering to remember: An investigation of simulated medication regimens. *Australian Journal of Ageing, 12*, 11–18.

Rendell, P. G., & Thomson, D. M. (1999). Aging and prospective memory: Differences between naturalistic and laboratory tasks. *Journals of Gerontology Series B: Psychological Sciences and Social Sciences, 54*, 256–269.

Reuter-Lorenz, P. A. (2002). New visions of the aging mind and brain. *Trends in Cognitive Sciences, 6*, 394–400.

Robbins, T. W., James, M., Owen, A. M., Sahakian, B. J., Lawrence, A. D., McInnes, L. et al. (1998). A study of performance on tests from the CANTAB battery sensitive to frontal lobe dysfunction in a large sample of normal volunteers: Implications for theories of executive functioning and cognitive aging. *Journal of the International Neuropsychological Society, 4*, 474–490.

Rolls, E. T., Hornak, J., Wade, D., & McGrath, J. (1994). Emotion-related learning in patients with social and emotional changes associated with frontal lobe damage. *Journal of Neurology, Neurosurgery and Psychiatry, 57*, 1518–1524.

Rowe, A. D., Bullock, P. R., & Polkey, C. E. (2001). "Theory of mind" impairments and their relationship to executive functioning following frontal lobe excisions. *Brain, 124*, 600–616.

Salthouse, T. A. (1985). *A theory of cognitive aging.* Amsterdam: North-Holland.

Salthouse, T. A. (1996). The processing-speed theory of adult age differences in cognition. *Psychological Review, 103*, 403–428.

Shallice, T. (1982). Specific impairments of planning. *Philosophical Transactions of the Royal Society of London, 298*, 199–209.

Shallice, T. (1988). *From neuropsychology to mental structure.* Cambridge University Press.

Shallice, T., & Burgess, P. W. (1991). Deficits in strategy application following frontal-lobe damage in man. *Brain, 114*, 727–741.

Shilling, V. M., Chetwynd, A., & Rabbitt, P. M. A. (2002). Individual inconsistency across measures of inhibition: An investigation of the construct validity of inhibition in older adults. *Neuropsychologia, 40*, 605–619.

Sprengelmeyer, R., Rausch, M., Eysel, U. T., & Przuntek, H. (1998). Neural structures associated with recognition of facial expressions of basic emotions. *Proceedings of the Royal Society of London B, 265*, 1927–1931.

Stone, V. E., Baron-Cohen, S., & Knight, R. T. (1998). Frontal lobe contributions to theory of mind. *Journal of Cognitive Neuroscience, 10*, 640–656.

Stuss, D. T., & Benson, D. F. (1986). *The frontal lobes.* New York: Raven Press.

Stuss, D. T., Gallup, G. G., & Alexander, M. P. (2001). The frontal lobes are necessary for "theory of mind." *Brain, 124*, 279–286.

Stuss, D. T., & Levine, B. (2002). Adult clinical neuropsychology: Lessons from studies of the frontal lobes. *Annual Review of Psychology, 53*, 401–433.

Sullivan, S., & Ruffman, T. (2004a). Emotion recognition deficits in the elderly. *International Journal of Neuroscience, 114*, 94–102.

Sullivan, S., & Ruffman, T. (2004b). Social understanding: How does it fare with advancing years? *British Journal of Psychology, 95*, 1–18.

Tisserand, D. J., & Jolles, J. (2003). On the involvement of prefrontal networks in cognitive ageing. *Cortex, 39*, 1107–1128.

Tombaugh, T. N., Kozak, J., & Rees, L. (1999). Normative data stratified by age and education for two measures of verbal fluency: FAS and animal naming. *Archives of Clinical Neuropsychology, 14*, 167–177.

Troyer, A. K., Graves, R. E., & Cullum, C. M. (1994). Executive functioning as a mediator of the relationship between age and episodic memory in healthy aging. *Aging and Cognition, 1*, 45–53.

Troyer, A. K., Moscovitch, M., & Winocur, G. (1997). Clustering and switching as two components of verbal fluency: Evidence from younger and older healthy adults. *Neuropsychology, 11*, 138–146.

Verhaeghen, P., & de Meersman, L. (1998). Aging and the Stroop effect: A meta-analysis. *Psychology and Aging, 13*, 120–126.

West, R., & Alain, C. (2000). Effects of task context and fluctuations of attention on neural activity supporting performance of the Stroop task. *Brain Research, 873*, 102–111.

West, R. L. (1996). An application of prefrontal cortex function theory to cognitive aging. *Psychological Bulletin, 120*, 272–292.

Wilson, B. A., Alderman, N., Burgess, P., Emslie, H., & Evans, J. (1996). *Behavioral assessment of the dysexecutive syndrome.* Bury St Edmunds, UK: Thames Valley Test.

Woodruff-Pak, D. D. (1997). *The neuropsychology of aging.* Oxford: Blackwell.

Yeudall, L. R., Fromm, D., Reddon, J. R., & Stefanyk, W. O. (1986). Normative data stratified by age and sex for 12 neuropsychological tests. *Journal of Clinical Psychology, 42*, 918–946.

Chapter 9

The gateway hypothesis of rostral prefrontal cortex (area 10) function

Paul W. Burgess, Jon S. Simons, Iroise Dumontheil, and Sam J. Gilbert

Abstract

One of the most fascinating puzzles in cognitive neuroscience concerns the functions of a large brain area known as the rostral prefrontal cortex (or Area 10). This is a sizeable brain region, which is especially large in humans compared with other animals, yet very little is known about what role it plays in cognition. This chapter contains three sections. The first reviews the existing empirical and theoretical evidence. The second presents a new theoretical account of its function that synthesises this evidence. The third describes a recent series of experiments in our laboratory, which demonstrate the plausibility of the theory. Rostral prefrontal cortex (rostral PFC) is identified as subserving a system that biases the relative influence of stimulus-oriented and stimulus-independent thought. This cognitive control function (and its product) is used in a wide range of situations critical to competent human behaviour in everyday life, ranging from straightforward "watchfulness" to complex activities such as remembering to carry out intended actions after a delay, multitasking, and aspects of recollection. In everyday terms, these are situations that require one to be particularly alert to the environment, to deliberately concentrate on one's thoughts, or involve conscious switching between these states.

Preparation of this chapter, and most of the work reported in it was supported by Wellcome Trust grant number 061171 to PWB. We would like to thank Dr Jiro Okuda for valuable discussions; Dr Laura Goldstein and Dr Vinod Goel for kindly supplying the scans for patients GN and PF in Figure 9.1; and Jordan Grafman, Chris Frith, Etienne Koechlin, Kalina Christoff, and Peter McLeod for their very helpful comments on an earlier draft.

Introduction

> Attempts to define . . . executive function encounter . . . a . . .
> difficulty: no single exemplary task or even subset of tasks
> provides an adequate ostensive definition. It is often necessary to
> fall back on consensus definitions drawn from the common sense
> of the "man in the street" or poll the collective wisdom of "distin-
> guished experts in the field" . . . these tend to be wide-ranging
> catalogues of examples of intelligent behaviour and to avoid
> entirely discussions of underlying process (Rabbitt, 1997, p. 30).

The part of the frontal lobes that is foremost in the brain has many
names. The most common of these are: "anterior prefrontal cortex" (anterior
PFC), "the frontal pole," "frontopolar cortex," and "rostral prefrontal cortex."
Of these, we favor the use of the term "rostral" since the term is equivalent to
others that are used to denote regions of the brain (e.g. caudal, dorsal, lateral,
medial, ventral). However these terms all refer to a region which broadly
corresponds to the cytoarchitectonic area known as Brodmann Area 10 (BA 10).
This is probably the region of the brain whose function is least understood,
although there is good reason for suspecting that it plays a critical role in
human cognition. For instance, this is a very large brain region in humans: in
volumetric terms probably the largest single architectonic region of the frontal
lobes (Christoff et al. 2001). Indeed, Area 10 of the human right hemisphere
alone (approx. 14,000 mm^3) makes up 1.2% of the *entire* brain volume
(Semendeferi et al. 2001). Given that the brain may consume as much as 20%
of the oxygen we extract from the air that we breathe (Raichle et al. 2001),
there must surely be some evolutionary advantage to having such a large brain
region (or rather, the capacities that it enables). Moreover, rostral PFC is in
relative terms twice as large in the human brain as in any of the great apes
(Semendeferi, Armstrong, Schleicher, Zilles, & Van Hoesen, 2001). And finally,
this region is possibly the last to achieve myelination, and it has been argued that
tardily myelinating areas engage in complex functions highly related to the
organism's experience (Fuster, 1997, p. 37). These are all good reasons to imagine
that the rostral PFC may support cognitive processing which is especially
important to humans.

However, very little is known about the functions of rostral PFC. There are
many reasons for this situation: animal studies of this region are problematic
since the very fact of the structural difference between humans and other animals creates doubt as to the transferability of findings from one species to
another. Moreover, animal lesion studies of this region are hindered by practical anatomical considerations. Other cognitive neuroscience methods also face

limitations. For instance, electrophysiological methods do not presently have the required spatial resolution to separate subregions of the frontal lobes, and transcranial magnetic stimulation studies of rostral PFC may be difficult for anatomical reasons. Thus virtually the only significant evidence one might call upon from methods other than functional imaging comes from human lesion studies. These however are difficult and costly: Area 10 lesions are not common, and typically do not produce "hard" neurological signs (such as hemiparesis, marked aphasia, etc.). So unless they are the result of trauma, rostral lesions are often not detected unless (or until) they are large, covering many other brain regions in addition to Area 10. This then raises the question of which of the symptoms can be attributable specifically to the rostral aspect of the lesion, usually necessitating a group study using the overlapping lesion method (see below). However since there is no straightforward pathology to lesion site correspondence, the pattern will typically be made more difficult by issues of the effects of different pathologies. These issues are not insurmountable (see for example, Burgess, Veitch, Costello, & Shallice, 2000; Burgess, Veitch, & Costello, submitted), but will necessitate careful and lengthy data collection and analysis, often taking several years. In this context, it is unsurprising that most data relevant to rostral PFC function comes from functional neuroimaging. However, there is a problem with the use of functional imaging as the sole source of data. Rostral PFC activation is found in such a wide variety of tasks that this provides relatively few constraints on theorizing. Local haemodynamic (e.g. blood-flow, blood oxygenation) changes occur in Area 10 during the performance of a very wide variety of cognitive tasks (Grady, 1999), from the simplest (e.g. conditioning paradigms; Blaxton et al. 1996) to highly complex tests involving memory and judgment (e.g. Burgess, Quayle, & Frith, 2001; Burgess, Scott, & Frith, 2003; Frith & Frith, 2003; Koechlin, Basso, Pietrini, Panzer, & Grafman, 1999) or problem-solving (e.g. Christoff et al. 2001). Indeed, one can find activation of the rostral PFC in just about any kind of task, for example, verbal episodic retrieval (Rugg, Fletcher, Frith, Frackowiak, & Dolan, 1996; Tulving, Markowitsch, Craik, Habib, & Houle, 1996); nonverbal episodic retrieval (Haxby et al. 1996; Roland & Gulyas, 1995); semantic memory (Jennings, McIntosh, Kapur, Tulving, & Houle, 1997; Martin, Haxby, Lalonde, Wigges, & Ungerleider 1995); language (Bottini et al. 1994; Klein, Milner, Zatorre, Meyer, & Evans, 1995); motor learning (Jenkins, Brooks, Nixon, Frackowiak, & Passingham, 1994); rule learning (Strange, Henson, Friston, & Dolan, 2001); shock/ tone conditioning (Hugdahl et al. 1995); nonverbal working memory (Gold, Berman, Randolph, Goldberg, & Weinberger, 1996; Haxby, Ungerleider, Horwitz, Rapoport, & Grady, 1995); verbal working memory (Petrides,

Alivisatos, Meyer, & Evans, 1993); spatial memory (Burgess, Maguire, Spiers, & O'Keefe, 2001); auditory perception (Zatorre, Halpern, Perry, Meyer, & Evans, 1996); object processing (Kosslyn et al. 1994; Kosslyn, Alpert, & Thompson, 1995); Tower of London Test (Baker et al. 1996); Wisconsin Card Sorting Test (Berman et al. 1995); reasoning tasks (Goel, Gold, Kapur, & Houle, 1997); intelligence tests such as Raven's Progressive Matrices (Christoff et al. 2001; Prabhakaran, Smith, Desmond, Glover, & Gabrieli, 1997).

Perhaps a meta-analysis of the tasks which most reliably produce rostral PFC activation would isolate the critical processing component supported by this region? Grady (1999) provides an excellent analysis of this sort. She reviewed 90 PET studies showing prefrontal rCBF changes, and concluded that the most heavily represented function of BA 10 is episodic memory, on the grounds that most of the experiments reporting BA 10 activation were using episodic memory paradigms. This was a very useful and carefully conducted review. However it did not take into account the predominance of episodic memory investigations in functional imaging studies. If one takes this into account, a quite different picture emerges. Thus 37/90 (41%) of the studies that Grady considered in her review investigated episodic memory, and 47/90 (52%) of the studies she considered implicated BA 10. However, only 68% of the episodic memory studies were found to cause BA 10 activations, and just 25 (53%) of the paradigms that caused BA 10 activations were episodic memory ones. Furthermore, 7/90 of the studies that Grady considered were investigations of "Working Memory" and 6 of these (86%) showed BA 10 activation. And finally, 6/90 studies investigated conditioning or motor learning, and all 6 (100%) reported BA 10 activation. Thus it is doubtful that, whatever role BA 10 functions play in cognition, they are any more active when people are involved in episodic memory tasks than when they are engaged in other sorts of tasks. As MacLeod, Buckner, Miezin, Petersen, & Raichle (1998) put it, "although . . . BA 10 is routinely activated by episodic memory tasks, it is not uniquely activated by episodic memory tasks" (p. 41; see also Duncan & Owen, 2000).

Theories of rostral PFC (area 10) function

Perhaps because of the widespread nature of the evidence from functional imaging, there are a number of extant theories, each of which seeks to explain some part of the findings. There are, broadly, four categories of these theories:

1. *Episodic memory accounts*: Notwithstanding the criticisms above, the idea that Rostral PFC (area 10) plays some particularly significant role in episodic memory is widespread. This is largely based on evidence from

functional imaging (e.g. Rugg et al. 1996; Tulving et al. 1996). For instance Buckner (1996, p. 156) suggests that "the common activation during episodic retrieval is highly localised, falling at or near Brodmann area 10."

2. *Metacognition*: The theories in this category hold that BA 10 supports processing that perhaps can best be described as "metacognition," that is reflecting on one's own thoughts, or thinking in a very controlled, conscious, or goal-directed mode (e.g. Johnson et al. 2002). For instance, Christoff & Gabrieli (2000, p. 183) describe the role of this region as of "evaluation, monitoring, or manipulation of internally generated information"; and others talk about states of awareness, for example, "felt-rightness" (Moscovitch & Winocur, 2002). Proponents of the "Theory of Mind" perspective, meanwhile, suggest that medial rostral PFC may be "engaged when we attend to our own mental states as well as the mental states of others" (Frith & Frith, 2003, p. 467).

3. *Sum processes*: There are two subcategories of these theories: processing and anatomical. The processing views maintain that rostral PFC supports processing involved in the coordination of potentially independent processing resources (e.g. Ramnani & Owen, 2004). For instance Koechlin and colleagues (e.g. Dreher, Koechlin, Ali, & Grafman, 2002; Koechlin et al. 1999; Koechlin, Ody, & Kouneiher, 2003) maintain that lateral rostral PFC "selectively mediates the human ability to hold in mind goals while exploring and processing secondary goals" (Koechlin et al. 1999, p. 148), with the frontal lobes organized along a posterior to anterior axis as the task being performed becomes more endogenously guided (Dreher et al. 2002). The highest level of this control is exerted by (lateral) rostral PFC when the task rules must be derived from a previous episode (Koechlin et al. 2003). Significantly, Etienne Koechlin was also one of the first people to demonstrate a possible medial–lateral dissocia-tion in rostral PFC function, with a study that implicated medial rostral regions in situations where a subject encounters predictable sequences of stimuli, and lateral polar regions where the subject is performing tasks in sequences contingent upon unpredictable events (Koechlin, Corrado, Pietrini, & Grafman, 2000). (We will return to the issue of lateral–medial functional distinctions later.) Fletcher & Henson (2001) outline an anatomically-based variant, suggesting that rostral PFC operates with other (frontal) brain regions to effect cognitive control, "selecting between processes or goals (rather than between information maintained in WM and stored in LTM). It can also be viewed as another type of monitoring, in which it is the interaction between ventrolateral frontal cortex (VLFC) and dorsolateral frontal cortex (DLFC) processes that is being monitored rather than the information being maintained/manipulated *per se*" (p. 876).

4. *The default mode hypothesis*: This influential account relates specifically to medial rostral PFC, and is motivated by the repeated finding of decreases in activation of medial area 10 relative, usually, to rest, that are found when people perform a wide range of demanding cognitive tasks (Christoff, Ream, & Gabrieli, 2004; Gusnard & Raichle, 2001). Raichle et al. (2001) argue that "when an individual is awake and alert and yet not actively engaged in an attention-demanding task, a default state of brain activity exists that involves . . . the [medial prefrontal cortices] . . . Information broadly arising in the external and internal milieu is gathered and evaluated. When focused attention is required, particularly if this activity is novel, activity within these areas may be attenuated. This attenuation in activity reflects a necessary reduction in resources devoted to general information gathering and evaluation" (p. 682; see also Gusnard, Akbudak, Shulman, & Raichle, 2001; Raichle, 1998).

These hypotheses are all extremely useful, and represent a staggeringly fast advance in our state of knowledge compared with five years or so ago, when virtually no accounts existed. However whilst they all account for some aspects of the empirical data, each of them is incomplete in some respect. This incompleteness takes two forms. First, they typically attempt to either explain medial or lateral rostral PFC functions, but not both, despite suggestions that these regions may work as a functional unit (e.g. Burgess et al. 2003; Koechlin et al. 2000). Second they are incomplete in that they (a) fail to explain all the functional imaging data, and (b) encounter severe problems when it comes to explaining the data from human lesion studies. We will examine the latter challenge below. But let us first consider the incompleteness of these theories from the point of view of the functional imaging data.

We have already shown the episodic memory accounts to be only partial accounts of the totality of the data: BA 10 seems to be involved in the performance of tasks that have no particular episodic memory component. The metacognition accounts are also problematic on two grounds. First there is the confusion concerning the location of the critical area. Thus, for instance Christoff & Gabrieli (2000) refer only to *lateral* regions, yet Zysset, Huber, Ferstl, & Von Cramon (2002), for instance, refer to *medial* rostral PFC as critical for "metacontrol" processes (p. 989). Second, these accounts do not explain why activations in these regions can be seen during tasks which have little obvious "metacognitive" component (e.g. motor learning, eyeblink conditioning). One might perhaps also consider Rabbitt's (1997) criticism here: there is no clear specification of which we are aware of what constitutes a task requiring "metacognitive" processing. Thus there does seem to be some confusion. For instance, would all theorists agree that "Theory of Mind" should be considered a metacognitive process (see Frith, 2002; Zysset et al. 2002)?

The "Sum Process" accounts are also incomplete accounts of the evidence. Lateral BA 10 activations can be seen during quite straightforward tasks, which do not obviously make great demands upon two processes at once. For instance Belin et al. (2002) report BA 10 activations provoked by a simple paradigm involving the detection of sounds of infrequent duration. Additionally, strong BA 10 activations are not always accompanied by strong activations in other parts of the frontal lobes (e.g. Burgess et al. 2003) as the Fletcher & Henson (2001) hypothesis might suggest. Finally, the Default Mode Hypothesis is problematic in that medial rostral PFC activity can differ between conditions that have similar requirements for goal-directed attention (e.g. Zysset et al. 2002). Further data relevant to this point will be presented below.

The hypothesis that we later outline maintains that all of these accounts are however essentially correct in what they cover, and attempts to unify them with one simple hypothesis. But first, we need to consider the constraints the data provide, which can form the basis for theorizing about the functions of Area 10 in humans.

Rostral PFC function: from data to theory

Burgess, Gilbert, Okuda, & Simons (in press) surveyed the available literature and came to the following conclusions:

1 There is very little data concerning the putative functions of rostral PFC other than from functional imaging and a small number of human lesion studies.

2 Functional imaging data provides few constraints on theorizing because rostral PFC activation is found in such a wide variety of tasks.

3 Human lesion data rules out many aspects of the theories from functional imaging.

4 The most promising approach for functional imaging is therefore to start with the possible explanations emerging from lesion data.

5 Functional imaging studies that start from this base suggest that the role of rostral PFC is in the attentional control between stimulus-independent and stimulus-oriented thought.

For full support for these contentions, readers are referred to Burgess et al. (in press). We will, however, cover in brief here aspects of points 3 and 4 before summarizing the constraints from empirical data that we have applied to our theorizing, and outlining in much more detail than in Burgess et al. (in press) an integrative theory of the role of rostral PFC processes in human cognition.

Human lesion data provides valuable constraints for theorizing

As already noted, functional imaging experiments implicate BA 10 in the performance of a very wide range of tasks. One obvious expectation therefore might be that damage to this area in humans would cause impairment on a wide range of cognitive tasks. However the available evidence shows emphatically that this is *not* the case. Consider for instance case AP from Shallice & Burgess (1991a), who was called "NM" when he was investigated by Metzler & Parkin (2000). AP was involved in a serious road-traffic accident when he was in his early twenties, and sustained an open head injury, leading to virtually complete removal of the rostral PFC. However on standard neuropsychological measures of intellectual functioning, memory, perception and even traditional tests of executive function, AP performs within the superior range (see Wood & Rutterford, 2004 for further evidence).

This is not however to say that AP was unimpaired in other regards (Metzler & Parkin, 2000; Shallice & Burgess, 1991a; Wood & Rutterford, 2004). The most noticeable impairment in everyday life was a marked multitasking problem. This manifested itself as tardiness and disorganization, the severity of which ensured that despite his excellent intellect and social skills, he never managed to make a return to work at the level he had enjoyed premorbidly. Shallice & Burgess (1991a) invented two new tests of multitasking to assess these problems. One was a real-life multitasking test based around a shopping exercise, the "Multiple Errands Test," and the second a multitasking test for use in the laboratory or clinic, the "Six Element Test." Despite excellent general cognitive skills, AP and the other cases reported by Shallice and Burgess all performed these tasks below the 5% level compared with age- and IQ-matched controls.

There are now a number of cases reported in the literature who show similar everyday behavioural impairments (see Burgess, 2000 for review) and there is a remarkably consistent finding of involvement of Area 10 amongst them. For instance, in the six cases reviewed by Burgess, all of them had rostral PFC involvement of either the left or right hemispheres (or both). Moreover, all cases to whom the Shallice/Burgess multitasking tests have been administered have failed at least one of them. In addition to these cases, we might now also add the recent case GT described by Bird, Castelli, Malik, Frith, & Husain (2004) who failed the Six Element Test.

Not only is there congruence in the tasks that patients with rostral damage fail, but there is congruence in the tasks that they pass. Most importantly, the data from single cases whose lesions invade rostral PFC (Bird et al. 2004; Eslinger & Damasio, 1985; Goldstein, Bernard, Fenwick, Burgess, & McNeil, 1993; Goel & Grafman, 2000; Shallice & Burgess, 1991a) categorically show that rostral PFC lesions need *not* cause impairments on a wide range of tests of executive function, such as the Wisconsin Card Sorting Test (Grant & Berg, 1948), the Tower of London planning test (and its variants; Shallice, 1982), the Cognitive Estimates Test (Shallice & Evans, 1978) or Stroop paradigms (see Figure 9.1).

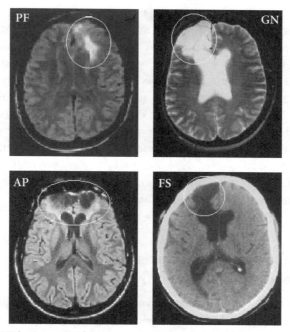

Fig. 9.1 MRI/CT brain scans of four neurological patients with rostral prefrontal damage. All patients achieved superior scores on IQ tests, and all achieved excellent scores on traditional executive tasks such as the Wisconsin Card Sorting and Verbal Fluency tests. However they all showed significant behavioural organization problems in everyday life. (PF: Goel Grafman, 2000; GN: Goldstein et al. 1993; AP and FS: Shallice & Burgess, 1991a. Site of rostral lesions are circled. The lesions are different colours because of their differing pathologies and the different methods used to image them. Some scans have been left-right transposed from the originals for ease of understanding, for example, left hemisphere is on the left of figure etc.)

Of course anatomical-behavioural associations made on the grounds of data from single case studies should be treated with caution, since individual cases might be anatomically atypical. However two recent group human lesion studies also convincingly demonstrate that patients with rostral PFC damage do *not* necessarily have widespread cognitive deficits. Thus Burgess et al. (2000) examined a series of 60 acute neurological patients (approximately three-quarters of whom were suffering from brain tumors) and 60 age- and IQ-matched healthy controls on a multitasking test called the Greenwich Test. In this test, subjects are presented with three different simple tasks and told that they have to attempt at least some of each of the tasks in 10 min, while following a set of rules. Despite being able to learn the task rules, form a plan, remember their actions, and say what they should have done, patients with left hemisphere rostral lesions showed a significant multitasking impairment: they were able to perform the individual subtasks perfectly well, but tended not to switch tasks, and when they did, showed a problem following the rules of the other tasks.

A further recent human group lesion study underlines these results (Burgess et al. submitted). In this study, a new version of the Burgess et al. (1996) Six Element Test (SET) of multitasking was given to sixty-nine acute neurological patients with circumscribed focal lesions and sixty healthy controls, using the administration framework of Burgess et al. (2000). The SET differs from the Greenwich Test in that there are more subtasks that have to be attempted (six rather than three), and fewer rules to follow. Compared with other patients, those whose lesions involved the rostral prefrontal regions of the right hemisphere made significantly fewer voluntary task switches, attempted fewer subtasks, and spent far longer on individual subtasks. They did not however make more rule-breaks.

Using human lesion data as a starting point for functional imaging studies

In this laboratory we have taken the constraints presented by human lesion data as a starting point for our functional imaging studies. The multitasking failures in our patients could be characterized as reflecting difficulty with carrying out delayed intentions (i.e. "prospective memory"; Brandimonte, Einstein, & McDaniel, 1996; see also Duncan, Emslie, Williams, Johnson, & Freer, 1996). Prospective memory (PM) tasks differ from working memory tasks principally in that they involve performance of an ongoing task during the delay period, which prevents continuous rehearsal (see Burgess et al. 2001 for a full description of PM task characteristics). The initial step toward understanding multitasking failures was therefore to investigate the brain regions involved in PM tasks as indicated by functional imaging. In the first study, Burgess et al. (2001) used PET to investigate regional cerebral blood flow changes in eight participants performing four different tasks, each under three conditions. The first condition (baseline) was subject-paced, and consisted of making judgments about two objects appearing together (e.g. which of two digits is the largest, or which of two letters comes nearer the start of the alphabet). The second condition consisted of the baseline task, but subjects were also told that if a particular combination of stimuli appeared (e.g. two vowels, two even numbers) they were to respond in a different way (press a particular key combination). However, in this condition ("expectation") none of these stimuli actually appeared. In the third condition participants were given the same instructions and stimuli as in the first, except that the expected PM stimuli did occur (after a delay, and on 20% of trials), and participants had the chance to respond to them ("execution" condition). In the terminology of prospective memory researchers, the last two conditions were PM conditions in that they involved a delayed intention (see Burgess et al. 2001 for an outline of the further characteristics of PM tasks).

Relative to the baseline condition, rCBF increases across the four tasks were seen in the frontal pole (BA 10) bilaterally when the participants were expecting to see a stimulus, even though it did not occur. There were no further increases in this region when the intention cues were seen and acted upon. This result corresponded well with that of Okuda et al. (1998), who were the first people to demonstrate a role for BA 10 in prospective memory using functional imaging. Thus there seems to be both within- and cross-method support for a role of BA 10 in PM functions. And the Burgess et al. (2001) study suggests that this role is material and stimulus nonspecific, and probably involved more with maintenance than execution of the delayed intention.

However, one possible explanation for the Burgess et al. (2001) findings is that the activations seen in the expectation condition could be due to task difficulty or increased stimulus processing demands rather than anything to do with delayed intentions *per se*. This hypothesis was examined in a second PET experiment (Burgess et al. 2003). Three different tasks were administered under four conditions: baseline simple RT; attention-demanding ongoing task only; ongoing task plus "unpracticed" delayed intention (i.e. the first block of this condition); ongoing task plus "practiced" delayed intention (i.e. the second block of this condition). Under prospective memory conditions, Burgess et al. (2003) found significant rCBF decreases in the superior medial aspects of the rostral prefrontal cortex (BA 10) relative to the baseline or ongoing task only conditions. However, more lateral aspects of area 10 (plus the medio-dorsal thalamus) showed the opposite pattern, with rCBF increases in the prospective memory conditions relative to the other conditions, with lowest rCBF in the ongoing task . These patterns were broadly replicated over all three tasks. Since both the medial and lateral rostral regions showed (a) instances where rCBF was higher in a *less* effortful condition (as estimated by RTs and error rates), and (b) there was no correlation between rCBF and RT durations or number of errors in these regions, a simple task difficulty explanation of the rCBF changes in the rostral aspects of the frontal lobes during PM tasks was rejected. Instead, the favored explanation concentrated upon the particular processing demands made by these situations irrespective of the precise stimuli used or the exact nature of the intention, in particular the requirement to hold a thought in mind (i.e. stimulus-independent thought) whilst carrying out other operations on the presented stimuli.

Constraints for theorizing about the role of rostral PFC in cognition

The data that we have reviewed so far provide some constraints on theorizing about the functions of rostral PFC. Specifically, we will take the phenomena listed in Tables 9.1 and 9.2 as a bare minimum of those for which a theory of rostral PFC function should account. The list is however: (a) far from being a complete summary of the findings that need to be explained; (b) partisan in that it favors findings from our own lab and emphasises results which show relative medial/lateral differences; and (c) a somewhat unrealistic view in that it ignores concomitant changes in other brain regions, which may be theoretically instructive. One also needs to make the caveat, in considering the imaging findings, that in most neuroimaging experiments stimuli are presented visually, with responses made manually or verbally. Thus the relationship with situations using other stimuli/response forms is not well-established.

Bearing in mind these caveats, however, we will proceed with the currently available evidence (or at least the evidence of which we are aware: we would be very interested in hearing from researchers who have further evidence which can add to, or modify the content of this list, or the supporting citations). Please note that for the sake of completeness, findings FI(g), (o), and (p) are included in Table 9.2, even though they actually emerged from our testing of the theory, which was originally derived with the other constraints listed in Table 9.2 in mind.

Implications of these constraints

Human lesion (HL) study point (A) removes the possibility that rostral PFC plays a *critical* role in the over-learned cognitive processing of specialized

Table 9.1 Constraints for theorizing about rostral PFC function derived from human lesion (HL) studies

A. Rostral PFC lesions need not markedly impair performance on standard tests of intelligence, especially those that measure "crystallized" intelligence (e.g. Burgess, 2000; Goel & Grafman, 2000; Shallice & Burgess, 1991a), or those involving the use of over-learned procedures (e.g. arithmetic).

B. Rostral PFC lesions need not impair simple episodic memory functions such as forced-choice recognition (Burgess, 2000; Goel & Grafman, 2000; Burgess, Veitch, & Costello, submitted).

C. Medial rostral PFC lesions need not cause impairments on "Theory of Mind" tasks (Bird et al. 2004).

D. Rostral PFC lesions do not necessarily cause impairments on many (structured) traditional tests of executive function, such as the Tower of London test (Shallice, 1982), Stroop paradigms, WCST, Verbal Fluency (e.g. Burgess, 2000; Goel & Grafman, 2000). Importantly however, people with lesions that *include* rostral damage but also extend elsewhere may often show impairments on some of these tests (and others), e.g. Burgess, Veitch, & Costello, submitted; Stuss et al. 1998, 2000).

E. However it seems likely that rostral PFC lesions *do* cause disruption of episodic memory functions which have a high meta-cognitive component (see Burgess & Shallice, 1996), such as initial learning of complex rules (Alexander, Stuss, & Fansabedian, 2003; Burgess, Veitch, & Costello, submitted; see also Strange et al. 2001 for congruent findings from functional imaging), and cause abnormal priming and false positive effects (e.g. Metzler & Parkin, 2000).

F. Rostral PFC lesions disproportionately impair performance in "ill-structured" situations (e.g. Burgess et al. 2001; Goel & Grafman, 2000; Grafman, 2002). In other words where the optimal way of behaving is not precisely signalled by the situation, so one has to impose one's own structure.

G. Rostral PFC lesions impair multitasking, both in the laboratory and in everyday life (e.g. Burgess et al. 1998, 2000; Burgess, Veitch, & Costello, submitted).

systems (e.g. semantic memory, calculation, reading), and HL(D) suggests that rostral PFC processes are not critical for dealing with novel situations where performance parameters are easily determined, for example, where the demands of the task are well-specified by the task instructions, and moment-by-moment feedback occurs (in the sense that it is quite obvious when one has made a mistake, or is performing poorly). The corollary is given by findings HL(F) and HL(G): Rostral PFC would seem to be most involved in situations for which there is not a well-rehearsed or well-specified way of behaving, and therefore where behavioural organization needs to be self-determined. These points support the suggestion of Dreher et al. (2002), on grounds of functional imaging data, of a posterior-to-anterior organization of PFC as tasks become more "endogenously guided." They also need to be balanced alongside the functional imaging (FI) finding (e), which argues

Table 9.2 Constraints for theorizing about rostral PFC (area 10) function from functional brain imaging (FI)

Rostral PFC	
a	Is not sensitive to the precise nature of stimuli (e.g. whether they are words, numbers, shapes, etc., see, for example, Burgess et al. 2001, 2003).
b	Is not sensitive to the precise nature of intended action (in prospective memory tasks, see Burgess et al. 2001, 2003).
c	Is not sensitive to precise response method (Burgess et al. 2001, 2003).
d	Is consistently implicated in tasks where one has to "bear something in mind" whilst doing something else, for example, voluntary task switching after a delay (e.g. Koechlin et al. 1999), prospective memory (Burgess et al. 2001, 2003; Okuda et al. 1998), and "monitoring" type tasks (e.g. MacLeod et al., 1998).
e	Haemodynamic changes in rostral PFC occur in a very wide variety of situations (e.g. Burgess et al. in press; Grady, 1999; MacLeod et al. 1998)
f	Rostral PFC activations are not necessarily concomitant with recognizing experienced events (Burgess et al. in press; Herron, Henson, & Rugg, 2004).
g	But do occur when one is remembering the thoughts one had about those events (Simons et al. in press a; in press b).
h	Activation in rostral PFC regions may be unrelated to "task difficulty," at least as it is indexed by changes in RTs and errors on a task (Burgess, Scott, & Frith, 2003; Gilbert et al. in press).
Lateral Rostral	
i	Lateral rostral regional cerebral blood flow (rCBF) increases can occur when targets are expected but not actually experienced (Burgess, Quayle, & Frith, 2001).
j	Lateral rostral PFC is sensitive to target frequencies or distributions (Herron et al. 2004; Okuda et al. in preparation).
k	Lateral rostral regions show increased activation in situations requiring the recollection or manipulation of the products of previous processing (Burgess, Dumontheil, Gilbert, Simons, & Frith, in preparation; Christoff et al. 2003; Simons et al. in press a, in press b).
Medial Rostral	
l	Medial rostral regions do *not* show easily predictable blood oxygen dependent (BOLD) responses to routinization or practice (Burgess, Scott, & Frith, 2003).
m	Medial rostral regions often show decreased activation in conditions that require goal-directed thought (Raichle, 1998; Raichle et al. 2001)
n	Medial rostral regions show BOLD increases associated with attending to stimuli in the external world (Janata et al. 2002; Small et al. 2003).
o	Medial rostral regions show BOLD increases when participants are viewing stimuli rather than imagining them (Gilbert, Frith, & Burgess, in press).
p	Medial rostral regions (relative to lateral rostral regions) show activations in conditions which require attention to external stimuli but "shallow" processing of them (Burgess, Dumontheil, Gilbert, Simons, & Frith, in preparation; Gilbert, Frith, & Burgess, in press; Gilbert, Simons, Frith, & Burgess, submitted).
q	Some medial rostral regions may show BOLD increases in a variety of situations that require stimulus-provoked introspection, such as recalling past thoughts one had about a stimulus when re-presented with it, or even thinking about the future when prompted to (Okuda et al. 2003; Simons et al. in press a, in press b; see also Zysset et al. 2002).

against a very task-specific interpretation (although there will be specific tasks which stress the processes supported by rostral PFC). This suggests that "rostral processes" (as we will refer to the cognitive processes, which are supported at least in part by the anterior parts of the PFC) operate at a "meta-representational" level, in other words are not tied tightly to one form or domain of representation (e.g. words, numbers, shapes, faces, actions, etc.). Support for this view comes also from findings HL(E), FI(a), (b), (c), (i), (l) and (m).

Thus the characterization of the rostral processing system as cross-domain (Burgess et al. 2003) and serving the purpose of guiding behaviour in situations where the optimal course of action is not obvious or established (Burgess, 2000; Goel & Grafman, 2000; Pollman, 2004) seems secure. This view is consistent with both that of Fletcher & Henson (2001) and Christoff and colleagues (e.g. Christoff, Ream, Geddes, & Gabrieli, 2003). Fletcher and Henson echo the suggestion by McIntosh (1999) that the role of BA 10 in cognition is governed by its interactions with anatomically related regions. More specifically, they suggest that anterior PFC controls ventrolateral PFC (VLPFC) and dorsolateral PFC (DLPFC) processes, and that its role is to select between processes or goals: "if VLPFC and DLPFC form a functional unit concerned with updating/maintenance and selection/manipulation/monitoring, respectively, then perhaps controlling influences from AFC (anterior frontal cortex) regions enable optimal switching between these processes in order to maximise task performance." (p. 876).

It is important to note at this stage that these views contain strong implicit views of how the cognitive system might operate, or be organized. Thus, there is the inherent assumption that some brain processing is "stimulus-independent" (McGuire et al. 1996) and therefore that some is stimulus-dependent. This is a critical distinction, which is adopted in the forthcoming characterization of rostral PFC processes.

Findings HL(B) and HL(C) together make it unlikely, however, that the role of rostral PFC is simply to support the "tonic" or "steady" state of either stimulus-oriented (SOT) or stimulus-independent thought (SIT), because lesions in this area need not impair performance on simple forced-choice recognition or Theory of Mind tasks: the former are by definition stimulus-oriented in form and "theory of mind" tasks require some component of stimulus-independent thought in that one has to consider possibilities not directly signalled by the current stimuli (see also finding FI(f)). Nevertheless, Findings FI(n), (o), and (p) do suggest that, in a number of situations, medial rostral PFC can be involved in stimulus-oriented (as contrasted with *goal-directed*) processing. Furthermore, finding FI(d) could be interpreted as suggesting a role for rostral PFC, especially for lateral BA 10, in stimulus-independent thought, since these experiments require subjects to maintain a thought in the face of potentially competing stimuli.

One possible resolution that potentially fits these findings obtains in particular from the situations provoking finding FI(d), but also HL(F) and (G). These are nonroutine situations, where one has to formulate a way of behaving, or "create a new schema" in the terminology of the Shallice and Burgess model, beyond that directly signalled by the stimuli (see Burgess, 1997 for an outline of the role of novelty in executive function). It was therefore at this point that our thinking turned to investigating formally the possible role of rostral PFC in the contrast between stimulus-independent and stimulus-oriented thought, and the switching between these states specifically in novel situations. These investigations led to findings FI (g), (h), (j), (k), (o), (p), and (q). We will now outline the general specification of the hypothesis that spawned these investigations, and then the empirical evidence used to test it.

The gateway hypothesis: model specification

Basic assumptions

We make three basic assumptions, which should be fairly uncontroversial for most cognitive neuroscientists. (1) At an information processing level, the cognitive system is composed of modules specialized for certain functions. (2) The cognitive system is arranged as a functional hierarchy for much complex novel behaviour, that is, that process A operates upon the products of the previously active process B. (3) "Thought" (i.e. the instantiation of mental representations) may occur without influence from neuronal activity provoked directly by stimuli external to the body.

Given these assumptions, we then adopt the general information processing framework outlined by Norman & Shallice (1980, 1986), and later expanded by Shallice and colleagues (e.g. Burgess et al. 2000; Shallice, 1988, 2002; Shallice & Burgess, 1991b, 1993, 1996; Stuss, Shallice, Alexander, & Picton, 1995).

A full description of this well-established theoretical framework is beyond the scope of the present chapter. However in brief, Shallice's Supervisory Attentional System theory is concerned with the role of the frontal lobes in the allocation of processing resources (Shallice, 1988) and describes a theory of behavioural organization and adaptation. There are four levels of increasing organization in this theory. The first level consists of "cognitive or action units," which correspond to basic abilities (e.g. reaching for an object, reading a word). The second level consists of "schemata." These are nests of cognitive or action units that have come to be closely associated through repetition. The third level is a process called "contention scheduling." This is the basic triggering interface between incoming stimuli, including thoughts, and the schemata. Its purpose is to effect the quick selection of routine behaviours in well-known situations. However of course many situations (or aspects of them) that we encounter are not well rehearsed. In this situation one has to decide consciously what one has to do. The cognitive system that effects this conscious deliberation is referred to as the "supervisory attentional system" (SAS), and processing critical to the function of this capacity is thought to be underpinned by structures in the PFC. More recent work has attempted to provide a finer level of specification of this model (Burgess et al. 2000; Shallice, 2002; Shallice & Burgess, 1996, 1998; Stuss et al. 1995).

The account developed below expands upon this model, by supposing that the information processing system supported at least in part by rostral PFC effects the biasing of the schemata operated upon by the contention scheduling process in two ways: (a) by biasing the relative activation of schemata in situations of low triggering input and also (b) by increasing the relative activation levels of schemata which are not currently receiving input via sensory input systems, in accordance with a higher-level goal representation. Thus the overall function of the system is to enable mental behaviour in situations where (1) no schema is sufficiently triggered by incoming stimuli (e.g. because there is no established way of behaving, the stimulus is entirely novel, or activation levels have reached asymptote) or (2) too many schema are being simultaneously activated (e.g. in a very difficult complex situation, or one where there are very many possible established behaviours without an obvious advantage to one of them).

The gateway hypothesis: specific proposals

In this way, we suggest that rostral PFC plays a role in the goal-directed *co-ordination* of SIT and SOT in situations where the established or predominant way of behaving would not achieve optimal outcome.

The stimulus-oriented and stimulus-independent distinction

All cognition can be classified as either stimulus-oriented, stimulus-independent, or more commonly perhaps, a combination of the two (often working together in different phases). By stimulus-oriented, we mean either *provoked by* something being experienced through the senses, or *oriented toward* something to be experienced through the senses. Examples of stimulus-provoked cognition are obvious (e.g. reading). Stimulus-oriented cognition is where one's attention is oriented toward input from the senses (or one of them), but there is an absence of the stimulus itself (e.g. a state of "watchfulness" or "readiness"). The precise relationship between stimulus-provoked and stimulus-oriented cognition is a moot point. But to simplify terminology, in the foregoing argument we will use the more general term "stimulus-oriented" to refer to any cognition, which is provoked by or oriented toward stimuli external to the body. This form can be contrasted with stimulus-independent thought, which is any cognition that has not been provoked by, or directed toward, an external stimulus. An obvious example is daydreaming or "zoning-out," but one might also include some forms of unprovoked rumination, introspection, or creative thought and the like.

As already stated, many examples of cognition lasting more than a few milliseconds will include aspects of both stimulus-oriented and stimulus-independent thought. For instance, remembering, in response to a question, a complex autobiographical event that occurred some time ago has aspects of stimulus-oriented cognition in that it is provoked by the stimulus question and is oriented toward that stimulus (e.g. to answer the question). Yet it also has a stimulus-independent component (the actual reconstruction of the memory; see Burgess & Shallice, 1996). In this way, it is most helpful perhaps to see these *in practice* as classificatory dimensions rather than absolutes.

Since there is only one set of central cognitive representations, there will be continuous attentional competition between SIT and SOT for activation of those representations. In many situations the relative attentional bias is determined automatically. For instance, a sudden unexpected stimulus will naturally "capture" attention, as would an expected stimulus congruent with the currently active goals which has a strong S–R relation (i.e. a sum if one were performing a mental arithmetic test). However in the absence of external stimuli, or where monotony has been achieved, SIT will tend to dominate (e.g. one's "mind will tend to wander"). SIT should also dominate when it is not obvious how one should behave (e.g. "ill-structured" situations); or where cognitive capacity has been exceeded to the point where behaviour starts to break down (e.g. one starts to notice a large number of errors and ruminative (i.e. self-generated) thoughts ensue).

As a first hypothesis, for the sake of parsimony, we do not suppose that rostral PFC plays any direct part in the actual information transformations involved in either stimulus-independent or oriented thought, but merely acts as a routing system, determining whether it is the outputs of current (internal) processing or input from currently available (new) stimuli, which will be the focus of further processing by the cognitive system. A simple analogy might be a railway track switch-point, where we imagine the train as representing packets of information within the brain, and the tracks as the pathways that carry that information. The switch-point will have no influence upon the train itself (i.e. does not effect an information transformation), but merely determines the direction of the flow. In this analogy, one "track" governed by the switch-point may lead back to the specialist regions from which the information came, and another governs the flow of information to and from basic input/output systems (e.g. visual processing, motor effector systems, speech and language systems, etc.) via central representations.

In a model of this type, there would be competition for activation of central representations between the two pathways (i.e. either input to central representations from more basic systems or reciprocal activation from currently active central representations), and much of cognition could occur naturally through this competition without influence from the processes supported by rostral PFC (including much "thought," for example, that required to generate a new plan, solve a crossword problem, etc.). It would only be when either one pathway needs to be consistently *biased*, or when there needs to be rapid switching between the bias of the two that influence from the "switch-point" would be needed (see Figure 9.2). This biasing would typically occur in situations that are novel or where a specific demand for it has been determined (e.g. "I must pay special attention to . . ."; "I must think about . . ."). It will also

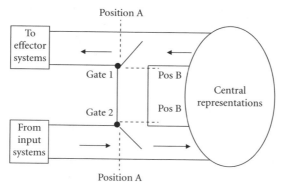

Fig. 9.2 Stylised representation of the "Gateway Hypothesis, Version 1.1" of rostral prefrontal function. Rostral regions are hypothesised to support a system, which biases the flow of information between basic systems and central representations (i.e. is equivalent to the adjustment of the position of the "Gates"). The gates are shown in the neutral position (= bias freely determined by context). If both gates are at position A, stimulus-independent thought is favored. If both gates are at position B, full engagement with (external) stimuli is effected. Other combinations have further experiential correlates, especially when one considers dynamic, moment-by-moment switching: part of the purpose of the diagram is to make the point that even a very simple switch system could effect a range of mental activity.

be used in spontaneous solution generation—perhaps, for example, the unprovoked thought "is there a better way of doing this?". In this way, this system is an important component of the "supervisory attentional system" (Shallice & Burgess, 1996). We assume, however, that much of the actual processing required in novel situations to determine a new course of action requires the additional operation of other prefrontal control systems (and the systems they control).

Direct empirical support for the gateway hypothesis

We have recently conducted a series of experiments, which lend support to this overall framework. These studies consistently find that areas of rostral PFC are involved in co-ordinating attention between externally-presented and internally-represented information.

Experiment 1: Evidence for the involvement of rostral PFC in switching between stimulus-independent and stimulus-oriented thought.
Gilbert, Frith, and Burgess (in press) asked subjects to perform three separate tasks in two conditions whilst undergoing functional magnetic resonance imaging (fMRI). In one condition subjects had to respond to stimuli presented visually, in the other subjects had to do the same tasks "in their heads." In task A, subjects tapped a response button in time with a visually-presented clock, or ignored the visual display (which now presented distracting information) and continued to tap at the same rate as before. Task B required subjects to navigate around the edge of a visually-presented shape, or to imagine the same shape and continue navigating as before. In task C, subjects performed a classification task on letters of the alphabet that followed a regular sequence. They either classified visually-presented letters, or mentally continued the sequence and classified the letters that they generated internally. Thus all three tasks alternated between phases where subjects attended to externally-presented information, and phases where they ignored this information and attended to internally-represented information instead. We investigated both the sustained neural activity that differed between two phases, and transient activity at the point of a switch between these two phases. Consistently, across all three tasks, medial rostral PFC exhibited sustained activity that differed between the two phases, in all three cases showing greater activity when subjects attended to externally-presented information. By contrast, right lateral rostral PFC exhibited transient activity when subjects switched between these phases, regardless of the direction of the switch (see Figure 9.3). This dissociation between medial and lateral rostral PFC regions was confirmed statistically in all three tasks. Thus, the results of the study strongly support the hypothesis that rostral PFC

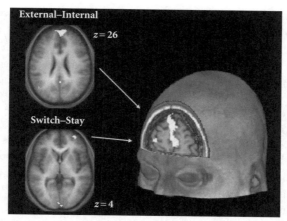

Fig. 9.3 Rostral brain regions identified as involved more in doing a task using stimuli one can currently see rather than doing the same task in one's head only (upper left-hand panel), and in switching between doing a task "in one's head" and doing the same task using stimuli one can currently see (the "Switch-Stay" contrast, lower panel).

supports selection between externally- and internally-oriented cognitive processes, and suggest dissociable roles of medial and lateral rostral PFC in this selection process.

Experiment 2: Medial rostral PFC is most active in low demand attentional situations.

In a follow-up study (Gilbert, Simons, Frith, & Burgess, submitted), we replicated the finding of greater medial rostral PFC activity during attention to externally-presented versus internally-represented information. In addition, however, we found that activity in this region was correlated on a trial-by-trial basis with faster reaction times (i.e. a negative correlation) in a simple-reaction-time (SRT) baseline task. This finding is important for two reasons. First, it rules out an explanation of the activity we observe in medial rostral PFC in terms of "daydreaming" during simple tasks. If this were the case, greater medial rostral PFC activity (and hence the occurrence of daydreaming) would reflect disengagement from the baseline task, and should show a positive correlation with RT. Second, this finding helps to constrain theorizing on the functional role of this brain region. By demonstrating that rostral medial PFC activity correlates with better performance in a SRT baseline task, we can point to a task requiring focussed attention (in this case, focussed attention toward intermittent visual targets) to which medial rostral PFC makes a functional contribution (see also Stuss et al. 2005, for evidence from a human lesion study). Thus, contrary to the default mode hypothesis (Raichle, 1998;

Raichle et al. 2001), it does not seem that any task requiring focussed attention will lead to "deactivation" of this area. Rather, we propose that this region plays a specific role in particular types of focussed attention tasks (i.e. deliberate biasing of attention toward externally-presented or internally-represented information), which it may also play during the state of conscious rest.

Experiment 3a and 3b: Evidence for the role of rostral PFC in stimulus-independent thought.
The suggestion from the studies of findings FI(d), (i) and (k) is that rostral PFC, especially lateral rostral PFC, plays a role in SIT. One example of a situation that involves SIT is where one is remembering the thoughts one had about a stimulus previously experienced (rather than the stimulus itself) or remembering other details of the context in which the stimulus was encountered. Simons, Owen, Fletcher, and Burgess (in press a) investigated this area of human cognition, with particular reference to understanding the anomaly that some functional imaging experiments of contextual recollection observed activation in BA 10 (e.g. Dobbins, Foley, Schacter, & Wagner, 2002; Rugg, Fletcher, Chua, & Dolan, 1999) whereas others did not (e.g. Henson, Shallice, & Dolan, 1999; Nyberg et al. 1996). One possible explanation is that the studies which did find BA 10 activation involved recollecting which of two tasks was undertaken with target items: "task context," whereas the other studies focused on externally-derived features of context (e.g. recollecting the position on a monitor screen where target items were presented: "position context").

Simons et al. (in press a) investigated the possibility that BA 10 might be differentially involved in recollecting internally-generated versus externally-derived contextual information by contrasting directly the recollection of task context and position context within participants. They observed a functional dissociation within rostral PFC, with lateral regions associated with recollection of both task- and position-based contextual details and a more medial region showing significantly greater activation during recollection of task context than position context. This lateral versus medial dissociation was apparent regardless of whether words or famous faces were being remembered, reinforcing the idea that the region is involved in central, stimulus-independent executive control processes (see findings FI(a)–(c)), and was unrelated to task difficulty as estimated by accuracy and reaction time. These findings show remarkable concordance with the regions identified as showing BOLD changes in prospective memory paradigms by Burgess et al. (2001, 2003; see Figure 9.4).

A follow-up study was conducted to contrast recollection of task context with another example of contextual detail—remembering the temporal context in which stimuli were presented (Simons, Gilbert, Owen, Fletcher, & Burgess, in press b). The principal results were very similar to those from

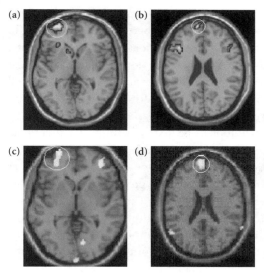

Fig. 9.4 Remarkable agreement between functional imaging method and study. Panels (a) and (b) show the rostral PFC regions identified as important for source memory using fMRI by Simons et al. (in press a). Panels (c) and (d) show the rostral brain regions identified as showing activation changes in prospective memory tasks using PET, by Burgess et al. (2001, 2003).

the previous experiment. Regions in lateral and medial rostral PFC were associated with significantly greater activation during task context than time context recollection. Just as before, the rostral PFC regions were not stimulus-specific, and were unrelated to task difficulty. An interesting further question concerned the stage of the retrieval process during which rostral PFC might be recruited: pre-retrieval cue specification or post-retrieval monitoring and verification, for example (Burgess & Shallice, 1996; Simons & Spiers, 2003). Simons et al. (in press b) addressed this question by presenting some retrieval cues (indicating whether the upcoming trial would involve task or time context recollection) on their own, without accompanying target stimuli. During such trials, which might be considered to involve pre-retrieval processes but no retrieval search or post-retrieval monitoring, significant activation was observed in the same lateral rostral PFC region that was associated with recollection of both task and time context, indicating that the role played by this region may be in pre-retrieval cue specification processes (see also Ranganath & Paller, 2000, for a similar view). Medial rostral PFC activation was not observed in this contrast, suggesting a role for this region in processes occurring after presentation of the target stimulus (e.g. relating to retrieval search or monitoring of retrieved information). This view was corroborated by evidence from timecourse analysis, in which activation in medial rostral PFC peaked significantly later than that in the more lateral region. In this way, the results echo strongly those of Gilbert et al. described above, in which activation in medial rostral PFC was also found to occur when coordinated attention between external stimuli and internal thoughts was required.

Experiment 4: Stimulus-oriented and stimulus-independent thought contrasted.
In a fourth experiment (Burgess, Dumontheil, Gilbert, Simons, and Frith, in preparation) we aimed to contrast directly the conditions which in Experiment 2 we had found to provoke medial BA 10 activations (low-demand attention to external stimuli) with the suggestion from Experiments 3a and 3b that lateral rostral PFC is involved in stimulus-independent processing (see also Christoff et al. 2003). In this fMRI experiment, two different tasks (numerical or spatial) were administered under four conditions. The first was a simple RT attentional baseline (press the left/right button on alternate trials as fast as you can each time a stimulus appears). The second made the same attentional demands as condition 1, but also required some basic stimulus processing (e.g. "press the button on the side of the largest of two numbers"). The third condition made the same demands as conditions 1 and 2 but additionally introduced a requirement of processing self-generated information. For instance, for the numbers task, participants were asked if the sum of two numbers currently being presented to them was larger or smaller than the sum of the last two numbers presented. Clearly however, this condition not only makes demands on processing self-generated information, but also requires Ss to remember information from one display to another. Therefore we had a fourth condition, which was a control for these demands. For instance, in the numerical task, participants were asked if the number on the left of the screen was larger or smaller than the number on the left of the previous screen. The results were as predicted by the Gateway Hypothesis: an area of medial BA 10 was more active in condition 1 (basic attention to external stimuli, no stimulus processing) than in condition 3 (stimulus-independent thought) as previously discovered (see experiment 2). And an area of lateral rostral PFC was more active in condition 3 compared with condition two (stimulus processing). Overall, the brain region by condition interaction was significant at $p < 0.001$. Moreover, the lateral BA 10 finding could not be due to the "working memory" or rehearsal demands of the task, since activation in this region was significantly greater in condition 3 than in condition 4 (although we do not contend that rehearsal has no SIT component whatsoever).

The gateway hypothesis and the medial *vs.* lateral rostral PFC distinction

The results of this series of studies strongly support a role of rostral PFC in co-ordinating internally- and externally-oriented information. There is also strong evidence for functional dissociations between medial versus lateral rostral PFC across a number of tasks (see also Burgess et al. 2003; Koechlin et al. 2000).

However the precise operating dynamics of this system have yet to be determined. There are many possibilities that will need to be resolved both conceptually and experimentally. For instance we have characterized on the basis of our experiments a function of medial BA 10 as "biasing attention toward current sensory input," and that of lateral BA 10 as being concerned with "biasing attention toward internally generated thought." For the most part we have contrasted these two functions. Yet since the purpose of both is to modulate the activity of currently selected schemata, there seems no need to exclude the possibility that both "streams" could work in concert in some situations. It is possible to conceive of such situations, but this possibility remains largely untested. Another possible avenue of enquiry concerns the possible U–shaped function for rostral PFC function that emerges from our characterization. According to this hypothesis SIT could be provoked on the one hand by a lack of stimulating input (e.g. one's mind wandering whilst performing a monotonous task) or on the other by too much sensory input (e.g. performing a very difficult task where one is making mistakes and starts to ruminate on one's failures). There are many other fascinating dynamic aspects which also remain to be discovered.

Summary

This chapter presents a new information processing hypothesis of rostral PFC function, and some empirical supporting evidence. The framework makes a distinction between stimulus-oriented (i.e. provoked by, or directed toward) and stimulus-independent thought, and suggests that rostral PFC acts as a "gateway," which biases the priority of information from each stream. The strength of this hypothesis is that it is a framework that (a) makes a small number of assumptions; (b) makes predictions that are more readily testable empirically than alternative theories; and (c) introduces a potentially unifying explanation of the previous findings involving both medial and lateral rostral PFC that is independent of "task difficulty." The account is in this sense a synthesis of the excellent previous work by, in particular, Kalina Christoff, Etienne Koechlin, Marcus Raichle, Vinod Goel, Jordan Grafman, Chris Frith, Don Stuss, and their colleagues, using a simple proposal to explain how these quite different previous accounts might be linked. We do not, however, suppose that we have as yet achieved anything like a full specification of how the rostral PFC system works. Indeed, we have pointed out some aspects of our own data which whilst very broadly fitting the overall framework, nevertheless test our knowledge of the dynamics of the system in certain situations, in particular the exact relative roles of the medial and lateral rostral PFC regions. For this reason, the hypothesis presented here has been termed "version 1.1." We will update these versions as progress allows.

If the "gateway hypothesis" is correct, it makes interesting predictions about the potential involvement of this brain region in psychological or psychiatric disorders. Thus one might suppose that some forms of dysfunction of a mechanism of this kind might contribute to an inability to distinguish between one's thoughts and one's experiences, which could be a plausible partial account of hallucinatory phenomena in schizophrenia. Similarly for instance, an account using this framework could be constructed for symptoms linked to unwanted (intrusive) thoughts. These speculations remain to be tested. For the moment, we have attempted to address a critical issue for our understanding of how the brain operates, and do so taking full heed of Pat Rabbitt's sage words.

References

Alexander, M. P., Stuss, D. T., & Fansabedian, N. (2003). California verbal learning test: Performance by patients with focal frontal and non-frontal lesions. *Brain*, **126**, 1493–1503.

Baker, S. C., Rogers, R. D., Owen, A. M., Frith, C. D., Dolan, R. J., Frackowiak, R. S. J., et al. (1996). Neural systems engaged by planning: A PET study of the Tower of London task. *Neuropsychologia*, **34**, 515–526.

Belin, P., McAdams, S., Thivard, L., Smith, B., Savel, S., Zilbovicius, Samson, S., et al. (2002). The neuroanatomical substrate of sound duration discrimination. *Neuropsychologia*, **40**, 1956–1964.

Berman, K. F., Ostrem, J. L., Randolph, C., Gold, J., Goldberg, T. E., Coppola, R., et al. (1995). Physiological activation of a cortical network during performance of the Wisconsin card sorting test: A positron emission tomography study. *Neuropsychologia*, **33**, 1027–1046.

Blaxton, T. A., Zeffiro, T. A., Gabrieli, J. D. E., Bookheimer, S. Y., Carrillo, M. C., Theodore, W. H., et al. (1996). Functional mapping of human learning: A positron emission tomography activation study of eyeblink conditioning. *Journal of Neuroscience*, **16**, 4032–4040.

Bottini, G., Corcoran, R., Sterzi, R., Paulesu, E., Schenone, P., Scarpa, P., et al. (1994). The role of the right hemisphere in the interpretation of figurative aspects of language. *Brain*, **117**, 1241–1253.

Brandimonte, M., Einstein, G. O., & McDaniel, M. A. (Eds.) (1996). *Prospective memory: Theory and applications*. Mahwah, NJ: Lawrence Erlbaum.

Bird, C. M., Castelli, F., Malik, O., Frith, U., & Husain, M. (2004). The impact of extensive medial frontal lobe damage on "Theory of Mind" and cognition. *Brain*, **127**, 914–928.

Buckner, R. L. (1996). Beyond HERA: Contributions of specific prefrontal brain areas to long-term memory retrieval. *Psychonomic Bulletin and Review*, **3**, 149–158.

Burgess, N., Maguire, E. A., Spiers, H. J., & O'Keefe, J. (2001). A temporoparietal and prefrontal network for retrieving the spatial context of lifelike events. *Neuroimage*, **14**, 439–453.

Burgess, P. W. (1997). Theory and methodology in executive function research. In P. Rabbitt (Ed.), *Methodology of Frontal and Executive Function* (pp. 81–111). Hove: Psychology Press.

Burgess, P. W. (2000). Strategy application disorder: The role of the frontal lobes in human multitasking. *Psychological Research, 63*, 279–288.

Burgess, P. W., Alderman, N., Evans, J., Emslie, H., & Wilson, B. A. (1998). The ecological validity of tests of executive function. *Journal of the International Neuropsychological Society, 4*, 547–558.

Burgess, P. W., Alderman, N., Evans, J. J., Wilson, B. A., Emslie, H., & Shallice, T. (1996). *The modified six element test.* Bury St. Edmunds, U.K.: Thames Valley Test Company.

Burgess, P. W., Dumontheil, I., Gilbert, S.J., Simons, J.S. and Firth, C. D. (in preparation). A test of the gateway hypothesis of rostral PFC function (Area 10) using FMRI.

Burgess, P. W., Gilbert, S. J., Okuda, J., & Simons, J. S. (In press). Rostral prefrontal brain regions (Area 10): A gateway between inner thought and the external world? In W. Prinz & N. Sebanz (Eds.), *Disorders of Volition.* Cambridge, MA: MIT Press.

Burgess, P. W., Quayle, A., & Frith, C. D. (2001). Brain regions involved in prospective memory as determined by positron emission tomography. *Neuropsychologia, 39*, 545–555.

Burgess, P. W., Scott, S. K., & Frith, C. D. (2003). The role of the rostral frontal cortex (area 10) in prospective memory: A lateral versus medial dissociation. *Neuropsychologia, 41*, 906–918.

Burgess, P. W., & Shallice, T. (1996). Confabulation and the control of recollection. *Memory, 4*, 359–411.

Burgess, P. W., Veitch, E., & Costello, A. (submitted). The role of the right rostral prefrontal cortex in multitasking: The six element test.

Burgess, P. W., Veitch, E., Costello, A., & Shallice, T. (2000). The cognitive and neuroanatomical correlates of multitasking. *Neuropsychologia, 38*, 848–863.

Christoff, K., & Gabrieli, J. D. E. (2000). The frontopolar cortex and human cognition: Evidence for a rostrocaudal hierarchical organization within the human prefrontal cortex. *Psychobiology, 28*, 168–186.

Christoff, K., Prabhakaran, V., Dorfman, J., Zhao, Z., Kroger, J. K., Holyoak, K. J., et al. (2001). Rostrolateral prefrontal cortex involvement in relational integration during reasoning. *Neuroimage, 14*, 1136–1149.

Christoff, K., Ream, J. M., & Gabrieli, J. D. E. (2004). Neural basis of spontaneous thought processes. *Cortex, 40*, 1–9.

Christoff, K., Ream, J. M., Geddes, L. P. T., & Gabrieli, J. D. E. (2003). Evaluating self-generated information: Anterior prefrontal contributions to human cognition. *Behavioral Neuroscience, 117*, 1161–1168.

Dobbins, I. G., Foley, H., Schacter, D. L., & Wagner, A. D. (2002). Executive control during episodic retrieval: Multiple prefrontal processes subserve source memory. *Neuron, 35*, 989–996.

Dreher, J. C., Koechlin, E., Ali, S. O., & Grafman, J. (2002). The roles of timing and task order during task switching. *Neuroimage, 17*, 95–109.

Duncan, J., Emslie, H., Williams, P., Johnson, R., & Freer, C. (1996). Intelligence and the frontal lobe: The organization of goal-directed behavior. *Cognitive Psychology, 30*, 257–303.

Duncan, J., & Owen, A. (2000). Consistent response of the human frontal lobe to diverse cognitive demands. *Trends in Neurosciences*, 23, 475–483.

Eslinger, P. J., & Damasio, A. R. (1985). Severe disturbance of higher cognition following bilateral frontal lobe ablation: patient EVR. *Neurology*, 35, 1731–1741.

Fletcher, P. C., & Henson, R. N. A. (2001). Frontal lobes and human memory: Insights from functional neuroimaging. *Brain*, 124, 849–881.

Frith, C. D. (2002). Attention to action and awareness of other minds. *Consciousness and Cognition*, 11, 481–487.

Frith, U., & Frith, C. D. (2003). Development and neurophysiology of mentalizing. *Philosophical Transactions of the Royal Society of London* B, 358(1431), 459–473.

Fuster, J. M. (1997). *The prefrontal cortex: Anatomy, physiology, and neuropsychology of the frontal lobe*. Philadelphia, PA: Lippincott-Raven.

Gilbert, S. J., Frith, C. D., & Burgess, P. W. (in press). Involvement of rostral prefrontal cortex in selection between stimulus-oriented and stimulus-independent thought. *European Journal of Neuroscience*.

Gilbert, S. J., Simons, J. S., Frith, C. D., & Burgess, P. W. (submitted). Performance-related activity in medial rostral PFC (Area 10) during low demand tasks.

Goel, V., Gold, B., Kapur, S., & Houle, S. (1997). The seats of reason? An imaging study of deductive and inductive reasoning. *Neuroreport*, 8, 1305–1310.

Goel, V., & Grafman, J. (2000). The role of the right prefrontal cortex in ill-structured problem solving. *Cognitive Neuropsychology*, 17, 415–436.

Gold, J. M., Berman, K. F., Randolph, C., Goldberg, T. E., & Weinberger, D. R. (1996). PET validation of a novel prefrontal task: Delayed response alternation. *Neuropsychology*, 10, 3–10.

Goldstein, L. H., Bernard, S., Fenwick, P. B. C., Burgess, P. W., & McNeil, J. (1993). Unilateral frontal lobectomy can produce strategy application disorder. *Journal of Neurology, Neurosurgery and Psychiatry*, 56, 274–276.

Grady, C. L. (1999). Neuroimaging and activation of the frontal lobes. In B. L. Miller & J. L. Cummings (Eds.), *The human frontal lobes: Function and disorders* (pp. 196–230). New York: Guilford Press.

Grafman, J. (2002). The structured event complex and the human prefrontal cortex. In D. T. Stuss & R. T. Knight (Eds.), *Principles of frontal lobe functions* (pp. 292–310). New York: Oxford University Press.

Grant, D. A., & Berg, E. A. (1948). A behavioral analysis of degree of reinforcement and ease of shifting to new responses in a Weigl-type card-sorting problem. *Journal of Experimental Psychology*, 38, 404–411.

Gusnard, D. A., Akbudak, E., Shulman, G. L., & Raichle, M. E. (2001). Medial prefrontal cortex and self-referential mental activity: Relation to a default mode of brain function. *Proceedings of the National Academy of Sciences, USA*, 98, 4259–4264.

Gusnard, D. A., & Raichle, M. E. (2001). Searching for a baseline: Functional imaging and the resting human brain. *Nature Reviews Neuroscience*, 2, 685–694.

Haxby, J. V., Ungerleider, L. G., Horwitz, B., Maisog, J. M., Rapoport, S. I., & Grady, C. L. (1996). Storage and retrieval of new memories for faces in the intact human brain. *Proceedings of the National Academy of Sciences, USA*, 93, 922–927.

Haxby, J. V., Ungerleider, I. G., Horwitz, B., Rapoport, S. I., & Grady, C. L. (1995). Hemispheric differences in neural systems for face working memory: A PET-rCBF study. *Human Brain Mapping*, 3, 68–82.

Henson, R. N. A., Shallice, T., & Dolan, R. J. (1999). Right prefrontal cortex and episodic memory retrieval: A functional MRI test of the monitoring hypothesis. *Brain*, 122, 1367–1381.

Herron, J. E., Henson, R. N., & Rugg, M. D. (2004). Probability effects on the neural correlates of retrieval success: An fMRI study. *Neuroimage*, 21, 302–310.

Hugdahl, K., Beradi, A., Thomson, W. I., Kosslyn, S. M., Macy, R., Baker, D. P., et al. (1995). Brain mechanisms in human classical conditioning: A PET blood flow study. *Neuroreport*, 6, 1723–1728.

Janata, P., Birk, J. L., Van Horn, J. D., Leman, M., Tillmann, B., & Bharucha, J. J. (2002). The cortical topography of tonal structures underlying Western music. *Science*, 298, 2167–2170.

Jenkins, I. H., Brooks, D. J., Nixon, P. D., Frackowiak, R. S. J., & Passingham, R. E. (1994). Motor sequence learning: A study with positron emission tomography. *Journal of Neuroscience*, 14, 3775–3790.

Jennings, J. M., McIntosh, A. R., Kapur, S., Tulving, E., & Houle, S. (1997). Cognitive subtractions may not add up: The interaction between semantic processing and response mode. *Neuroimage*, 5, 229–239.

Johnson, S. C., Baxter, L. C., Wilder, L. S., Pipe, J. G., Heiserman, J. E., & Prigatano, G. P. (2002). Neural correlates of self-reflection. *Brain*, 125, 1808–1814.

Klein, D., Milner, B., Zatorre, R. J., Meyer, E., & Evans, A. C. (1995). The neural substrates underlying word generation: A bilingual functional-imaging study. *Proceedings of the National Academy of Sciences, USA*, 92, 2899–2903.

Koechlin, E., Basso, G., Pietrini, P., Panzer, S., & Grafman, J. (1999). The role of the anterior prefrontal cortex in human cognition. *Nature*, 399, 148–151.

Koechlin, E., Corrado, G., Pietrini, P., & Grafman, J. (2000). Dissociating the role of the medial and lateral anterior prefrontal cortex in human planning. *Proceedings of the National Academy of Sciences, USA*, 97, 7651–7656.

Koechlin, E., Ody, C., & Kouneiher, F. (2003). The architecture of cognitive control in the human prefrontal cortex. *Science*, 302, 1181–1185.

Kosslyn, S. M., Alpert, N. M., & Thompson, W. L. (1995). Identifying objects at different levels of hierarchy: A positron emission tomography study. *Human Brain Mapping*, 3, 107–132.

Kosslyn, S. M., Alpert, N. M., Thompson, W. L., Chabris, C. F., Rauch, S. L., & Anderson, A. K. (1994). Identifying objects seen from different viewpoints. A PET investigation. *Brain*, 117, 1055–1071.

MacLeod, A. K., Buckner, R. L., Miezin, F. M., Petersen, S. E., & Raichle, M. E. (1998). Right anterior prefrontal cortex activation during semantic monitoring and working memory. *Neuroimage*, 7, 41–48.

McGuire, P. K., Paulesu, E., Frackowiak, R. S. J., & Frith, C. D. (1996). Brain activity during stimulus independent thought. *NeuroReport*, 7, 2095–2099.

McIntosh, A. R. (1999). Mapping cognition to the brain through neural interactions. *Memory*, 7, 523–548.

Martin, A., Haxby, J. V., Lalonde, F. M., Wigges, C. L., & Ungerleider, L. G. (1995). Discrete cortical regions associated with knowledge of color and knowledge of action. *Science*, **270**, 102–105.

Metzler, C., & Parkin, A. J. (2000). Reversed negative priming following frontal lobe lesions. *Neuropsychologia*, **38**, 363–379.

Moscovitch, M., & Winocur, G. (2002). The frontal cortex and working-with memory. In D. T. Stuss & R. T. Knight (Eds.), *Principles of frontal lobe function* (pp. 189–209). Oxford: Oxford University Press.

Norman, D. A., & Shallice, T. (1980). *Attention to action: Willed and automatic control of behavior. Center for Human Information Processing* (Tech. Rep. No. 99). (Reprinted in revised form in R. J. Davidson, G. E. Schwartz, & D. Shapiro [Eds.] [1986] *Consciousness and self-regulation* [Vol. 4]. New York: Plenum Press.)

Nyberg, L., McIntosh, A. R., Cabeza, R., Habib, R., Houle, S., & Tulving, E. (1996). General and specific brain regions involved in encoding and retrieval of events: What, where, and when. *Proceedings of the National Academy of Sciences, USA*, **93**, 11280–11285.

Okuda, J., Simons, J. S., Gilbert, S. J., Frith, C. D., & Burgess, P. W. (in preparation). Target probability effects in prospective memory: a trade-off between ongoing- and target-related activities as revealed by functional magnetic resonance imaging.

Okuda, J., Fujii, T., Ohtake, H., Tsukiura, T., Tanji, K., Suzuki, K., et al. (2003). Thinking of the future and past: The roles of the frontal pole and medial temporal lobes. *Neuroimage*, **19**, 1369–1380.

Okuda, J., Fujii, T., Yamadori, A., Kawashima, R., Tsukkiura, T., Fukatsu, R., et al. (1998). Participation of the prefrontal cortices in prospective memory: Evidence from a PET study in humans. *Neuroscience Letters*, **253**, 127–130.

Petrides, M., Alivisatos, B., Meyer, E., & Evans, A. C. (1993). Functional activation of the human frontal cortex during the performance of verbal memory tasks. *Proceedings of the National Academy of Sciences, USA*, **90**, 878–882.

Pollmann, S. (2004). Anterior prefrontal cortex contributions to attention control. *Experimental Psychology*, **51**, 270–278.

Prabhakaran, V., Smith, J. A., Desmond, J. E., Glover, G. H., & Gabrieli, J. D. (1997). Neural substrates of fluid reasoning: An fMRI study of neocortical activation during performance of the Raven's Progressive Matrices test. *Cognitive Psychology*, **33**, 43–63.

Rabbitt, P. M. A. (1997). Methodologies and models in the study of executive function. In P. Rabbitt (Ed.), *Methodology of Frontal and Executive Function* (pp. 1–38). Hove, UK: Psychology Press.

Raichle, M. E. (1998). Behind the scenes of functional brain imaging: A historical and physiological perspective. *Proceedings of the National Academy of Sciences, USA*, **95**, 765–772.

Raichle, M. E., MacLeod, A.-M., Snyder, A. Z., Powers, W. J., Gusnard, D. A., & Shulman, G. L. (2001). A default mode of brain function. *Proceedings of the National Academy of Sciences, USA*, **98**, 676–682.

Ramnani, N., & Owen, A. M. (2004). Anterior prefrontal cortex: Insights into function from anatomy and neuroimaging. *Nature Reviews Neuroscience*, **5**, 184–194.

Ranganath, C., & Paller, K. A. (2000). Neural correlates of memory retrieval and evaluation. *Cognitive Brain Research*, **9**, 209–222.

Roland, P. E., & Gulyas, B. (1995). Visual memory, visual imagery, and visual recognition of large field patterns by the human brain: Functional anatomy by positron emission tomography. *Cerebral Cortex*, **5**, 79–93.

Rugg, M. D., Fletcher, P. C., Chua, P. M. L., & Dolan, R. J. (1999). The role of the prefrontal cortex in recognition memory and memory for source: An fMRI study. *Neuroimage*, **10**, 520–529.

Rugg, M. D., Fletcher, P. C., Frith, C. D., Frackowiak, R. S. J., & Dolan, R. J. (1996). Differential activation of the prefrontal cortex in successful and unsuccessful memory retrieval. *Brain*, **119**, 2073–2084.

Semendeferi, K., Armstrong, E., Schleicher, A., Zilles, K., & Van Hoesen, G. W. (2001). Prefrontal cortex in humans and apes: A comparative study of area 10. *American Journal of Physical Anthropology*, **114**, 224–241.

Shallice, T. (1982). Specific impairments of planning. *Philosophical Transactions of the Royal Society of London B*, **298**, 199–209.

Shallice, T. (1988). *From neuropsychology to mental structure*. Cambridge, U.K.: Cambridge University Press.

Shallice, T. (2002). Fractionation of the supervisory system. In D. T. Stuss & R. T. Knight (Eds.), *Principles of frontal lobe functions* (pp. 261–277). New York: Oxford University Press.

Shallice, T., & Burgess, P. W. (1991a). Deficits in strategy application following frontal lobe damage in man. *Brain*, **114**, 727–741.

Shallice, T., & Burgess, P. W. (1991b) Higher-order cognitive impairments and frontal lobe lesions in man. In H. S. Levin, H. M. Eisenberg, & A. L. Benton (Eds.), *Frontal lobe function and dysfunction* (pp. 125–138). New York: Oxford University Press.

Shallice, T., & Burgess, P. W. (1993). Supervisory control of action and thought selection. In A. Baddeley & L. Weiskrantz (Eds.), *Attention: Selection, awareness and control: A tribute to Donald Broadbent* (pp. 171–187). Oxford: Clarendon Press.

Shallice, T., & Burgess, P. W. (1996). The domain of supervisory processes and temporal organisation of behaviour. *Philosophical Transactions of the Royal Society of London B*, **351**, 1405–1412.

Shallice, T., & Burgess, P. W. (1988). The domain of supervisory processes and temporal organisation of behaviour. In A. C. Roberts, T. W. Robbins & L. Weiskrantz (Eds.), *The Prefrontal Cortex: Executive and Cognitive Functions* (pp. 22–35). Oxford: Oxford University Press.

Shallice, T., & Evans, M. E. (1978). The involvement of the frontal lobes in cognitive estimation. *Cortex*, **14**, 294–303.

Simons, J. S., Owen, A. M., Fletcher, P. C., & Burgess, P. W. (in press a). Anterior prefrontal cortex and the recollection of-contextual information. *Neuropsychologia*.

Simons, J. S., Gilbert, S. J., Owen, A. M., Fletcher, P. C., & Burgess, P. W. (in press b). Distinct roles for lateral and medial anterior prefrontal cortex in the control of contextual recollection. *Journal of Neurophysiology*.

Simons, J. S., & Spiers, H. J. (2003). Prefrontal and medial temporal lobe interactions in long-term memory. *Nature Reviews Neuroscience*, **4**, 637–648.

Small, D. M., Gitelman, D. R., Gregory, M. D., Nobre, A. C., Parrish, T. B., & Mesulam, M. M. (2003). The posterior cingulate and medial prefrontal cortex mediate the anticipatory allocation of spatial attention. *Neuroimage*, **18**, 633–641.

Stuss, D. T., Alexander, M. P., Hamer, L., Palumbo, C., Dempster, R., Binns, M., et al. (1998). The effects of focal anterior and posterior brain lesions on verbal fluency. *Journal of the International Neuropsychological Society, 4*, 265–278.

Stuss, D. T., Alexander, M. P., Shallice, T., Picton, T. W., Binns, M. A., Macdonald, R., et al. (2005). Multiple frontal systems controlling response speed. *Neuropsychologia. 43*, 396–417.

Stuss, D. T., Levine, B., Alexander, M. P., Hong, J., Palumbo, C., Hamer, L., et al. (2000). Wisconsin card sorting test performance in patients with focal frontal and posterior brain damage: Effects of lesion location and test structure on separable cognitive processes. *Neuropsychologia, 38*, 388–402.

Stuss, D. T., Shallice, T., Alexander, M. P., & Picton, T. W. (1995). A multidisciplinary approach to anterior attentional functions. *Annals of the New York Academy of Sciences, 769*, 191–212.

Strange, B. A., Henson, R. N., Friston, K. J., & Dolan, R. J. (2001). Anterior prefrontal cortex mediates rule learning in humans. *Cerebral Cortex, 11*, 1040–1046.

Tulving, E., Markowitsch, H. J., Craik, F. I. M., Habib, R., & Houle, S. (1996). Novelty and familiarity activations in PET studies of memory encoding and retrieval. *Cerebral Cortex, 6*, 71–79.

Wood, R. Ll., & Rutterford, N. A. (2004). Relationships between measured cognitive ability and reported psychosocial activity after bilateral frontal lobe injury: An 18-year follow-up. *Neuropsychological Rehabilitation, 14*, 329–350.

Zatorre, R. J., Halpern, A. R., Perry, D. W., Meyer, E., & Evans, A. C. (1996). Hearing in the mind's ear: A PET investigation of musical imagery and perception. *Journal of Cognitive Neuroscience, 8*, 29–46.

Zysset, S., Huber, O., Ferstl, E., & Von Cramon, D. Y. (2002). The anterior frontomedian cortex and evaluative judgment: An fMRI study. *Neuroimage, 15*, 983–991.

Chapter 10

Prefrontal cortex and Spearman's *g*

John Duncan

Abstract

This chapter addresses one of Pat Rabbitt's enduring concerns—the basis for general intelligence or Spearman's *g*. I begin with a striking finding from functional brain imaging: In specific regions of frontal and parietal cortex, there is a pattern of similar activation for many different cognitive demands. Plausibly, this pattern of multiple-demand (MD) activity could reflect functions basic to *g*. A related finding comes from monkey studies: In the lateral prefrontal cortex, neurons produce a dense, selective representation of information relevant to a current task, whatever that task may be. This representation is reminiscent of a basic idea from artificial intelligence—task modeling in working memory— and I suggest that *g* could largely be a reflection of this task modeling function. Moving on to behavioural studies, I show how competition in a task model can result in loss of vulnerable task components. This "goal neglect" is closely related to *g*. I finish with evidence from an ongoing study of human brain lesions. Though MD damage is associated with *g* deficits, such deficits can also be produced by large lesions elsewhere. Plausible though it is to link *g* to MD functions, many questions remain over this hypothesis.

Introduction

In the winter term of 1972 I had eight weekly tutorials with Pat Rabbitt on the subject of "human skills." Certainly there were some of the standard props for initiation of the novice—we wore flowing black robes—I ascended to the meetings on the dark staircase of an imposing College—we thumbed weekly through a volume of many worn pages (Broadbent's *Decision and Stress*, 1971), which as a matter of fact Pat did refer to as the Bible—and periodically a bottle would be brought forth from a cupboard, in a reasonable simulation of Mass. But more than any of these, it was Pat's personal charisma that produced the standard impact, and by the end of term I was converted—to human experimental psychology, information processing, and choice reaction time. Heaven knows how this happens . . . the malleability of the 18-year-old mind is a remarkable thing.

More than 30 years later, I seem still to be addressing some of Pat's central concerns. In this chapter I focus on two of these—the functions of prefrontal cortex (PFC), and the nature of "general intelligence" or Spearman's g (Spearman, 1904). After prefrontal lesions there can be a broad disorganization of behaviour. The normal, goal-directed structure of thought and action can be disrupted, both by omission of important stages, and by insertion of irrelevant or inappropriate material (Luria, 1966). In formal testing, deficits can appear in almost every conceivable task domain, including perception, memory, response choice, problem-solving, and many others. The results suggest impairment in some fundamental process of shaping behaviour to satisfy task requirements (Bianchi, 1922). Meanwhile, the concept of g was originally proposed to account for universal positive correlations between tests of different abilities (Spearman, 1904). To account for this observation, Spearman proposed some general or g factor contributing to success in all manner of different activities. Factor analysis can be used to identify the best tasks for measuring g. These will be tasks with the strongest overall pattern of positive correlation with others. Empirically, they turn out to be tests of novel problem-solving, using spatial, verbal, or other materials (e.g. see Marshalek, Lohman, & Snow, 1983). Their broad ability to predict success in other tasks, including educational and career achievements, accounts for their use as tests of "general intelligence."

My interest in these problems derives originally from a study of London Transport bus drivers, run in 1980–81 at their training school in Chiswick (see McKenna, Duncan, & Brown, 1986). In a (failed) attempt to understand individual differences in driving ability, we administered a series of cognitive tests to over 150 driver trainees. Among others, we used the Embedded Figures Test (Witkin, Oltman, Raskin, & Karp, 1971) to measure "field dependence," and a rather complex dichotic listening test (Gopher & Kahneman, 1971) to measure selective attention. Both had previously been related to accident involvement. We also included a standard test of Spearman's g, Cattell's Culture Fair (Institute for Personality and Ability Testing, 1973).

The most interesting observation from this study began as an annoyance—fairly consistently, there would be subjects who understood the instructions for the dichotic listening test, repeated them back after a few practice trials, but then completed the whole task incorrectly. Subjectively, this behaviour had a rather striking appearance, as if the subject knew what *ought* to be done, but somehow failed to use this knowledge to focus on the errors that were being made and attempt to correct them. This sort of mismatch between knowledge and behaviour—which later we called *goal neglect* (Duncan, Emslie, Williams, Johnson, & Freer, 1996)—is occasionally reported in frontal lobe patients (Luria, 1966; Milner, 1963). It seemed that, in the dichotic listening test, we were seeing a similar phenomenon even in people from the normal population.

This became much more interesting when later we realized who these people were. First, they very often did conspicuously badly on the Embedded Figures Test. Second, they also tended to score poorly on the Culture Fair. A search of the literature soon showed that, rather than measuring a separate construct, the Embedded Figures Test was closely correlated with general intelligence measures (McKenna, 1984). The results suggested the idea that Spearman's *g* might be largely a reflection of frontal lobe function—with some central role at the interface between task demands or goals and effective behaviour.

As I said, these issues are closely related to Pat's own concerns in the study of aging. At the time of the London Transport study, I was very much impressed by a paper that Pat had just written on age deficits in choice reaction time tasks (Rabbitt, 1981). His argument was that, over and above the "basic" operations of stimulus identification and response selection, even these simple tasks involve a complex structure of additional, perhaps more peripheral cognitive operations—adjusting the balance between speed and accuracy, setting expectancies based on preceding trials, directing attention to relevant regions of a display, and so on. Rather reminiscent of our goal neglect, Pat suggested that the problems of the elderly often arose from a failure to implement parts of this complex task control structure. In subsequent work, much attention has been given to the possibility of frontal lobe deficits in old age (e.g. see Phillips & Henry, this volume). And as Pat has also documented, measures of Spearman's *g*—in particular those based on novel problem-solving—are an excellent index of age-related deficits (Rabbitt, 1993; see also Parkin & Java, 1999). For many tasks, indeed, age-related declines can be almost completely explained by the measured change in *g*.

In this chapter I present a newer version of the idea that *g* is a reflection of frontal lobe function. In the first section I consider functional imaging data, and the finding that, in specific regions of frontal and parietal cortex, there is a pattern of similar recruitment for diverse task demands. Plausibly, this pattern of multiple-demand (MD) activity might indicate functions that are basic to *g*. In the second section, I review single unit recording data from the behaving monkey. Characteristically, I suggest, the lateral prefrontal cortex produces a dense, selective representation of information relevant to a current task—whatever that task may be. This representation is reminiscent of a basic idea from artificial intelligence—task modeling in working memory—and in the third section, I suggest that this task modeling may be a useful way to conceive of "control processes" and *g*. In the fourth section, I return to goal neglect, and show how competition in a task model results in loss of vulnerable task components. Finally I review recent lesion data, and the hypothesis that lesions to MD regions should predict *g* impairment.

Multiple-demand activity in frontoparietal cortex

My starting point is a striking set of findings from functional imaging. Over the past 15 years, functional imaging studies have revealed many brain systems recruited by specific kinds of mental operation. But there is also another striking finding. In regions of frontal and parietal cortex, many different task demands produce a very similar pattern of activation. Here I call this the multiple-demand (MD) pattern.

Three illustrations of this MD pattern appear in Figure 10.1. Figure 10.1(a), extended from Duncan and Owen (2000), shows activations associated with five different cognitive demands. For this exercise, we searched the literature for studies that, as clearly as possible, had manipulated a single cognitive demand in the context of an otherwise unchanged task. We found useful data for five demands—response conflict, task novelty, number of elements in working memory, working memory delay, and perceptual difficulty. In each case we listed peak activations for a contrast of high minus low demand—strong minus weak response conflict, early in practice minus late in practice for the same task, long minus short working memory list, long minus short delay, and difficult minus easy stimulus identification. In the original paper (Duncan & Owen, 2000) we were concerned just with activations within PFC. Figure 10.1(a), however, shows all peak cortical activations from the 20 separate studies included in our review.

The first striking result is the clustering of activations from these very different studies. On the lateral surface, one major cluster focuses around the posterior part of the inferior frontal sulcus, with some points spreading further forward toward the frontal pole, and some further back into premotor cortex. A second cluster, especially evident in the right hemisphere, appears just anterior to the lateral fissure; though plotted here on the lateral surface, these points in fact spread inward along the frontal operculum and become continuous with activations in the anterior insula. A third cluster is evident in the parietal lobe, extending along both banks of the intraparietal sulcus. On the medial surface is the most striking cluster of all, in the dorsal part of the anterior cingulate and adjacent supplementary motor area. Also evident are scattered activations

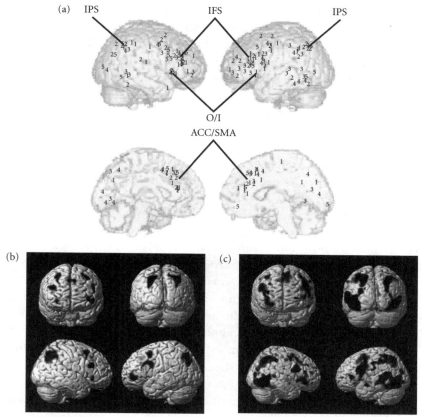

Fig. 10.1 MD (multiple-demand) network in functional imaging. (a) Cortical activation foci from 20 studies examining: (1) response conflict; (2) task novelty; (3) number of elements in working memory; (4) working memory delay; and (5) perceptual difficulty. IFS—inferior frontal sulcus; O/I—operculum/insula; ACC/SMA—anterior cingulate/supplementary motor area; IPS—intraparietal sulcus. (b) Activation (black) for standard test of *g* (Culture Fair) minus sensorimotor control. (c) Activation (black) for attended minus unattended visual events.

in higher visual cortex, doubtless reflecting the visual content of most of the tasks studied (and absent for those few nonvisual studies).

The second striking result is lack of cognitive specificity. For all five of the demands reviewed, results were essentially similar, with joint activations around the inferior frontal sulcus, operculum/insula, intraparietal sulcus, and dorsal anterior cingulate.

Figure 10.1(b) comes from a recent fMRI study of the Culture Fair test of *g* (Bishop, Bor, & Duncan, unpublished data; see also Duncan et al. 2000). The Culture Fair is a problem-solving test of the sort often used to measure *g*.

For our experiment, we adapted materials from one of its subtests, with an odd-one-out format. Each problem had four abstract figures, and the subject was to find which figure in some sense did not belong with the others. Blocks of these problems were compared with blocks of a low-level sensorimotor control, in which subjects simply chose which figure was not identical to the other three. Though this is just one study making one task comparison, its results (Figure 10.1(b)) are remarkably similar to the whole MD pattern from the Duncan and Owen (2000) review.

Perhaps most striking of all are the data in Figure 10.1(c). In this experiment (Hon, Duncan, Epstein, & Owen, 2004), we gave subjects no task whatsoever. Instead we examined activity associated with simple awareness of a visual event. Subjects saw a repeatedly flashing display containing two four-letter words, one white and one black. To ensure central fixation, both words were centerd on the screen, one printed horizontally and the other vertically. For a whole scanning block, subjects were simply told either to watch the horizontal words, or to watch the vertical words, but with no decisions to be taken or responses to be made. Occasionally as the display flashed, either the horizontal or the vertical word would change, then remaining the same for the next few flashes until the next change occurred. At the end of the experiment, a surprise recognition test confirmed that subjects obeyed instructions, showing memory just for the words they had been told to attend to. Figure 10.1(c) shows the contrast between brain activity associated with attended/seen and unattended/unseen changes. Again, visual activity associated with seen changes is accompanied by prominent activity in dorsal and ventral parts of the lateral frontal surface, the anterior cingulate, and the intraparietal sulcus.

Together, these data suggest a revised version of the idea that g may be a reflection of frontal lobe function. The key idea of g is that some common factor or process may be important in many different kinds of cognitive activity. Functional imaging data suggest the MD pattern not for the whole of frontal cortex, but for specific regions—the lateral surface, especially around the posterior part of the inferior frontal sulcus, the operculum/anterior insula, and the dorsal anterior cingulate. Similar activations spread into premotor cortex, and outside the frontal lobe, along the intraparietal sulcus. One good way to see the MD pattern is certainly to use a standard intelligence test, though interestingly, the Hon et al. (2004) data show similar results even for simple awareness of an attended visual event, with minimal additional task demand. In the following sections I go on to consider the functions of MD regions, and how these may relate to cognitive control and g.

Single cell physiology

Of course, only limited conclusions can be drawn from functional imaging. Limited spatial resolution, for example, could be partially responsible for the impression of similar activation patterns associated with different cognitive demands. For this reason, it is useful to move from global results of imaging studies to the properties of single neurons. In this section I consider one component of the MD network illustrated in Figure 10.1—the lateral PFC.

Many studies have recorded responses of prefrontal neurons in the behaving monkey. Many different tasks have been used—with visual, auditory and somaesthetic inputs, manual and oculomotor responses, with and without memory delays between presentation of stimulus information and its use, and with many different task structures and rules. For largely practical reasons, the most common recording site has been the lateral frontal surface, in particular the cortex in and around the principal sulcus. Together, these experiments suggest some fairly striking general conclusions.

First, *many* cells in the lateral prefrontal cortex will respond to critical events in the task the animal is performing. Even when neurons are randomly selected on the lateral prefrontal surface, and even though the animal is carrying out an arbitrary task designed just for the purposes of a particular experiment, task-related responses are the rule rather than the exception. For a fairly lax criterion, such as significantly different response between any task event and baseline, "task-related" activity can be found in 90% of cells or more (e.g. Asaad, Rainer, & Miller, 2000). Even a much stricter criterion, such as significant discrimination between two relevant stimulus events, can easily be satisfied by 20% of cells or more (e.g. Everling, Tinsley, Gaffan, & Duncan, 2002; Freedman, Riesenhuber, Poggio, & Miller, 2001).

Second, these task-related responses are of many different kinds. They can reflect the occurrence or identity of stimuli in visual and other modalities (e.g. Funahashi, Bruce, & Goldman-Rakic, 1989; Fuster, Bauer, & Jervey, 1985; Romo, Brody, Hernández, & Lemus, 1999), be related to responses (e.g. Watanabe, 1986), carry information across working memory delays (e.g. Funahashi et al. 1989), or describe task rules (e.g. Wallis, Anderson, & Miller, 2001) and rewards (Watanabe, 1996). All these different kinds of response are found closely intermingled, and broadly distributed across the recording area (e.g. Niki & Watanabe, 1979; Wallis et al. 2001).

Third, there is selective attention to task-relevant information—the same information is coded much more strongly when it is relevant to the animal's decision than when it is not. This applies to the different features of a visual stimulus (Lauwereyns et al. 2001; Sakagami & Niki, 1994), to different objects in a display (Rainer, Asaad, & Miller, 1998), to the information preserved in working memory (Rao, Rainer, & Miller, 1997), and to alternative categorizations of the same object (Freedman et al. 2001). An example (Everling et al. 2002) is shown in Figure 10.2. In this study (Figure 10.2(a)), the animal was trained to monitor a series of pictures, waiting for a specified target (fish). When the target appeared, the animal immediately fixated it for reward. In the unilateral task, stimuli appeared just to left or right of fixation; in the bilateral task, stimuli appeared simultaneously on both sides, but with the animal instructed just to watch for the target on one side or the other. Even in the unilateral task, the data showed tuning of neural responses by task relevance. Around a quarter of all cells discriminated the target (fish) from nontarget objects (hamburger and teddy bear). In contrast, essentially no cells made the irrelevant discrimination between one nontarget and the other. Task relevance was also a key influence in the bilateral task. Target-selective cells responded strongly to the fish on the attended side, but little if at all to a fish on the unattended side (Figure 10.2(b)).

Together, these results suggest what I have called an *adaptive coding* principle of prefrontal function (Duncan, 2001; see also Miller & Cohen, 2001). According to this principle, even single neurons of PFC have no fixed functional properties. Instead, they have the potential to respond to many different kinds of input, reflecting the rich connections that exist from other brain regions into the frontal lobe, and between one frontal region and another (Pandya & Yeterian, 1996). For any given task, neurons adapt to emphasize information of current relevance—producing a dense, distributed representation of this task's inputs, outputs, rules, rewards, etc. This is why so many task-related neurons, coding many different task features, are found broadly distributed across PFC.

Though this flexibility of function is certainly much stronger in PFC than in many other regions (e.g. Nieder & Miller, 2004), few direct comparisons have been made. In particular, data are needed for other MD regions. Though much of parietal cortex, for example, is traditionally associated with spatial functions, neurons code nonspatial object properties when these are relevant to the monkey's task (Toth & Assad, 2002). Meanwhile, the conclusion for one particular MD region seems clear. As required by a role in *g*, neurons of the lateral PFC are involved in a wide range of different cognitive operations. Even single neurons, indeed, can carry very different information in different contexts—selectively emphasizing information of relevance to current behaviour.

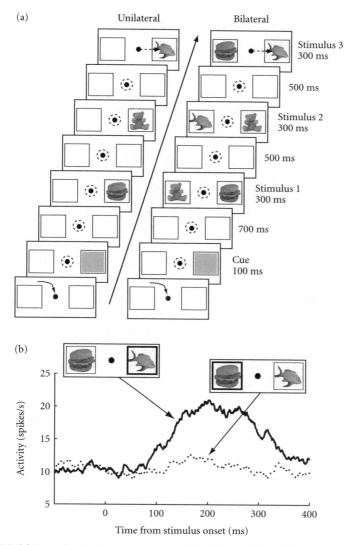

Fig. 10.2 (a) Example stimulus sequences from Everling et al. (2002). Each trial began when the monkey fixated (curved arrow) a small dot in the center of the screen. A cue (filled square) appeared to left or right, followed by a stream of stimuli in just the cued location (unilateral condition) or in both locations (bilateral condition). Central fixation (dotted circle) was to be maintained until a target (fish) appeared at the cued location, at which point an immediate saccade (dotted arrow) to this target was required.
(b) Mean responses for 33 target-selective cells in the bilateral task. Data are for displays containing a target (fish) on one side, accompanied by a nontarget on the opposite side. Attended location is shown by heavy box (not present in actual display). A strong response to an attended target (solid line) was eliminated (dotted line) when attention was focused on the opposite side. Adapted with permission from Everling et al. (2002).

Working memory and cognitive control

Evidently PFC plays some role in the control of thought and behaviour—but what does "control" mean? In this section I express some doubts over the attempt to separate cognition into "control" and "noncontrol" processes. Instead, I suggest a view that seems more compatible both with the overall structure of goal-directed behaviour, and with the neurophysiological data outlined in the previous section.

In fact, I can illustrate these doubts over the concept of "control processes" with some of the experiments Pat supervised in my DPhil. This work was concerned with response selection in spatial choice reaction time. It used stimulus-response mappings like the one shown in Figure 10.3. Each stimulus is a single vertical line, presented at one of four possible positions in a row across a computer screen. Each response is a keypress, made on one of four keys also arranged in a horizontal row. For the inner two lines, the correct response is spatially "corresponding"—the position of the stimulus in the stimulus array matches the position of the response in the response array. For the outer two lines, the correct response is "opposite"—it can be obtained by reflecting the stimulus position about the midline. What the data showed was that response selection in such tasks proceeds in two stages. First, there is selection of the appropriate spatial transformation, "corresponding" or "opposite." Second, this transformation is applied to the stimulus to produce the correct response. For example, the common error is to apply the wrong transformation to the right stimulus (e.g. Figure 10.3, inner left line to inner right key; see Duncan, 1977).

In a sense, selection of a spatial transformation certainly seems like a "control process". It is a higher-level process that guides how responses should be computed on this trial. On the other hand, transformation selection also

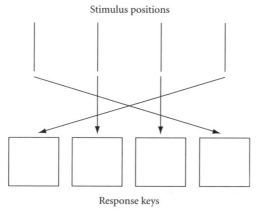

Stimulus positions

Response keys

Fig. 10.3 Stimulus-response mapping from Duncan (1977).

seems to have much in common with any choice based on a stimulus and an arbitrary rule. Suppose that a person must remember that the correct response to the stimulus letter A is to press a response key on the left. Though this might not be called a "control process," is it different in principle from remembering that the correct transformation for an outer left stimulus is "opposite?"

The problem is even more obvious and acute as soon as one looks beyond simple laboratory tasks to the structure of everyday behaviour. As many people have pointed out (e.g. Miller, Galanter, & Pribram, 1960), action planning develops by unpacking higher-order goals into more and more detailed subgoals. Figure 10.4, for example, shows the sort of structure that might be needed to organize travel from Australia to Oxford. In a scheme of this sort, each selected subgoal acts as an additional constraint on the action plan, guiding its more detailed development (Sacerdoti, 1974). For example, once the decision is made to drive to the airport, this combines with knowledge of driving to implement a process of searching for car keys. Once the decision is made to feel in one's pocket for keys, this indicates selection of a corresponding set of arm and hand movements. In a structure of this sort, there is no possible distinction between "control" and "controlled." Instead, every decision acts to shape or direct further stages of plan development.

In my opinion, there are many ideas about "control processes" and prefrontal function that cannot really be applied to complex, real-life action structures of this sort. For example, many experiments over the past 10 years

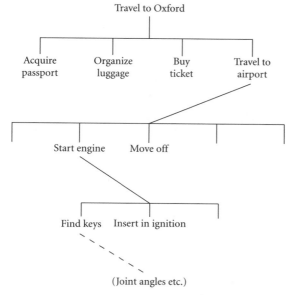

Fig. 10.4 Goal–subgoal hierarchy in everyday action.

have addressed the problem of "task switching." In the typical experiment (e.g. Rogers & Monsell, 1995), one cue (e.g. position of a stimulus on a screen) tells the subject which "task" to perform, while another (e.g. a letter or number) is the "stimulus" for this task. In a sense this is very close to my hierarchical spatial task, with separate stages of choosing a rule, then applying it to choose the response. Often, task/rule choice is seen as an executive control process that is different in kind from simple response selection. From the perspective of a structure like the one in Figure 10.4, however, these decisions are just two hierarchically-arranged components of the action plan; obviously it would not be possible to draw a line across Figure 10.4 such that decisions above the line were "task" choices, while decisions below were choices within a task. In experiments like these, the "switch costs" measured when the "task" changes from one trial to the next are simply the effects of one particular set of changes to the overall action structure. Much the same can be said about the idea that PFC sets cognitive "context" for lower-level decisions (Cohen & Servan-Schreiber, 1992). In a Stroop experiment, for example, the "context" might be the instruction to name colours or read words; "lower-level" processes are then enabled based on the prefrontal representation of this task instruction. A structure like Figure 10.4 suggests something different—there is no real distinction between "context" and other things, but rather, every selected component of the plan provides additional context guiding further choices.

How are such structures created? In artificial intelligence systems like ACT* (Anderson, 1983), and SOAR (Newell, 1990), each stage of plan development proceeds by building a temporary model of some aspect of the world, the goal states to be achieved in that model, and hence the actions to be undertaken. The subgoal of starting the car engine, for example, combines with knowledge of the world (e.g. car-starting procedures) and sensory input (e.g. presence or absence of keys on the table) to indicate that keys are required, where they are or may be, what procedures are needed to obtain them and so on. As this model builds up in the program's working memory, it provides the information that guides or controls the system's further choices and actions. Control here is not a matter of abstract "control processes"—it is a representation of detailed task content that determines how further progress should be made.

Many human and animal experiments have addressed the role of frontal and parietal cortex in "working memory" (Goldman-Rakic, 1988). In the typical experiment, stimulus information must be remembered through a brief delay before it is used to select a response. In the sense of systems like SOAR and ACT*, however, working memory involves far more than simple information storage. It is a system controlling action planning by constructing an on-line model of task-relevant knowledge. In line with the physiological data reviewed in the previous section, I would suggest that lateral PFC—probably in conjunction with the other parts of the MD network—is responsible for "control" through exactly this kind of on-line representation of task events, rules, and information (Kimberg & Farah, 1993; for related ideas see Dehaene, Sergent, & Changeux, 2003; Miller & Cohen, 2001).

Leading on from this, I would suggest that *g* may largely reflect the efficiency of this task modeling function. Various authors have proposed that *g* is related to properties of working memory—for example, simple memory capacity, or ability to exclude distracting or task-irrelevant information (see Engle, Kane, & Tuholski, 1999). As Pat pointed out in his 1981 Attention and Performance paper, the complete internal model for any task is likely to include a complex set of operations designed to control and optimize performance. Variable efficiency in constructing such models is a plausible explanation for universal positive correlations between performance and *g*. In the following section, I turn to evidence that *g* is indeed associated with competition in a task model, and with loss of vulnerable task components.

Goal neglect

In this section I return to goal neglect, or apparent mismatch between what is known of a task's requirements, and what is actually carried out. As I noted earlier, striking examples are occasionally reported in frontal lobe patients. Konow and Pribram (1970), for example, describe a patient who drew an A when asked to draw a square. Her comment was, "That's not a square—I guess I'll draw you an A." As described at the start of the chapter, early observations with a rather complex dichotic listening test suggested that, under the right task conditions, a similar goal neglect could sometimes be observed in people from the normal population. In particular, it seemed associated with low scores on a standard test of *g*. In subsequent work, we have moved to a visual version of the task. The results repeatedly confirm the occurrence of goal neglect, its association with *g*, and the importance of competition in a complex task model.

The task we have most commonly used is illustrated in Figure 10.5 (Duncan et al. 1996). On each trial, a series of letter and number pairs is shown one after the other at the centre of a computer screen. Each pair is presented for 200 ms, with a further 200 ms blank interval between one pair and the next. The task is to watch just the characters on one side, left or right, and on that side, to ignore numbers but repeat letters aloud. Two cues tell the subject which side to watch. At the start of the trial, there is a verbal instruction WATCH LEFT or WATCH RIGHT. In the example shown in Figure 10.5, for example, the subject is told WATCH LEFT and repeats E, L . . . while ignoring X, P . . . Then, immediately before the last three pairs, there is a second side cue. This time it is a symbol, either + or −, also flashed for 200 ms in the

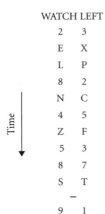

WATCH LEFT

Time

Fig. 10.5 Stimuli from Duncan et al. (1996). The task is to repeat just letters from the attended side. For the last part of each trial, side is indicated by a brief central symbol: + for right, − for left.

center of the screen. A + means that, for the final three pairs, the subject should watch right, while a − means watch left. In the example, the subject sees −, stays on the left, and repeats M, K. A +, however, would have called for a switch to the right, and repetition of A, B.

In this task, it is the +/− cue that is sometimes neglected. Most commonly, the subject completes the whole task as if these cues simply did not exist, always continuing to report letters from the starting side until the trial finishes. Several things are striking about this behaviour (Duncan et al. 1996). First, the actual task requirements are always well remembered. Asked at the end of the task, all subjects can repeat what they were told to do. Second, there is no absolute inability to follow instructions, for example, because the task is too fast. In various experiments, we have examined what happens if, after a first block of trials, subjects are given various kinds of prompt to focus on the +/− cue. One especially effective prompt is simply to point out errors after every trial. Almost always, a few such reminders are sufficient for neglect to disappear. Third, questions at the end of the experiment elicit comments such as, "I realize now that I have not been looking out for the plus or minus," or, "I have been letting those go over my head." Though initially understood, the +/− requirement is somehow inactive in controlling behaviour. Fourth, and in line with our original observations in dichotic listening, neglect is very closely related to g. Typically we have used the Culture Fair as our g measure. When the Culture Fair score is more than one standard deviation below the population mean, there is almost complete goal neglect in the letter monitoring task. For people more than one standard deviation above the population mean, neglect is essentially absent. Apparently, the simple tendency to neglect one part of a complex task reflects very much the same thing as a standard problem-solving test of *g*.

Is competition between task requirements an important consideration in neglect? If so, neglect of the $+/-$ cue should depend on the other requirements to be satisfied. In various experiments (Duncan, Parr, Bright, Cox, & Bishop, unpublished data), we have studied different aspects of task structure. Though neglect indeed depends on competition from other task requirements, this competition takes a rather surprising form.

One obvious hypothesis could depend on the real-time demands of performance. Subjectively, paying attention to letters could distract the subject from monitoring for side cues. In one relevant experiment, we manipulated the demand of letter monitoring. For half the subjects, we used the standard task, with characters flashed in pairs as in Figure 10.5. For the remaining subjects, we increased the number of characters/display from two to four, two to the left and two to the right. The two characters on each side were either both numbers, or one letter and one number. Under these circumstances, letters on the cued side were appreciably harder to find and report; in the first part of the trial, before the $+/-$, the proportion of letters correctly repeated fell from 0.97 for subjects with two characters/display to 0.83 for subjects with four. We asked whether this increase in letter monitoring demand led to a corresponding increase in $+/-$ neglect.

The results are shown in Figure 10.6(a). In this figure, subjects have been sorted into bins using Culture Fair scores, here expressed as *z*-scores. The lowest bin in each panel, for example, includes all subjects with a score more than 0.5 standard deviations below the population mean (taken from published norms; see Institute for Personality and Ability Testing, 1973). For subjects in each bin, the figure shows mean goal neglect score, with 0.5 indicating complete neglect of the $+/-$ cue (across trials, equal probability of reporting letters from correct and incorrect side), and 0 indicating perfect performance (letters from correct side on every trial). In this experiment, the close relationship between neglect and *g* is actually less evident than in most of the experiments we have run. For present purposes, however, the key result is that 2- and 4-character displays lead to essentially the same level of performance on $+/-$ cues. Apparently, neglect is rather insensitive to real-time demands of the letter monitoring task—a result we have confirmed with other kinds of demand manipulation.

What neglect does depend on, however, is complexity of the entire set of requirements specified in task instructions. A new version of the task establishing this point is shown in Figure 10.7. Again, pairs of characters are

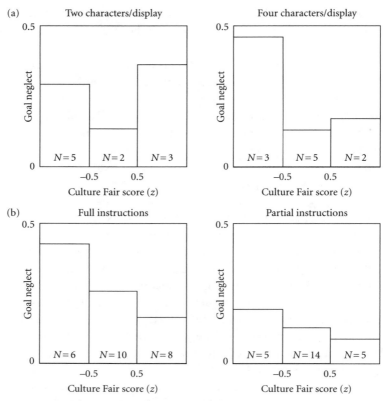

Fig. 10.6 Goal neglect score as a function of Culture Fair score in comparison of (a) 2- vs. 4-character displays, (b) full vs. partial instructions for pure blocks of letter and number tasks. In each panel, mean goal neglect score (chance = 0.5, perfect performance = 0) is shown for subjects with Culture Fair scores $z < -0.5$, $z = -0.5$ to $z = 0.5$, and $z > 0.5$. N shows number of subjects falling into each bin.

presented one after the other, at the same rate as before. Now, the trial is split into three segments, separated by pairs of astrisks flashing for the same duration as other character pairs. After each pair of asterisks come two more pairs—either two pairs of letters, or two pairs of numbers. As we have found that it makes little difference, this time we have replaced the $+/-$ cue with an arrow pointing directly to the side to watch for the last part of the trial. For letter trials, the task is the same as before—simply to repeat letters from the attended side. For each segment of a number trial, the task is to add the two successive numbers from the attended side, and to state the result. Thus for the number trial in Figure 10.7, the correct answer would be "four, nine, ten."

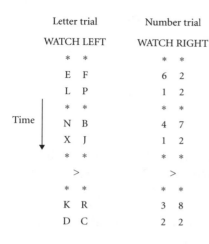

Letter trial		Number trial	
WATCH LEFT		WATCH RIGHT	
*	*	*	*
E	F	6	2
L	P	1	2
*	*	*	*
N	B	4	7
X	J	1	2
*	*	*	*
>		>	
*	*	*	*
K	R	3	8
D	C	2	2

Time

Fig. 10.7 Stimuli for comparison of full and partial instructions in goal neglect. Within each trial, asterisk pairs serve as place-markers separating one trial segment from the next. For letter trials, the task is to repeat all letters from the attended side. For number trials, the task is to add together the two attended numbers in each segment.

Again there were two groups of subjects, differing only in the way instructions were given. For subjects with full instructions, everything was explained at the outset. These subjects were told about the character streams, the letter task, the number task, and finally the arrow cues. Then, before performance began, they were told that the first block of eight trials would involve either just letters (half the subjects in this group), or just numbers (the other half). Eight trials with the specified task were followed by a warning that the materials would now change, then eight more trials of the other kind. For subjects with partial instructions, only one task, letters or numbers, was described at the outset. After eight trials with this task, the other materials were introduced, and eight trials given with those. In terms of the actual performance required, subjects in the two groups were identical. The only difference lay in the way that task requirements were introduced, either in a single block at the outset, or in two parts.

In terms of letter and number performance, subjects in the two groups were very similar. In the first part of the trial, before the arrow cues, proportion of correct responses was 0.93 for full-instruction subjects, compared with 0.96 for partial instructions. As shown in Figure 10.6(b), however, arrow neglect was much more common with full instructions. With more to bear in mind, full-instruction subjects were much more likely to lose one task component. In both groups, furthermore, the data this time showed the usual close relationship between neglect and *g*.

Certainly these goal neglect data are well explained by the task modeling idea of *g*. They suggest that, in low *g* subjects, competition in a task model leads to loss of a vulnerable task component. Subjectively, it "slips the subject's mind" and fails to trigger when required. More generally, it has often been proposed that g is increasingly important as tasks are made more "complex" (e.g. Marshalek et al. 1983). Competition in a task model provides a plausible explanation. As more task components are added, there is an increasing chance that one or more will be lost from the model and fail in its control of behaviour.

Lesion studies

Lastly I want to consider some problematic findings. In two small early studies, we found that both g and goal neglect were selectively sensitive to frontal lobe lesions (Duncan, Burgess, & Emslie, 1995; Duncan et al. 1996). In a current study we are conducting a more extensive comparison of frontal and posterior lesions (Duncan, et al. unpublished data). Our prediction is that deficits in g should reflect damage to MD regions. To date, however, we are unable to separate MD damage from simple lesion volume; even more fundamentally, the whole attempt to predict g deficits is weakened because, very often, similar lesions lead to very different cognitive outcomes.

We currently have data for 55 patients, 29 with lesions strictly confined to the frontal lobe, and 26 with posterior lesions. All have chronic lesions, with behavioural testing and MRI at least six months post-onset. To measure g we are combining performance from the Culture Fair and a second test of problem solving using letter strings (Letter Sets from the Kit of Factor-Referenced Cognitive Tests; Ekstrom, French, Harmon, & Derman, 1976). Scores are expressed as a discrepancy from the score expected based on the patient's age and an assessment of premorbid function (the National Adult Reading Test; Nelson, 1982), greater negative scores indicating greater discrepancy or impairment.

To assess MD damage, we use the complete set of peak activation coordinates from the 20 studies included in the Duncan and Owen (2000) review. To define frequently-activated regions, we smoothed each coordinate, added the smoothed results, and thresholded to give three continuous regions in each hemisphere—a lateral frontal region encompassing both posterior IFS and the operculum/insula, a dorsomedial frontal region encompassing the anterior cingulate/supplementary motor area, and a parietal region based around the intraparietal sulcus. In Figure 10.8(a), discrepancy scores for combined frontal and posterior patients are plotted against total volume of damage in these MD regions. Though the correlation is significant, $r(53) = -0.30$, it is certainly modest. In fact, a somewhat better prediction is obtained just from total lesion volume, irrespective of where in the brain the damage occurs, $r(53) = -0.36$ (Figure 10.8(b)).

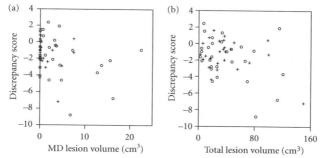

Fig. 10.8 Discrepancy scores as a function of (a) summed volume of lesion in MD regions; (b) total lesion volume. For each patient, Culture Fair discrepancy (obtained score minus predicted score) is divided by standard deviation of these discrepancies in a control sample. The same procedure is followed for Letter Sets. Plotted discrepancy is the sum of these two values. o — frontal lesion; + — posterior lesion.

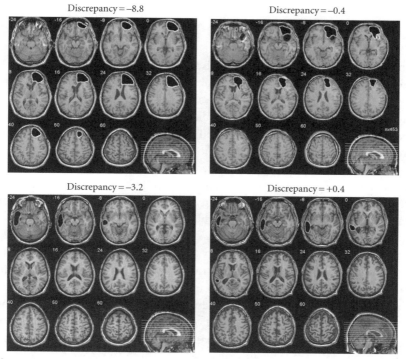

Fig. 10.9 Normalized MRIs (horizontal slices, left of slice is left of brain) for pairs of patients with (a) similar frontal lobe lesions, (b) similar temporal lobe lesions. Lesion tracing in black. Numbers for each slice show *z*-levels in space of Montreal Neurological Institute template brain; slice levels are shown for each patient on medial brain view at bottom right. Discrepancy scores as Figure 10.8.

It is also worth emphasizing how closely similar lesions can produce very different behavioural results. Two examples are shown in Figure 10.9. In Figure 10.9(a) are two patients with frontal lobe lesions. Though the lesions are so similar, the patient on the left has a major impairment, while the patient on the right has little or none. In Figure 10.9(b) are two patients with temporal pole lesions. Surely, based on functional imaging evidence (Figure 10.1(b)), the temporal pole should not be closely involved in tests like the Culture Fair. Though the patient on the right shows the expected preservation of function, the patient on the left is very impaired.

It is too soon to draw strong conclusions from these data. To dissociate MD damage from overall lesion size, we need more cases with large lesions outside the MD regions. To understand the variability in the data, we may need functional imaging in patients with apparently similar lesions but very different cognitive outcomes. Meanwhile, though, these data show some of the difficulties of using lesion data to test the MD hypothesis.

Conclusions

In this chapter I have presented a revised and extended version of the simple idea that g may be a measure of prefrontal function. According to this revised hypothesis, the MD pattern—activation by a broad range of cognitive demands—reveals cortical processes underlying g. In the frontal lobe, the MD pattern is strongest around the inferior frontal sulcus, in the operculum/insula, and in the dorsal anterior cingulate. Single unit data for one MD region—the lateral PFC—show a flexible, distributed representation of task-relevant information, suggestive of a "working memory" used to build a model of the current task's structure, events and requirements. Variable efficiency in such task modeling would certainly provide a plausible account of g, and indeed, g is strongly associated with a tendency to neglect vulnerable aspects of a task's requirements.

Of course, there are many questions over these ideas. Most important are the lesion data, showing that damage far outside MD regions can sometimes produce major deficits in tests like the Culture Fair. A second significant question concerns the generality of the task modeling account. The proposal is that something akin to goal neglect in internal task models accounts for universal correlations between task performance and g. In the tasks we have studied, neglect of one component is particularly transparent in the data, but usually this is not true—though many internal operations or task components contribute to successful performance, their contributions cannot be clearly separated in behaviour. This makes the general idea of neglected task components hard to assess. A third question concerns the detailed function of the frontal and parietal regions that we have linked to the task modeling function. Do the inferior frontal sulcus, operculum/insula, anterior cingulate, and intraparietal cortex make essentially similar, parallel contributions to this function, or can their roles be differentiated? And how do these regions, commonly activated by the simple demands of most imaging studies, relate to other regions of prefrontal cortex, for example, more anterior parts of the lateral surface (Koechlin, Ody, & Kouneiher, 2003)?

Evidently, much remains open. As a student, I worked on choice reaction time because Pat was working on choice reaction time. Subsequently, he has spent much time working on frontal lobe functions, and I have done the same thing. He has spent much time working on general intelligence; so have I. Recently, I looked at the acknowledgments page of my DPhil to discover: "The careful student could doubtless find much of the best in this thesis between the lines of three papers published by my supervisor, Pat Rabbitt (Rabbit & Vyas, 1970, 1973; Rabbitt, Vyas, & Fearnley, 1975)."

I remember quite well why I put it this way. I had once asked Pat exactly what he meant by a comment in a recent paper. He replied that he regarded his Discussion sections as a Rorschach test for psychologists. Perhaps I can best sum up the work in this chapter as . . . still working on those blots . . .

References

Anderson, J. R. (1983). *The architecture of cognition*. Cambridge, MA: Harvard University Press.

Asaad, W. F., Rainer, G., & Miller, E. K. (2000). Task-specific neural activity in the primate prefrontal cortex. *Journal of Neurophysiology, 84*, 451–459.

Bianchi, L. (1922). *The mechanism of the brain and the function of the frontal lobes*. Edinburgh: Livingstone.

Broadbent, D. E. (1971). *Decision and stress*. London: Academic Press.

Cohen, J. D., & Servan-Schreiber, D. (1992). Context, cortex, and dopamine: A connectionist approach to behavior and biology in schizophrenia. *Psychological Review, 99*, 45–77.

Dehaene, S., Sergent, C., & Changeux, J.-P. (2003). A neuronal network model linking subjective reports and objective physiological data during conscious perception. *Proceedings of the National Academy of Sciences USA, 100*, 8520–8525.

Duncan, J. (1977). Response selection rules in spatial choice reaction tasks. In S. Dornic (Ed.), *Attention and performance VI* (pp. 49–61). Hillsdale, NJ: Erlbaum.

Duncan, J. (2001). An adaptive coding model of neural function in prefrontal cortex. *Nature Reviews Neuroscience, 2*, 820–829.

Duncan, J., Burgess, P., & Emslie, H. (1995). Fluid intelligence after frontal lobe lesions. *Neuropsychologia, 33*, 261–268.

Duncan, J., Emslie, H., Williams, P., Johnson, R., & Freer, C. (1996). Intelligence and the frontal lobe: The organization of goal-directed behavior. *Cognitive Psychology, 30*, 257–303.

Duncan, J., & Owen, A. M. (2000). Common regions of the human frontal lobe recruited by diverse cognitive demands. *Trends in Neurosciences*, **23**, 475–483.

Duncan, J., Seitz, R. J., Kolodny, J., Bor, D., Herzog, H. et al. (2000). A neural basis for general intelligence. *Science*, **289**, 457–460.

Ekstrom, R. B., French, J. W., Harmon, H. H., & Derman, D. (1976). *ETS kit of factor-referenced cognitive tests*. Princeton, NJ: Educational Testing Service.

Engle, R. W., Kane, M. J., & Tuholski, S. W. (1999). Individual differences in working memory capacity and what they tell us about controlled attention, general fluid intelligence and functions of the prefrontal cortex. In A. Miyake & P. Shah (Eds.), *Models of working memory: Mechanisms of active maintenance and executive control* (pp. 102–134). Cambridge: Cambridge University Press.

Everling, S., Tinsley, C. J., Gaffan, D., & Duncan, J. (2002). Filtering of neural signals by focused attention in the monkey prefrontal cortex. *Nature Neuroscience*, **5**, 671–676.

Freedman, D. J., Riesenhuber, M., Poggio, T., & Miller, E. K. (2001). Categorical representation of visual stimuli in the primate prefrontal cortex. *Science*, **291**, 312–316.

Funahashi, S., Bruce, C. J., & Goldman-Rakic, P. S. (1989). Mnemonic coding of visual space in the monkey's dorsolateral prefrontal cortex. *Journal of Neurophysiology*, **61**, 331–349.

Fuster, J. M., Bauer, R. H., & Jervey, J. P. (1985). Functional interactions between inferotemporal and prefrontal cortex in a cognitive task. *Brain Research*, **330**, 299–307.

Goldman-Rakic, P. (1988). Topography of cognition: Parallel distributed networks in primate association cortex. *Annual Review of Neuroscience*, **11**, 137–156.

Gopher, D., & Kahneman, D., (1971). Individual differences in attention and the prediction of flight criteria. *Perceptual and Motor Skills*, **33**, 1335–1342.

Hon, N., Duncan, J., Epstein, R., & Owen., A. (2004). On the role of the frontoparietal network: Attention, task or awareness. *NeuroImage*, **22**, S51.

Institute for Personality and Ability Testing. (1973). *Measuring intelligence with the Culture Fair tests*. Champaign, Illinois: The Institute for Personality and Ability Testing.

Kimberg, D. Y., & Farah, M. J. (1993). A unified account of cognitive impairments following frontal lobe damage: The role of working memory in complex, organized behavior. *Journal of Experimental Psychology: General*, **122**, 411–428.

Koechlin, E., Ody, C., & Kouneiher, F. (2003). The architecture of cognitive control in the human prefrontal cortex. *Science*, **302**, 1181–1185.

Konow, A., & Pribram, K. H. (1970). Error recognition and utilization produced by injury to the frontal cortex in man. *Neuropsychologia*, **8**, 489–491.

Lauwereyns, J., Sakagami, M., Tsutsui, K.-I., Kobayashi, S., Koizumi, M., & Hikosaka, O. (2001). Responses to task-irrelevant visual features by primate prefrontal neurons. *Journal of Neurophysiology*, **86**, 2001–2010.

Luria, A. R. (1966). *Higher cortical functions in man*. London: Tavistock.

Marshalek, B., Lohman, D. F., & Snow, R. E. (1983). The complexity continuum in the radex and hierarchical models of intelligence. *Intelligence*, **7**, 107–127.

McKenna, F. P. (1984). Measures of field dependence: Cognitive style or cognitive ability. *Journal of Personality and Social Psychology*, **47**, 593–603.

McKenna, F. P., Duncan, J., & Brown, I. D. (1986). Cognitive abilities and safety on the road: A re-examination of individual differences in dichotic listening and search for embedded figures. *Ergonomics*, **29**, 649–663.

Miller, E. K., & Cohen, J. D. (2001). An integrative theory of prefrontal function. *Annual Review of Neuroscience*, **24**, 167–202.

Miller, G. A., Galanter, E., & Pribram, K. H. (1960). *Plans and the structure of behavior*. New York: Holt, Rinehart, and Winston.

Milner, B. (1963). Effects of different brain lesions on card sorting. *Archives of Neurology*, **9**, 90–100.

Nelson, H. E. (1982). *National Adult Reading Test (NART)*. *Test Manual*. Windsor, UK: NFER-Nelson.

Newell, A. (1990). *Unified theories of cognition*. Cambridge, MA: Harvard University Press.

Nieder, A., & Miller, E.K. (2004). A parieto-frontal network for visual numerical information in the monkey. *Proceedings of the National Academy of Sciences, USA*, **101**, 7457–7462.

Niki, H., & Watanabe, M. (1979). Prefrontal and cingulate unit activity during timing behavior in the monkey. *Brain Research*, **171**, 213–224.

Pandya, D. N., & Yeterian, E. H. (1996). Comparison of prefrontal architecture and connections. *Philosophical Transactions of the Royal Society of London Series B*, **351**, 1423–1432.

Parkin, A. J., & Java, R. I. (1999). Deterioration of frontal lobe function in normal aging: Influences of fluid intelligence versus perceptual speed. *Neuropsychology*, **13**, 539–545.

Rabbitt, P. M. A. (1981). Cognitive psychology needs models for changes in performance with old age. In J. Long & A. D. Baddeley (Eds.), *Attention and performance IX* (pp. 555–573). Hillsdale, NJ: Erlbaum.

Rabbitt, P. M. A. (1993). Does it all go together when it goes? The nineteenth Bartlett memorial lecture. *Quarterly Journal of Experimental Psychology*, *46A*, 385–434.

Rabbitt, P. M. A., & Vyas, S. (1970). An elementary preliminary taxonomy for some errors in laboratory choice RT tasks. In A. F. Sanders (Ed.), *Attention and performance III* (pp. 56–76). Amsterdam: North-Holland.

Rabbitt, P. M. A., & Vyas, S. (1973). What is repeated in the "repetition effect"? In S. Kornblum (Ed.), *Attention and performance IV* (pp. 327–342). London: Academic Press.

Rabbitt, P. M. A., Vyas, S., & Fearnley, S. (1975). Programming sequences of complex responses. In P. M. A. Rabbitt & S. Dornic (Eds.), *Attention and performance V* (pp. 395–417). London: Academic Press.

Rainer, G., Asaad, W. F., & Miller, E. K. (1998). Selective representation of relevant information by neurons in the primate prefrontal cortex. *Nature*, **393**, 577–579.

Rao, S. C., Rainer, G., & Miller, E. K. (1997). Integration of what and where in the primate prefrontal cortex. *Science*, **276**, 821–824.

Rogers, R. D., & Monsell, S. (1995). Costs of a predictable switch between simple cognitive tasks. *Journal of Experimental Psychology: General*, **124**, 207–231.

Romo, R., Brody, C. D., Hernández, A., & Lemus, L. (1999). Neuronal correlates of parametric working memory in the prefrontal cortex. *Nature*, **399**, 470–473.

Sacerdoti, E. D. (1974). Planning in a hierarchy of abstraction spaces. *Artificial Intelligence*, **5**, 115–135.

Sakagami, M., & Niki, H. (1994). Encoding of behavioral significance of visual stimuli by primate prefrontal neurons: Relation to relevant task conditions. *Experimental Brain Research*, **97**, 423–436.

Spearman, C. (1904). General intelligence, objectively determined and measured. *American Journal of Psychology*, **15**, 201–293.

Toth, L. J., & Assad, J. A. (2002). Dynamic coding of behaviourally relevant stimuli in parietal cortex. *Nature*, **415**, 165–168.

Wallis, J. D., Anderson, K. C., & Miller, E. K. (2001). Single neurons in prefrontal cortex encode abstract rules. *Nature*, **411**, 953–956.

Watanabe, M. (1986). Prefrontal unit activity during delayed conditional go/no-go discrimination in the monkey. II. Relation to go and no-go responses. *Brain Research*, **382**, 15–27.

Watanabe , M. (1996). Reward expectancy in primate prefrontal neurons. *Nature*, **382**, 629–632.

Witkin, H. A., Oltman, P. K., Raskin, E., & Karp, S. A. (1971). *Manual for embedded figures test, children's embedded figures test, and group embedded figures test*. Palo Alto, CA: Consulting Psychologists Press.

Memory and age

Chapter 11

On reducing age-related declines in memory and executive control

Fergus I. M. Craik

Abstract

Are age-related declines in cognitive functions inevitable? Although there are wide individual differences in the extent to which intellectual capacities become less efficient in the course of normal aging, the general answer appears to be in the affirmative. Cognitive abilities depend on the brain, and the brain—like other bodily organs—becomes less efficient as we age. Two major factors make the picture less negative. The first is that age-related declines are highly task-dependent, and performance on some tasks holds up well. The second is that certain manipulations and conditions can serve to counteract the typical effects of aging. The present chapter describes some experiments that address this second factor. In the area of memory, the studies show that relatedness benefits older adults differentially; strategy instructions also boost recall in older adults, but at considerable cost in processing resources. Context reinstatement is a further factor that boosts recognition memory in older adults. Finally, some recent work is described showing that bilingualism in older adults is associated with higher levels of executive control. It seems then that cognitive decline in old age is modifiable in various ways, and this conclusion should encourage the development of techniques to offset the negative effects of aging on cognitive performance.

Introduction

I am delighted to contribute this chapter to the Festschrift for Patrick Rabbitt; I have known Pat for more years than either of us care to remember (or indeed *can* remember at this point), and I have admired and been influenced by his

The studies reported in this chapter were supported by grants to Fergus Craik from the Natural Sciences and Engineering Research Council of Canada, and to Ellen Bialystok and Fergus Craik from the Canadian Institutes of Health Research.

work over this lengthy period. Pat's ideas and findings have had a huge impact on the field of cognitive aging, and on the experimental psychology of memory, attention, and skilled performance. His work continues the tradition of British experimental psychology initiated by such figures as Bartlett, Broadbent, and Welford, and his ideas have typically been put forward in ways that cut to the heart of the matter. Tales of Pat's trenchant remarks at conferences and other gatherings are the stuff of legend, although many of the stories are unfortunately not appropriate for a family-oriented volume such as the present one. He is one of the people I most enjoy having a drink with, and coming from a Scotsman that is the highest possible praise.

To honour a retiree it seemed appropriate to emphasize the positive aspects of work on cognitive aging, so I will describe three sets of experiments that demonstrate ways in which age-related decrements in memory and executive control can be reduced. I was simply a collaborator on all three experiments, so I would first like to acknowledge the principal investigators of the studies—Moshe Naveh-Benjamin, Astrid Schloerscheidt, and Ellen Bialystok—and thank them for their permission to include accounts of the experiments in this chapter.

It is generally agreed that cognitive performance reflects both automatic and controlled aspects (e.g. Schneider & Shiffrin, 1977; Shiffrin & Schneider, 1977) and that in the course of normal aging the automatic aspects hold up well, but the controlled aspects decline in effectiveness (Salthouse, 1991; Welford, 1958). This decline in the efficiency of control processes is likely attributable (at least in part) to the declining efficiency of frontal lobe functions (Craik & Grady, 2002; Raz, 2000; West, 1996). There is also general agreement that age-related declines in memory and other cognitive functions are highly variable, with performance on some tasks (such as free recall, paired-associate learning, and source memory) showing large age-related decrements, whereas performance on other tasks (such as priming and recognition memory) shows very little change with age (see Craik & Jennings, 1992; Zacks, Hasher, & Li, 2000 for reviews). One major factor contributing to this differential pattern is the role that the external environment plays in different cognitive functions and abilities. I have previously suggested (Craik, 1983, 1986) that effective processing in tasks such as recognition memory is greatly aided by the fact that the stimuli to be recognized are re-presented at the time of test—that is, performance is helped by environmental support. When the environmental context does *not* provide such support, as in free recall, participants must "self-initiate" the necessary processes, and my suggestion was that the production of such self-initiated mental activities requires attentional resources, and that the availability of these processing resources declines in the course of normal aging. Past learning can also serve to support relevant

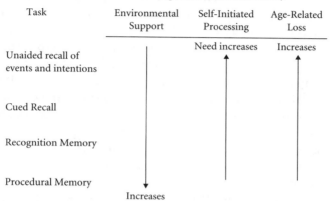

Age-related memory loss is a function of:

1. PERSON unable to execute controlled processing
   (self-initiated activity; frontal inefficiency)
2. TASK requires self-initiated processing
3. ENVIRONMENT fails to compensate (via cues, context)

Task	Environmental Support	Self-Initiated Processing	Age-Related Loss
		Need increases	Increases
Unaided recall of events and intentions			
Cued Recall			
Recognition Memory			
Procedural Memory			
	Increases		

Fig. 11.1 Schematic diagram relating environmental support and self-initiated processing to age-related memory loss.

cognitive activities, and therefore tasks that can rely on such "schematic support" (Bäckman & Herlitz, 1990; Craik & Bosman, 1992) will also hold up well in older people. A schematic representation of these ideas is shown in Figure 11.1; the basic premise is that levels of performance can be understood in terms of interactions among differences in personal characteristics, task characteristics, and the contributions of past learning and the external environment (see also Jenkins, 1974, 1979).

The three experiments that I will describe to illustrate the beneficial effects of various forms of cognitive support on performance in older adults, involve various manipulations. In the first study (Naveh-Benjamin, Craik, Guez, & Kreuger, 2005) we varied both the relatedness of word pairs in a cued recall paradigm, and also examined the effects of giving strategy instructions to half of the participants. The attentional costs of encoding and retrieval were also measured by means of a concurrent tracking task. In work with Astrid Schloerscheidt we studied relations between aging and context—both recall of encoded context and the effects of varying context reinstatement on recognition memory. Finally, a third study (Bialystok, Craik, Klein, & Viswanathan, 2004) explores the effects of bilingualism on executive control in younger and older participants. The overall message is the heartening one that although aging is typically associated with declining efficiency of many cognitive functions, there are ways in which such declines can be reduced.

Effects of strategy and relatedness on memory

One purpose of this study by Naveh-Benjamin, et al. (2005) was to examine the effects of varying relatedness in a paired-associate cued-recall paradigm on age-related differences in memory performance. On the assumptions that older adults do not spontaneously encode information so richly and elaborately as young adults do, and that aging is associated with a reduced likelihood of "going beyond the information given," we expected that the increased relatedness would be particularly beneficial to older participants. In a second manipulation, half of the participants were given explicit strategy instructions; they were told that memory performance can be improved by relating members of each word pair meaningfully, either by creating a sentence linking the words or by forming an interactive image of the two words. Participants in this condition (both younger and older adults) were strongly urged to use this type of strategy. The prediction here was less clear. On the one hand it could be argued that if older adults do not engage in elaborative processing spontaneously, they would show greater benefits than their younger counterparts from the use of an encoding strategy; on the other hand, if older people have fewer attentional resources (Craik & Byrd, 1982) then perhaps *younger* adults would be in a position to take greater advantage of more effective encoding operations. The other major purpose of the experiment was to measure the attentional costs of encoding and retrieval in younger and older adults, and how these costs would be affected by changes in relatedness and strategy. Costs were measured by means of a continuous visual tracking task. Each participant performed this task alone as well as concurrently with encoding and retrieval; the attentional cost of these memory processes was taken to be the difference (for each participant separately) between the task performed alone and together with the memory task. Each word pair was encoded and retrieved within a 6 s interval, so attentional costs were measured as the discrepancy between the visual target and the participant-controlled "chaser" over the averaged 6 s encoding and retrieval intervals.

In the encoding experiment, groups of 32 younger (mean age = 20.6 years) and older adults (mean age = 70.4 years) learnt and recalled lists of 12 pairs of nouns. Half of the participants in each group were given strategy instructions; the remaining participants were given no special instructions apart from "learn the word pairs for a later cued recall test." Within each of the resulting four groups, half of the lists contained unrelated word pairs and the other half contained semantically related pairs. Finally, all participants learnt and retrieved half of the lists under single-task conditions, and *encoded* the other half while also performing the tracking task; retrieval was under single-task conditions in all cases. A second experiment (with 64 different participants) replicated the design exactly, but with the difference that encoding was under full attention (single-task conditions) in all cases, but *retrieval* was performed under either single- or dual-task conditions.

The main results are shown in Figures 11.2 and 11.3. Figure 11.2(a) shows memory performance for the young and older groups, as a function of relatedness, strategy, and whether encoding was carried out under single or dual-task conditions. The results show that younger adults remembered more than their older counterparts in all conditions, related pairs were better remembered than unrelated pairs, the groups who had been given strategy

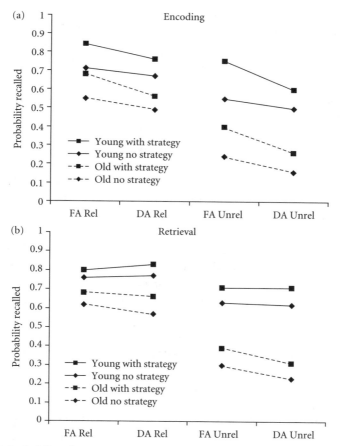

Fig. 11.2 Probability of cued recall as a function of age and condition. (a) and (b) are the encoding and retrieval manipulations respectively. FA = full attention; DA = divided attention; Rel = related pairs; Unrel = unrelated pairs. Data from Naveh-Benjamin et al. (2005).

instructions performed better than groups without such instructions, and single-task performance was higher than dual-task performance. Figure 11.2(a) also shows one significant interaction—between age and relatedness. As predicted, older adults benefitted more than the young groups from relatedness, but interestingly there was no interaction between age and strategy; in this case both groups benefitted equally. Finally, both groups performed less well under dual-task conditions, but this divided attention condition did not penalize either group differentially.

Figured 11.2(b) shows a similar pattern of performance when the tracking task was performed at retrieval. Again there were main effects of age, relatedness, and strategy, although in this case there was no significant effect of divided attention; performance was as good under dual-task conditions at retrieval as under single-task conditions, with the exception of the older group in the unrelated condition. As with encoding, age and relatedness interacted; the older group benefitted more from the related materials.

Figure 11.3(a) and (b) shows tracking costs when attention was divided at encoding and retrieval, respectively. There were no strong effects of relatedness at either encoding or retrieval, so costs are collapsed over this variable. Figure 11.3(a) shows that tracking costs first rise and then fall over the 6 s encoding interval; attentional demands are highest over the first 2–3 s as participants attempt to associate or integrate members of each pair. Tracking costs are substantially higher for the older groups, especially for the group given strategy instructions. We thus concluded that the benefit to memory performance associated with relatedness was achieved with little or no extra attentional costs—the benefit stems from "schematic support" or past learning. The benefit associated with strategy was costly, however, for the older groups at least. Figure 11.3(b) shows the comparable results for divided attention at retrieval. Again, older participants required substantially more attention (above their own baseline) to retrieve the word pairs, and again retrieval costs were higher for the strategy group. Comparing Figures 11.3(a) with (b), it is seen that attentional costs for the older groups were particularly high during retrieval; this result confirms previous findings by Anderson, Craik, and Naveh-Benjamin (1998).

The results are discussed at greater length by Naveh-Benjamin, et al. (2005), but some main implications may be discussed briefly here. First, divided attention during encoding reduced later memory performance substantially and equivalently for both age groups. In contrast, divided attention at retrieval had no effect on memory performance in the young group although it did reduce performance in the elderly. The lack of an effect of divided attention at retrieval in young adults is in line with previous findings (Baddeley, Lewis,

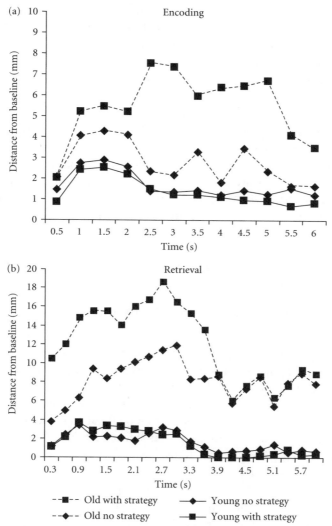

Fig. 11.3 Tracking costs at (a) encoding and (b) retrieval as a function of age and strategy instructions. Note the different scales for encoding and retrieval. Data from Naveh-Benjamin et al. (2005).

Eldridge, & Thomson, 1984; Craik, Govoni, Naveh-Benjamin, & Anderson, 1996) although it should be noted that effects of divided attention at retrieval *are* found if the secondary task involves verbal materials similar to those in the memory task (Fernandes & Moscovitch, 2000). Second, there were interesting differences between the beneficial effects of increased relatedness on the one hand and strategy instructions on the other. Relatedness interacted with age—that is, older adults benefitted more from the more meaningful pairs—whereas strategy instructions benefitted both groups to the same extent. The performance boost from relatedness was relatively cost-free (as shown by tracking costs) whereas the use of strategy was costly, especially for older participants.

In terms of theory, the results further illustrate the difficulties that older adults have with "self-initiated activities" (Craik, 1983, 1986), represented here by the costs required to utilize strategy instructions. This age-related difference contrasts with the *better* use that older adults can make of environmental support or, more precisely in this case, the "schematic support" from past learning associated with enhanced meaningfulness. The second theoretical point illustrated by the present results is the difficulty that older adults have with associative information (Naveh-Benjamin, 2000; Naveh-Benjamin, Guez, Hussain, & Bar-On, 2003). Encoding and retrieving associative information is costly for older people; the better news is that there are ways in which this associative deficit may be ameliorated.

Aging, context, and recognition memory

According to Naveh-Benjamin (2000), older adults have difficulty in remembering associative information. Typically, memory for associative information is studied by providing participants with lists of unrelated words, pictures, letters, or numbers to learn, but in real life associations are more typically formed between events and their contexts of occurrence. It would be expected that older adults would have greater difficulty in binding events and contexts, and indeed older people are less able to remember where and when an event occurred, and less able to recollect the source of information they have acquired (McIntyre & Craik, 1987; Schacter, Kaszniak, Kihlstrom, & Valdiserri, 1991). On the other hand, if older participants profit more from environmental and schematic support (Craik, 1983, 1986) it might be supposed that their ability to recognize previously encountered events might also profit (perhaps more so than young adults) from a reinstatement of the event's initial context of occurrence. If this pattern holds, it would yield the interesting and somewhat paradoxical outcome that, relative to young adults, older adults are less able to recall initial context, yet are more dependent on contextual support for success in recognition memory. These issues were explored in recent experiments by Schloerscheidt, Craik, & Kreuger (2005).

The paradigm used to study these issues was one in which either pictures of common objects or the verbal labels for these objects were presented superimposed on rich pictorial scenes (photographs of city scenes and landscapes downloaded from the Internet). On each trial, one pictured object or one word was presented on a background scene, and participants were instructed to try to make a connection between the object and its background, and to remember the pairing for a later memory test. The pictured objects and words were different on each trial, but the scenes were repeated. In the first experiment to be reported here, groups of 24 younger (average age = 20.5 years) and 24 older (average age = 70.5 years) adults of equivalent educational backgrounds were shown eight pictured objects with each of 10 background scenes. After this study session, participants were given a recall test followed by a recognition test. In the recall test, participants were shown 20 of the original objects, two from each of the 10 scenes, and asked to recall the scene associated with each object. The recall probabilities for younger and older groups were 0.72 and 0.35, respectively ($p < 0.001$). This result illustrates the difficulty that older adults have in recalling the context in which events occurred.

In the recognition test, the remaining 60 objects were shown again; 20 paired with their original background scene, 20 paired with a different scene but switched from the initial pairing, and 20 paired with one of 10 completely new scenes. The test was to say whether the object-scene *pair* was one that appeared in the study phase; it was thus a test of associative recognition. The results are shown in Table 11.1. The older group performed as well as their younger counterparts at recognizing original pairings, but made many more false alarms to switched pairings. Younger participants made very few false alarms to new scenes, but older participants made 10% false alarms in this condition. The ability to discriminate original from switched pairings was 0.65 in the case of young adults and a much lower 0.36 in older adults, a highly significant difference. The results give strong support to the idea developed by Jacoby and others (e.g. Hay & Jacoby, 1999; Jennings & Jacoby, 1993, 1997) that recognition memory in older adults is driven strongly by feelings of global familiarity, and less by the more analytic processes of recollection. Thus older adults' recognition performance is helped by reinstatement of the original context, but they are often misled by

Table 11.1 Probabilities of endorsing an object-scene pair as "old" as a function of age group and condition (SDs in brackets)[a]

Age Group	Context		
	Original	Switched	New
Young	0.85 (0.08)	0.20 (0.15)	0.01 (0.02)
Old	0.87 (0.09)	0.51 (0.23)	0.10 (0.12)

[a] Responses to "original" are hits, and responses to "switched" and "new" are false alarms.

the presence of a familiar context, even although it was not the context paired initially with the object in question.

In a second experiment, the paradigm was expanded to include not only original, switched and new contexts, but also a no-context condition. In this experiment the task was simply to recognize the object itself as old or new, regardless of the context presented at test; it therefore focused more precisely on the question of how much older adults rely on context reinstatement in recognition memory. In this experiment, half of the stimuli presented were pictured objects as before, but half were the words representing these objects; this manipulation was carried out between subjects. Our hypothesis was that pictures drive such a good encoding that item recognition would be at a high level, and would not be much affected by changes in context, but that words require more deliberate and strategic encoding, making them more dependent on context reinstatement, and perhaps more vulnerable to the effects of aging (e.g. see Craik & Byrd, 1982; Nelson, Reed, & McEvoy, 1977; Weldon & Roediger, 1987).

Four groups of subjects participated in the study. In the picture-object condition (referred to here as "pictures") groups of 32 younger (mean age = 20.8 years) and 32 older (mean age = 68.0 years) adults of comparable educational background performed the task. In the verbal label condition (referred to here as "names"), groups of 25 younger (mean age = 19.6 years) and 25 older adults (mean age = 67.7 years) participated in the experiment. In all cases, subjects studied a list of 120 object-scene pairs (either pictures or names of the objects) for a later memory test. Ten scenes were each paired with 12 different pictured objects or names. The recognition list comprised 180 items, of which 60 were identical to the studied pictures or names, 60 were *similar* to the remaining 60 presented items (e.g. a picture of a different hat, or a high associate of a presented word), and 60 were completely new pictured objects or names that had not been seen at study. Each set of 60 objects was distributed over four context conditions; original context, switched context, no context, or new context. Ten completely new scenes were used repeatedly in the new context condition. The purpose of including similar pictures and names was to assess the degree to which older adults would be misled by familiarity to make false positive responses to such items. In outline, this result was found (see also Koutstaal, 2003; Koutstaal & Schacter, 1997) but will not be discussed further in the present chapter.

The main results are shown as recognition performance (in terms of hits minus false alarms to new items) in Figure 11.4. Recognition levels are high for picture recognition—note that the older adults have slightly *higher* scores in this condition. Statistically, the original context yielded performance levels that were higher than those in the other three conditions, that did not differ.

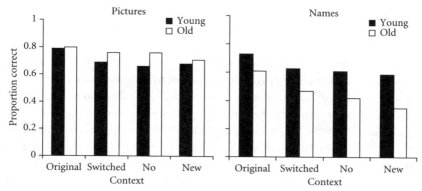

Fig. 11.4 Probability of correct recognition performance as a function of age, material, and context condition. Data from Schloerscheidt et al. (2005).

Picture recognition is thus apparently little affected by context change and immune to the effects of aging (see also Craik & Byrd, 1982; Grady, McIntosh, Rajah, Beig, & Craik, 1999). Results for name recognition are quite different. Now there are reliable effects of age (young better than old) and context, as well as an age by context interaction. This last effect was further analyzed to show that for young subjects, the original context was associated with higher levels of recognition than the other three conditions, which did not differ. For older subjects, however, there is a graded effect of context reinstatement, with significant differences between all pairs of conditions.

These results illustrate the point that the obtained age-related differences in memory performance depend on the test in question (e.g. recall or recognition), the materials used (e.g. pictures or words), and the conditions at test (e.g. the degree of context reinstatement). I take the view that recognition performance is good when pictures are used as materials because pictures drive a rich, elaborate, and meaningful encoded representation without much cognitive effort; older adults benefit particularly from these conditions. Words, on the other hand, require more conscious cognitive effort to achieve such good encodings, and such encodings are achieved less effectively by older adults. This encoding deficit can be ameliorated by the presence of good environmental support at retrieval (e.g. reinstatement of the original context) but exacerbated by the presence of misleading support—by presenting a completely new context at test.

Aging, bilingualism, and executive control

The third study illustrating factors that attenuate the detrimental effects of normal aging on cognitive function takes a rather different approach. Whereas the first two sets of experiments described manipulations that benefitted older adults, in some cases to a greater extent than young adults, the present study investigated the effects of an individual difference—bilingualism—on aspects of cognitive control. The study was an extension of a program of research in cognitive development carried out by Ellen Bialystok and her colleagues. In a series of studies, Bialystok has demonstrated that bilingual children have a processing advantage over their monolingual peers on certain cognitive tasks (Bialystok, 1993, 2001). The basic argument is that bilingual children must develop special control processes to manage fluent production of their two languages. In particular, one language system must be inhibited while the other is being used. What Bialystok has found is that this hypothesized greater degree of cognitive control in bilingual children generalizes to other cognitive tasks that necessitate the inhibition of one set of responses in order to carry out the appropriate response more effectively (see Bialystok, 2001 for a review). It is obviously of great interest to discover whether the processing advantage found in bilingual children persists into adulthood and old age. Perhaps bilingualism may even offer some protection against certain types of cognitive decline in the elderly. These questions were investigated by Bialystok et al. (2004).

We chose the Simon task to explore the effects of normal aging on cognitive control. The Simon task (see Lu & Proctor, 1995 for a review) is one in which one of two coloured patches appears either on the left or right side of a computer screen. Each colour was associated with a response key that was also on one of the two sides of the keyboard, aligned with the two stimulus positions. The task is to press the appropriate key when a colour patch appears, regardless of its side of presentation. Previous work has shown that reaction times (RTs) in the congruent condition (in which the stimulus and response key are on the same side) are faster than in the incongruent condition (stimulus and response key on opposite sides). The difference in RTs between congruent and incongruent conditions is the Simon effect. The size of the effect reflects the difficulty of overcoming the automatic tendency to make a same-side response when the stimulus appears; the further assumption is that better cognitive control is associated with an enhanced ability to ignore the misleading effects of the incongruent spatial information, and is therefore associated with a smaller Simon effect.

Four conditions were included in the experiment to be described (Bialystok et al. 2004, study 2) in an attempt to specify the locus of the bilingual advantage. The first condition was a control condition in which one of two coloured patches appeared in the centre of the screen, thereby eliminating the spatial conflict. The second condition was the standard Simon condition with one of two coloured squares appearing unpredictably on one side or the other. In the third and fourth conditions, four coloured squares were used as stimuli to check whether bilinguals would show an RT advantage over monolinguals in a situation with a high working memory demand—the necessity to hold four stimulus-response rules in mind. Two of the colours mapped to one key, and the other two colours mapped to the second key. In the third condition, one of the four colour patches appeared centrally, and in the fourth condition the stimulus appeared on the side, again either congruently or incongruently with the correct response. Each condition started with a few practice trials and continued with 48 scored trials in two blocks of 24 trials.

There were 94 participants in all, comprising two age and two language groups. The younger group ($n = 64$) ranged in age from 30 to 58 years (mean age = 42.6 years) and the older group consisted of 30 people ranging in age from 60 to 80 years (mean age = 70.3 years). Half of the participants in each age group were bilingual speakers—defined as people who were educated in both languages from the age of 6 years, and who had continued to use both languages daily. In the young group, the bilinguals were either speakers of English and Tamil or speakers of English and Cantonese; in the older group, the bilinguals were either speakers of English and Tamil or English and French. Typically, the language they had spoken at home as children was Tamil, Cantonese, or French, and their English was learnt when they first went to school at age six. The monolinguals were English speakers in both age groups, and did not have functional command of any other language. All four groups were matched on the Cattell Culture Fair Intelligence Test (Cattell & Cattell, 1960), a nonverbal test of general intelligence.

The main results are shown in Figure 11.5. Figure 11.5(a) shows the mean RTs for monolingual and bilingual participants broken down by age in decade groups in the condition with two stimuli presented centrally. Subjects in their sixties and seventies took longer to respond, but there is no hint of a difference between language groups. This null result is reassuring in that it confirms that the bilingual participants were not simply faster and more efficient generally; there is no reason for a bilingual advantage in a straightforward 2-choice RT task. Figure 11.5(b) shows the Simon effect (measured here as the average of the RT difference between congruent and incongruent trials for both 2-colour and 4-colour conditions) as a function of age and language group, and these data now show a strong bilingual advantage (i.e. a smaller Simon effect) that increases dramatically in the sixties and seventies. Figure 11.5(c) shows "working memory costs"—that is, the average difference between the 2-colour and 4-colour conditions (i.e. mean of conditions 3 + 4 minus the mean of conditions 1 + 2). The figure shows that these costs are also greater

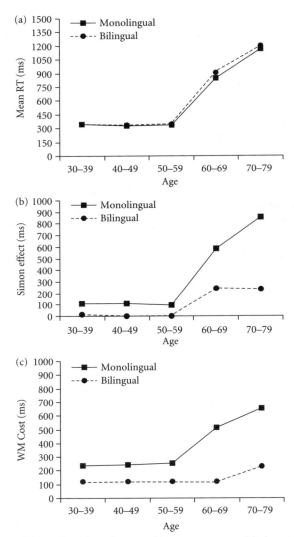

Fig. 11.5 Mean RT as a function of age and language group. (a) shows RTs in the control condition (2-central); (b) shows Simon effect costs; (c) shows working memory costs. Data from Bialystok et al. (2004).

for monolingual than for bilingual subjects, and that the size of the bilingual advantage again increases in the older age groups.

These rather dramatic results suggest several conclusions. First, bilingualism appears to confer an advantage in overcoming the competing response tendencies inherent in the Simon task, and this advantage increases in older age groups. In line with Bialystok's (2001) findings with children, the extended practice of inhibiting the language system not currently in use confers a benefit in the processing of nonverbal stimuli. It also seems that the bilingual advantage decreases from children to young adults, and then reappears strongly in older adults (Martin & Bialystok, 2003). The advantage cannot easily be attributed to a sampling difference between the two language groups given first that the groups were matched on the Cattell test, and second that there were no group differences in 2-choice RT when there was no competing spatial information (Figure 11.5(a)). The bilingual advantage in working memory costs (Figure 11.5(c)) was unexpected. It suggests that the processing advantage associated with bilingualism is not confined to tasks that involve inhibition, but may appear in all tasks requiring complex cognitive control. In our view, the rule for the 2-choice RT could be kept in mind rather easily, whereas the arbitrary mapping of four colours onto two response keys involved a greater working memory load. Speculatively then, central executive functions may be enhanced rather generally through the experience of lifelong bilingualism, although this conclusion requires confirmatory evidence from further studies.

Conclusion

Although normal aging is associated with poorer performance on many cognitive tasks, the work described in the present chapter shows that there are ways of counteracting these age-related declines. Older adults benefit differentially when the task involves well-learnt familiar materials (as in the related word pairs studied by Naveh-Benjamin, et al. 2005) and when the original context is reinstated in recognition memory (as in the word names condition studied by Schloerscheidt, et al. 2005). In theoretical terms, the cognitive performance of older adults benefits substantially from an enhancement of both external environmental support and internal schematic support (Bäckman & Herlitz, 1990; Craik, 1983; Craik & Bosman, 1992). Older adults also profit from explicit strategy instructions (Naveh-Benjamin, et al. 2005) although whether they benefit more, less, or to the same extent as young adults, probably depends on the materials and other aspects of the task. Finally, the work on bilingualism (Bialystok et al. 2004) suggests the intriguing possibility that certain long-lasting experiences can yield cognitive benefits in older adults.

What is it exactly that declines in the course of normal aging? One general description is "executive control," most likely mediated by the declining efficiency of the frontal lobes (Craik & Grady, 2002; West, 1996). I have talked about "declining attentional resources" in many previous publications (e.g. Craik & Byrd, 1982) although the precise definition of what constitutes a "resource" has remained rather vague. A better description might be an age-related decline in *processing power*, drawing an analogy between the loss of brain cells and neural connectivity that occurs in the course of normal brain aging (e.g. Raz, 2000) and the decreased processing power and consequent slowing that occurs in computers whose functional capacity has been decreased by too much "spam" or by viral infections.

In any event, the results of the present experiments are proffered to Pat Rabbitt as reassurance that his impressive intellectual powers *need* not decrease as he enters the phase of partial retirement. It may be too late for him to become a fluently bilingual Tamil speaker, but perhaps other results in the present chapter will provide him with some degree of cognitive comfort. I have admired his many past contributions, and look forward to his further keen insights into aspects of cognitive aging.

References

Anderson, N. D., Craik, F. I. M., & Naveh-Benjamin, M. (1998). The attentional demands of encoding and retrieval in younger and older adults: I. Evidence from divided attention costs. *Psychology and Aging, 13*, 405–423.

Bäckman, L., & Herlitz, A. (1990). The relationship between prior knowledge and face recognition memory in normal aging and Alzheimer's disease. *Journal of Gerontology: Psychological Sciences, 45*, 94–100.

Baddeley, A. D., Lewis, V., Eldridge, M., & Thomson, N. (1984). Attention and retrieval from long-term memory. *Journal of Experimental Psychology: General, 13*, 518–540.

Bialystok, E. (1993). Metalinguistic awareness: The development of children's representations of language. In C. Pratt & A. Garton (Eds.), *Systems of representation in children: Development and use* (pp. 211–233). London: Wiley.

Bialystok, E. (2001). *Bilingualism in development: Language, literacy, and cognition.* New York: Cambridge University Press.

Bialystok, E., Craik, F. I. M., Klein, R., & Viswanathan, M. (2004). Bilingualism, aging, and cognitive control: Evidence from the Simon task. *Psychology and Aging, 19*, 290–303.

Cattell, R. B., & Cattell, A. K. S. (1960). *The individual or group Culture Fair Intelligence Test.* Champaign, IL: Institute for Personality and Ability Testing.

Craik, F. I. M. (1983). On the transfer of information from temporary to permanent memory. *Philosophical Transaction of the Royal Society of London, Series B, 302*, 341–359.

Craik, F. I. M. (1986). A functional account of age differences in memory. In F. Klix & H. Hagendorf (Eds.), *Human memory and cognitive capabilities, mechanisms and performance* (pp. 409–422). Amsterdam: North Holland.

Craik, F. I. M., & Bosman, E. A. (1992). Age-related changes in memory and learning. In H. Bouma & J. A. M. Graafmans (Eds.), *Gerontechnology* (pp. 79–92). Amsterdam: IOS Press.

Craik, F. I. M., & Byrd, M. (1982). Aging and cognitive deficits: The role of attentional resources. In F. I. M. Craik and S. E.Trehub (Eds.), *Aging and cognitive processes* (pp. 191–211). New York: Plenum Press.

Craik, F. I. M., Govoni, R., Naveh-Benjamin, M., & Anderson. N. D. (1996). The effects of divided attention on encoding and retrieval processes in human memory. *Journal of Experimental Psychology: General*, 125, 159–180.

Craik, F. I. M., & Grady, C. L. (2002). Aging, memory, and frontal lobe functioning. In D. T. Stuss & R. T. Knight (Eds.), *Principles of frontal lobe function* (pp.528–540). New York: Oxford University Press.

Craik, F. I. M., & Jennings, J. J. (1992). Human memory. In F. I. M. Craik & T. A. Salthouse (Eds.), *The handbook of aging and cognition* (pp. 51–110). Hillsdale, NJ: Erlbaum.

Fernandes, M. A., & Moscovitch, M. (2000). Divided attention and memory: Evidence of substantial interference effects at retrieval and encoding. *Journal of Experimental Psychology: General*, 129, 155–176.

Grady, C. L., McIntosh, A. R., Rajah, M. N., Beig, S., & Craik, F. I. M. (1999). The effects of age on the neural correlates of encoding. *Cerebral Cortex*, 9, 805–814.

Hay, J. F., & Jacoby, L. L. (1999). Separating habit and recollection in young and older adults: Effects of elaborative processing and distinctiveness. *Psychology and Aging*, 14, 122–134.

Jenkins, J. J. (1974). Remember that old theory of memory? Well, forget it! *American Psychologist*, 29, 785–795.

Jenkins, J. J. (1979). Four points to remember: A tetrahedral model of memory experiments. In L. S. Cermak & F. I. M. Craik (Eds.), *Levels of processing in human memory* (pp. 429–446). Hillsdale, NJ: Erlbaum.

Jennings, J. M., & Jacoby, L. L. (1993). Automatic versus intentional uses of memory: Aging, attention, and control. *Psychology and Aging*, 8, 283–293.

Jennings, J. M., & Jacoby, L. L. (1997). An opposition procedure for detecting age-related deficits in recollection. Telling effects of repetition. *Psychology and Aging*, 12, 352–361.

Koutstaal, W. (2003). Older adults encode—but do not always use—perceptual detail: Intentional versus unintentional effects of detail on memory judgments. *Psychological Science*, 14, 189–193.

Koutstaal, W., & Schacter, D. L. (1997). Gist-based false recognition of pictures in older and younger adults. *Journal of Memory and Language*, 37, 555–583.

Lu, C.-H., & Proctor, R. W. (1995). The influence of irrelevant location information on performance: A review of the Simon and spatial Stroop effects. *Psychonomic Bulletin and Review*, 2, 174–207.

Martin, M. M., & Bialystok, E. (2003, October 24–26). *The development of two kinds of inhibition in monolingual and bilingual children: Simon vs. Stroop*. Poster session presented at the meeting of the Cognitive Development Society, Park City, Utah.

McIntyre, J. S., & Craik, F. I. M. (1987). Age differences in memory for item and source information. *Canadian Journal of Psychology*, 41, 175–192.

Naveh-Benjamin, M. (2000). Adult-age differences in memory performance. Tests of an associative deficit hypothesis. *Journal of Experimental Psychology: Learning, Memory and Cognition*, 26, 1170–1187.

Naveh-Benjamin, M., Craik, F. I. M., Guez, J., & Kreuger, S. (2005). Divided attention in younger and older adults: Effects of strategy and relatedness on memory performance and secondary task costs. *Journal of Experimental Psychology: Learning, Memory and Cognition*, (in press).

Naveh-Benjamin, M., Guez, J., Hussain Z., & Bar-On, M. (2003). Adult-age differences in episodic memory: Further support for an associative deficit hypothesis. *Journal of Experimental Psychology: Learning, Memory and Cognition, 29*, 826–837.

Nelson, D. L., Reed, V. S., & McEvoy, C. L. (1977). Learning to order pictures and words. A model of sensory and semantic encoding. *Journal of Experimental Psychology: Human Learning and Memory, 3*, 485–497.

Raz, N. (2000). Aging of the brain and its impact on cognitive performance: Integration of structural and functional findings. In F. I. M. Craik & T. A. Salthouse (Eds.), *The handbook of aging and cognition* (2nd ed., pp. 1–90). Mahwah NJ: Erlbaum.

Salthouse, T. A. (1991). *Theoretical perspectives on cognitive aging*. Hillsdale, NJ: Erlbaum.

Schacter, D. L., Kaszniak, A. W., Kihlstrom, J. F., & Valdiserri, M. (1991). The relation between source memory and aging. *Psychology and Aging, 6*, 550–568.

Schloerscheidt, A. M., Craik, F. I. M., & Kreuger, S. (2005). The influence of aging and context on the recognition of pictures and words. Manuscript submitted for publication.

Schneider, W., & Shiffrin, R. M. (1977). Controlled and automatic human information processing: I. Detection, search, and attention. *Psychological Review, 84*, 1–66.

Shiffrin, R. M., & Schneider, W. (1977). Controlled and automatic human information processing II: Perceptual learning, automatic attending, and a general theory. *Psychological Review, 84*, 127–190.

Welford, A. T. (1958). *Ageing and human skill*. London: Oxford University Press.

Weldon, M. S., & Roediger, H. L. (1987). Altering retrieval demands reverses the picture superiority effect. *Memory and Cognition, 15*, 259–280.

West, R. L. (1996). An application of prefrontal cortex function theory to cognitive aging. *Psychological Bulletin, 120*, 272–292.

Zacks, R. T., Hasher, L., & Li, K. Z. H. (2000). Human memory. In F. I. M. Craik & T. A. Salthouse (Eds.), *The handbook of aging and cognition* (pp. 293–358). Mahwah, NJ: Lawrence Erlbaum.

Chapter 12

Working memory and aging

Alan Baddeley, Hilary Baddeley,
Dino Chincotta, Simona Luzzi,
and Christobel Meikle

Abstract

This chapter falls into two parts. The first describes the effect of Pat Rabbitt's influence in encouraging the first author (AB) to use the increasingly sophisticated methods of aging research, to answer questions about the fundamental characteristics of working memory, together with reflections on why so little of this work reached publication. This is followed by a brief review of the literature on working memory and aging, followed by an account of more recent work in which we attempt to apply the traditional method of experimental dissociation to research on normal aging and Alzheimer's Disease. We suggest that even such simple methods can throw light on both the processes of aging and the understanding of working memory.

Introduction

Pat Rabbitt gives good talks. Lots of them: and if like me you are a fan, you get to learn a great deal about two topics, reaction times and aging.[1] You are also likely to hear about exciting new methods and techniques, and leave thinking that it would be nice to use them yourself.

In the case of Pat's research on reaction times such enthusiasm was for me relatively harmless. As a percent correct man, who only occasionally feels the temptation to use a stopwatch, the whale-shaped RT distributions and the subtle error monitoring strategies he describes are safely out of my technological reach.

---

[1] This chapter combines two components, personal views and speculations, which are the responsibility of AB, and are expressed in the first person, and accounts of both published and unpublished empirical evidence. The unpublished data on task switching and AD was collected in association with HAB, task switching in normal aging with DC and CM, and the data on the immediate recall of sentences jointly with SL. The support of MRC Grant G9423916 is gratefully acknowledged.

Alas, talks on aging are another matter. For virtually all my research career, I have continued to do experiments on aging, tempted in turn by Brinley plots, multiple regression, structural equation modeling and other arcane practices that Pat manages to make seem straightforward and enlightening. I did my first aging experiment over forty years ago, and have still not produced anything publishable. So, if the editors and the referees are kind, this will be a first.

I propose to speculate on why I have been so spectacularly unsuccessful in an area in which a very large number of people achieve sound and publishable work, and will try to persuade you that, by pulling together a series of studies, some published and some new, I might possibly make a positive though limited contribution to both the study of aging and the understanding of normal cognition. I will begin with some thoughts on possible reasons for my previous lack of success.

Ruminations on aging

For an interested spectator like myself, there seem to be a number of different approaches to aging, stemming from different aims and profiting from different methodologies. First of all, the study of aging is extremely important for both theoretical and practical reasons. Initially, a simple description of the effects of aging on cognition was a reasonable goal, but given the huge amount of good work directed at this problem, I suspect this descriptive stage is largely over, leading to the need to focus on a theoretical understanding of the effects and mechanisms whose changes underlie the process of aging. As Pat, and others have pointed out, our general concepts of cognition typically assume a static adult system, and are not well attuned to detecting progressive changes that in all probability differ in rate and form from one cognitive function to the next. This is of course, exactly the same problem as faces the study of child development. It is best addressed through sustained longitudinal studies of the sort associated for many years with Pat's own work, rather than the limited cross-sectional studies that I myself have attempted.

My own theoretical work has been based on the study of normal adult function, together with its neuropsychological impairments, which typically result in a relatively stable pattern of performance deficits. The analysis of such deficits has of course, contributed greatly to our understanding of normal function across a whole range of cognitive functions from perception through memory to attention and language. My own attempts to study aging have principally been concerned to try to use the deficits of age in a similar way, attempting to use dissociations between deficits in hypothetically different cognitive components to understand the underlying cognitive architecture. Given that this strategy has worked well in the case of amnesia, why not (for me at least) in the case of aging?

In my own opinion, one major difference lies in the problem of collinearity. As we get older, most physical and mental functions deteriorate to some extent. One simply does not find the "good experiment of nature" such as are provided by the classic amnesic syndrome where a single important cognitive function such as episodic memory, is grossly impaired, while the rest of cognition is spared. We are thus driven to depend on relative sparing, which immediately results in a range of further issues. How many functions need to be measured? How different do they have to be to provide a convincing dissociation? And how do we allow for the fact that very different functions need different measures, which are probably not linearly related? It is the attempted solution to these problems that I have found so intriguing but frustrating over the years.[2]

Let me begin with a method, encountered through hearing Pat talk, that I initially found particularly elegant and satisfying, the Brinley plot. This expresses the relationship between the performance on a range of tasks of young and old subjects, one axis of the graph representing the performance on a given task of a group of young subjects, while the other represents the performance on that same task of an older group. A range of tasks across which performance is known to vary is sampled, for example, simple two-choice, four-choice and eight-choice reaction times. On a Brinley plot, the points invariably seem to lie along a straight line, often with the young and the old falling along the same line, with a huge amount of the variance captured by a single line. I was very impressed with the way in which this apparently simple technique could simplify and summarize data from a complex series of experiments (e.g. Brinley, 1965; Cerella, 1985). My admiration gradually began to migrate in the direction of scepticism as Brinley plots appeared from all directions, apparently all accounting for some phenomenal amount of variance, even in the case of my own rather amateurish attempt at aging research. Could there be a problem? In my own case there were two.

The first problem concerns exactly what such plots reveal. This remains a highly controversial issue (see Cerella, 1994; Fisk & Fisher, 1994; Perfect, 1994; Perfect & Maylor, 2000), but my own strong suspicion is that this is a measure in which large differences between conditions are represented in a way which swamps potentially smaller age effects, leading to a form of analysis that makes subtle but theoretically important age differences very difficult to detect. The analysis typically plots data from a small number of conditions, based on data aggregated across groups of subjects, a process that tends to lead to exaggerate correlations (Fienberg, 1971), and minimize potentially important deviations from the broad overall picture.

---

[2] In this respect, aging resembles traumatic brain injury in constituting a problem of considerable practical significance which rarely results in "pure" cognitive deficits.

My second problem reflects a personal preference, as it concerns the type of solution that I would find most interesting and theoretically productive. If your primary interest is in giving an account of aging, then presumably, the simpler that account the better. Hence, the enthusiasm for theoretical accounts of the cognitive psychology of aging in terms of single factors such as speed or inhibition, which are discussed below. If however, like myself you are interested in using the cognitive deficits of aging to prise apart the components of cognition, a single general function is likely to produce the least interesting and productive account. So the solution that might seem to represent the Holy Grail to some of my colleagues in the psychology of aging, reduces to a rather boring null hypothesis from my own viewpoint, and I note from that of Perfect and Maylor (2000), who refer to it as "the dull hypothesis."

Ever the optimist, I persuaded myself that there could be a compromise solution, indeed a third way. Perhaps, although there are major and pervasive cognitive changes that underpin aging, there are also discontinuities that can be used to dissociate different sub-components of cognition. While at the Medical Research Council Applied Psychology Unit (APU), in Cambridge, I managed to convince a number of my colleagues of this possibility (Maylor, Godden, Ward, Robertson, & Baddeley, unpublished), and set out to attempt to use the processes of normal aging to fractionate the central executive component of working memory. This was assumed to be a limited capacity attentional system that played a central role in controlling working memory (Baddeley & Hitch, 1974).

The distinctions that we chose to investigate were those I had earlier proposed (Baddeley, 1996) as logically necessary features of any plausible attentional control system, namely the capacity to focus attention, to divide attention, and to switch from one focus to another. We designed a series of tasks to pull apart these hypothetical functions, and duly collected our data from young and elderly subjects. The question then arose as to how to remove the hypothetical broad general aging factor or factors.

There seemed to be two strong candidates at the time, Pat Rabbitt's suggestion that aging is best seen as a reduction in general intelligence, (G) and Tim Salthouse's proposal that the crucial underlying factor is speed of processing. We decided to statistically factor out both of these. Removing both by multiple regression left us a small but significant source of age-related variance associated with conditions in which subjects had to respond to one stimulus and ignore a distracter presented in the same modality. A second study using a somewhat different set of tasks appeared to replicate this. By this time I had moved from Cambridge to Bristol, and set out to perform a further replication using a conceptually equivalent though somewhat different set of tasks. The results were puzzling, but by this time, structural equation modeling had filtered down to my level and with the help from a colleague, Dan Wright, I tiptoed into this to me rather murky field. We followed up with a fourth experiment which, far from solving the mystery suggested yet further complexities. At this point, I did what I should have done at the start, and tried to understand just what the multiple regression methods were doing.

Consider first the two covariates we chose, IQ and speed. By definition, IQ is something that is highly correlated with performance on a wide range of tasks. This in turn will depend on the reliability of the measure. Hence it is entirely possible for the relative predictive power of two variables to switch, simply by increasing the number of observations, and hence the reliability of one of them, leading to a very different structural equation model. Intelligence tests are developed bearing this in mind and tend to have a very high level of reliability compared to components of novel cognitive tasks based on a relatively small number of observations. Hence, a measure like IQ may be soaking up a great deal of the available variance, without necessarily being itself a unitary variable, potentially swamping other purer but less reliable measures. Indeed, the essence of a test like the WAIS is that it samples a wide range of cognitive capacities, in order to produce a single reliable but potentially high complex index.

A similar argument can be applied to using speed as a covariate. Speed measures tend to be based on a relatively large number of simple observations, hence increasing their reliability. Furthermore it is possible to combine speed measures from a wide range of tasks to increase reliability yet further. Finally, I would question whether decline in *speed* is any more plausible as an explanation of the decline of cognitive function with age than is decrease in *percentage correct*. Neither is meaningful except with respect to specific tasks.

At about this stage in my ruminations, I began to read the work of the Baltes group from Berlin, who were asking similar questions to those raised by Pat Rabbitt and Tim Salthouse, but coming up with somewhat different answers (Baltes & Lindenberger, 1997). They found that their best and most reliable predictors of cognitive decline in the elderly were sensory measures based on visual and auditory discrimination, on percent correct indeed. Then an even better predictor seemed to emerge in the form of dynamic grip strength (Lindenberger & Pötter, 1998). Should we therefore be statistically removing IQ, speed, visual acuity, auditory acuity, and grip strength before looking for our interesting cognitive dissociations? I attended my first and only Atlanta Aging Meeting and publicly expressed my misgivings. Happily for my credibility a similar point was made more elegantly and quantatively at the same meeting by Ullman Lindenberger who suggested that we had simply been neglecting the basic principle that correlation does not mean causation, concluding that "the decision to entertain the hypothesis that a certain variable mediates the causal effect of another should be based on theoretical considerations, and not on the outcome of hierarchical linear regression analysis." (Lindenberger & Pötter, 1998, p. 227).

So where does that leave the cognitive psychologist with a naive enthusiasm for exploiting the aged and infirm in his pursuit of cognitive theory? I reverted to the role of an interested if by now somewhat sceptical observer. I have however, continued to apply dissociational techniques in an attempt to understand Alzheimer's Disease. The recent invitation to take part in Pat's Festschrift, prompted me to think again about aging, and to realize that, if I went back to the simple idea of applying the sort of dissociation that has proved fruitful in neuropsychology to data that we had already collected from our elderly control subjects, then it might be possible to draw such interesting conclusions, not with certainty, but perhaps with an increasing degree of confidence. Admittedly our data are based on single rather than the double dissociations which have been regarded as the strongest form of evidence for separating subsystems. Furthermore, the interpretation even of double dissociations can be questioned. My own view, which forms part of a series of discussions published in Cortex (Baddeley, 2003) is that neither correlations nor dissociations are ever likely to provide irrefutable evidence, but that they do however place constraints on theoretical interpretations. Double dissociations place stronger constraints on theory than single dissociations, which in turn tend to offer more powerful evidence than positive associations, particularly in data sets with strong collinearity among the variables, as is typical of studies of aging. In what remains of the paper therefore I will attempt to use the method of dissociation as means of casting light on the structure of memory in general, and working memory in particular.

Age and the components of memory

Long-term memory

This very important aspect of aging has of course been studied in considerable detail, yielding some very clear dissociations. For example, while measures of episodic long-term learning show clear and growing deficits from early middle age onwards (Craik & Salthouse, 1992), semantic memory as reflected in vocabulary score, for example, continues to improve (Light, 1992), although speed and reliability of access shows progressive impairment (Burke, Mackay, Worthley, & Wade, 1991). Another exception to the general decline of memory with age is the recency effect in immediate free recall. It is typically preserved despite a clear deficit in performance on the recall of items from earlier in the list (Craik, 1968; Spinnler, Della Sala, Bandera, & Baddeley, 1988).

Data from long-term memory thus support the idea of dissociations between (1) recency and long-term memory; (2) semantic and episodic memory, and (3) preserved semantic storage and impaired retrieval. In none of

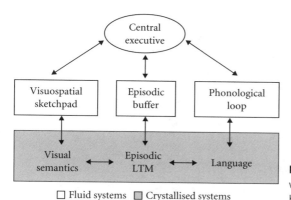

Fig. 12.1 The model of working memory proposed by Baddeley (2000).

these cases does the study of aging provide the only, or indeed the most powerful evidence for such dissociations, but it does make a valuable contribution to the range of data supporting these distinctions.

Working memory and aging

Let me begin by proposing a multi-component framework that has proved useful in accounting for data from normal adults, normal and learning disabled children, and neuropsychological patients. My current version of the original Baddeley and Hitch (1974) model is shown in Figure 12.1. It comprises the original three components of an attentional control system, the central executive, aided by the two subsystems, the visuospatial sketchpad and the phonological loop. Driven principally by evidence implicating the loop in the acquisition of language, a link between these components, and long-term memory is now included. Thus, the phonological loop is assumed to play an important role in the acquisition of language, while knowledge of language in turn supports the immediate retention of verbal material (Baddeley, Gathercole, & Papagno, 1998). We hypothesise a similar link between the sketchpad and visual semantics, although this has not so far been investigated.

A fourth component, the episodic buffer has recently been proposed (Baddeley, 2000). This is assumed to serve three major functions. The first is to provide storage capacity that allows the integration of a range of different codes into a unitary multi-dimensional representation. This provides an account of the observed interaction between the phonological loop system and visual similarity (Logie, Della Sala, Wynn, & Baddeley, 2000). The episodic buffer is assumed to act as a mental workspace, which is accessible to retrieval through the medium of conscious awareness (Baddeley, 2000). This framework is of course only one way of conceptualizing short-term and working memory (See Miyake & Shah, 1999 for other views). It is used here as an organizing framework for data, which we suggest are relevant to an understanding of working memory in the elderly, regardless of whether this particular set of assumptions is made.

What follows is not a comprehensive review of the extensive literature in this area, but represents rather an attempt to pull together evidence from a range of our own studies that have applied broadly comparable measures to groups of young and elderly subjects. In some cases, supplementary information on the same tasks is available from the study of matched subjects suffering from Alzheimer's Disease (AD).

The phonological loop

There is typically a small decrement in digit span attributable to age. Parkinson (1982) obtained a mean span of 6.6 digits in his young student subjects, and 5.8 in his elderly group, while Spinnler et al. (1988) found that span dropped from a mean of 4.67–4.3. Digit span in Italian is typically lower than in English, presumably because of the difference between monosyllabic English and disyllabic Italian digit names: (Naveh-Benjamin & Ayres, 1986). There is also typically a small age deficit in immediate serial recall of unrelated words (Wingfield, Stine, Lahar, & Aberdeen, 1988).

Visuospatial sketchpad

There appears to have been less work on visuospatial serial recall in the elderly, but the data from Spinnler et al. (1988) suggests a relatively modest deficit, with young subjects having a Corsi block tapping span of 5.14 on average, compared to a span of 4.74 in a group of elderly subjects, and 3.66 in the AD patients.

Central executive

In contrast to the reasonably coherent picture of preserved recency and modest immediate memory decline with age, the pattern for executive function proves more complex. It is certainly the case that adding further processing demands to immediate memory tasks can increase their sensitivity to the effects of age, and indeed Welford (1958) in his classic book, suggested that problems in holding and manipulating information may play a crucial part in the decline in cognition with age. Craik (1986) devised a task in which subjects were presented with a sequence of words, which they were required to hold and repeat back, either in the order presented, for example, hear *dog arm cat*, recall *dog arm cat*, or in alphabetic order, for example, hear *dog arm cat*, recall *arm cat dog*. He found little evidence of an age deficit for simple word repetition, but a clear effect when the additional alphabetic manipulation was required.

Further evidence of the vulnerability of the processing component of complex span tasks came from a series of studies by Craik, Morris, and Gick (1990). Old and young subjects were presented with a sequence of unrelated words, followed by a sentence which must be verified as true or false, which in turn was followed by the requirement to remember the words. Increasing the number of words to be stored and recalled impaired performance to an equivalent degree in young and elderly subject, whereas increasing sentence complexity had a greater effect on the performance of the elderly, again suggesting that processing could show a greater effect of aging than does storage. Although encapsulated in unitary task, both of Craik's studies required subjects to combine the storage and manipulation of information.

Daneman and Carpenter (1980) have suggested that the dual requirement of processing and storage is the hallmark of working memory, in contrast to the simple retention of information over a brief period, which is characteristic of standard STM tasks. The working memory span task devised by Daneman and Carpenter involves processing a sequence of sentences and then recalling the last word of each. It might therefore be expected to be highly sensitive to age effects. Evidence on this issue is somewhat mixed. An attempt to investigate this issue by Baddeley, Logie, Brereton, and Nimmo-Smith (1985) began as a study of the effects of age on working memory span, but in the absence of convincing age effects turned into a replication and extension of the original Daneman and Carpenter study. More recently May, Hasher, and Kane (1999) have cast more detailed light on the issue, finding a difference between their young and the elderly groups that was reduced by inserting a brief delay between successive trials, suggesting an interpretation in terms of the greater susceptibility of the elderly to the effects of a proactive interference (PI). Further evidence of this view came from an experiment in which subjects either began with short sequences and gradually increased number of sentences until span was reached, or began with long sequences, with the subsequent tests decreasing in length. May et al. argued that PI would build-up throughout the session at a faster rate for the older subjects, who would hence be penalized by the standard practice of starting with short sequences and working gradually up to crucial span length rather than starting at span. As predicted, the elderly performed better when they started with long sequences.

In general then, data from complex span studies are themselves complex, reinforcing the view that although executive function clearly declines with age, the detailed nature of the deficit or deficits is far from clear. The bad news is that it becomes harder to give a simple account on effects of age on working memory. The good news is that this very diversity offers the possibility that age may offer a means of fractionating executive processes.

Executive processing and aging

The study of attention is diverse in its methods, its data and its theories. For present purposes, we will maintain the view that the aspect of attention that is most centrally relevant to working memory it that concerned with the attentional control of action (Norman & Shallice, 1986). In an attempt to structure study of the central executive, Baddeley (1996) suggested that any such attentional control system would need to be able to do three things, (1) Focus attention, (2) Divide attention, and (3) Switch attention. In addition it would need to provide an interface between long-term and working memory.

The sections that follow describe a series of studies carried out within this framework, using the standard neuropsychological technique of looking for dissociations between the relevant sub-components as possible clues to fractionating the executive system. There are of course a number of objections to drawing strong conclusions from simple dissociations. We attempt to take account of these both through the use of replication and converging operations, and through the contrasts with Alzheimer's Disease. Four functions will be discussed in turn.

Aging and focused attentional capacity

There appears to be a general tendency for performance on tasks that depend on attentional capacity to show clear age deficits. Indeed Craik and colleagues have argued that the pattern of results obtained from elderly subjects may be effectively simulated by simply reducing the attentional capacity of younger subjects by means of a secondary task (Anderson, Craik & Naveh-Benjamin, 1988; Craik 1986). In our own data, clear effects are found for simple reaction time, where the subject merely responds to a target signal, with larger age effects for the attentionally more demanding choice reaction time, a classic finding in the literature (Baddeley, Chincotta, & Adlam, 2001). We found similarly robust age effects in visual search for letter Zs embedded in either curvilinear or more potentially confusing angular nontarget letters, and when subjects were searching for pictogram targets. In both cases, the age effect was reflected in both speed and error measures (Baddeley et al. 2001).

Although such effects are pervasive within the aging literature, their precise interpretation remains equivocal. As mentioned earlier, an explanation purely in terms of "speed" may provide a simple way of summarizing large bodies of data, but does not in itself offer an explanation. It can of course be referred back to the assumed efficiency of basic neuronal systems, but unless these can be identified and measured, this does not seem to offer a very fruitful way ahead.

General attentional capacity offers a somewhat more satisfactory concept, since it can be manipulated independently, for example, by using secondary tasks (Anderson et al. 1988). One variant of the limited capacity concept is the proposal of Hasher and Zacks (1988) that older subjects are less good at inhibiting irrelevant information. There are a number of studies that appear to confirm this, including a reduced capacity to read text against a visually noisy background (Hasher & Zacks, 1988; Zacks & Hasher, 1988) and the previously described study by May et al. (1999) showing that much of the decrement observed in performance on working memory span tasks may be due to the greater susceptibility of older subjects to proactive interference. Whatever is the precise interpretation, however, there does seem to be evidence for some kind deficit in the capacity of older subjects to bring to bear attention on the task in hand.

Divided attention and aging

The capacity to split attention between two concurrent tasks is classically regarded as one of the functions of the frontal lobes, with apparently supportive evidence both from neuropsychological studies of patients with lesions, and from neuroimaging studies. For example, patients with frontal lobe damage often have difficulty in attentional control, particularly when it is necessary to keep in mind a number of potentially competing tasks (Shallice, 1988) while neuroimaging studies have also been interpreted as suggesting that the frontal lobes are responsible for executive control (Henson, 2001; Posner & Di Giralamo, 2000). Given the frequent assertion that functions depending on the frontal lobes are particularly susceptible to aging (Foster, Black, Buck, & Bromskill, 1997), one might predict a clear problem of division of attention in the elderly.

This literature is in fact apparently conflicting. As the recent review by Riby Perfect and Stollery (2004) indicates, there are many studies that appear to show a clear tendency for dual task performance to decline more sharply with age then does the performance on the constituent single tasks. However, most of these studies involve combining two tasks under conditions whereby both constituent task show age effects. If one adds two tasks at which elderly participants are disadvantaged, it is surely hardly surprising that an even greater decrement is observed.

A better design is to titrate the load imposed by each of the tasks, so that in the single task condition the groups are performing equally efficiently. I and my colleagues have attempted this approach across a series of studies in which we use groups of young, elderly healthy, and elderly subjects suffering from Alzheimer's Disease. In many of our studies we have combined a visuo-spatial tracking task with immediate serial recall of auditory digits. These tasks allow us to equate performance across groups by varying the speed of the target in tracking, and the length of digit sequence. We find that both young and elderly subjects can combine these relatively demanding tasks very effectively, in contrast to AD patients who show impairment when required to combine the two. We have replicated this finding using a range of tasks, including a number in which one of the tasks was self-paced, allowing subjects to adjust their performance as the task becomes more difficult. Using this paradigm we have found similar results when tracking was combined with the task of crossing out a chain of printed boxes (Della Sala, Baddeley, Papagno, & Spinnler, 1995; Green, Hodges, & Baddeley, 1995), or when visual search is combined with auditory detection of a spoken town name (Baddeley et al. 2001).

Despite these numerous replications, it is still possible that the difference might stem from a limitation in total processing capacity, perhaps because the relationship between capacity and performance is nonlinear. If the relationship is an accelerating function, then we might conceivably be simply revealing the fact that this function is rather steeper in patients than in elderly or young subjects. Logie, Cocchini, Della Sala, and Baddeley (in press) therefore attempted to provide a more stringent test of the hypothesis that the dual task results obtained might be explained in terms of single capacity limitation. Three tests were made. The first of these involved only a single task, either tracking or memory load. The demands for each task was varied from substantially easier than the level typically chosen for the dual task studies, to substantially harder. Again, young, normal elderly, and AD subjects were tested. If the previous results simply reflected differences in overall processing capacity, then one might expect the three groups to diverge as load increased, with AD patients showing deterioration relative to the other two groups initially, with older subjects diverging from the young at a higher load. The results are shown in Figure 12.2, from which it is clear that, provided the three groups are equated in median performance, they respond identically to increases or decreases in task demand.

A second study was concerned with the question of whether the dual task deficit shown by the patients would disappear if the tasks were made simpler. Level of demand for the tracking task was reduced to 25% of the typical speed, and memory load was two items below each subject's span. Unsurprisingly, neither of the two normal groups showed any dual task decrement, whereas the AD group performed significantly less well when the two tasks were combined.

Our final study involved holding one of the tasks constant, while varying the demands of the second task from substantially below to substantially above the standard demand level. Once again, there was a clear effect of AD, but not age, on the capacity to combine the two tasks. The AD deficit was, however, no greater when level of difficulty was high, than when it was low.

In conclusion, while we would not wish to argue that the elderly will not show a dual task deficit under any conditions, our evidence suggests that this in itself is not a major deficit, provided that the level of difficulty of the

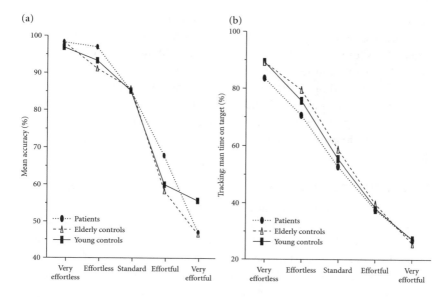

Fig. 12.2 Single task performance of young, normal elderly, and AD patients as a function of the level of demand imposed by a single task. (a) shows accuracy of immediate digit recall and; (b) shows tracking performance. Data from Logie et al. (in press).

individual tasks is equated between young and old subjects. While this point is of theoretical importance however, it is important to bear in mind that in everyday life, elderly people are constantly required to combine tasks on which their performance level is lower than that of the young, for example, driving and searching for a directional road sign. Under these conditions, deficits are likely to be increased by the need to combine tasks.

In an attempt to throw light on the anatomical basis of the dual task deficit observed in AD patients, Baddeley, Della Sala, Gray, Papagno, and Spinnler (1997) studied dual task performance in a group of patients with known frontal lobe lesions. Patients were independently rated on the behavioural signs of dysexecutive syndrome, and in addition were tested on the Wisconsin Card Sorting Test, and on verbal fluency, two tests that characteristically show impaired performance in patients with frontal lobe damage. Approximately half of the patients were categorized as showing dysexecutive everyday behaviour in their everyday life as reflected in blind interview with a carer. Only these patients showed impaired capacity for dual task coordination. This was not simply a general function of severity of impairment, since the group as a whole showed clear evidence of deficits on both card sorting and fluency, neither of which was associated with dysexecutive behaviour or dual task performance deficit. While not directly concerned with aging, the study has implications for interpretations of aging in terms of the more rapid deterioration of the frontal lobes (Foster et al. 1997; Parkin, 1997). As these and a range of other findings indicate (Stuss & Knight, 2002), the frontal lobes are far from uniform; while dual task performance probably does depend on the functioning of the frontal lobes, the system in question appears to be dissociable from other "frontal" tasks, and to be comparatively preserved in the elderly.

Task switching and aging

Another executive function that I assumed to be potentially separable is the capacity to switch attention from one task to another (Baddeley, 1996). However, the evidence that switching capacity is disproportionately sensitive to the effect of age remains sparse. The problem stems partly from the fact that this aspect of attention is still not well understood. After some classic work by Jersild (1927), the topic was largely ignored for the next 60 years, apart from isolated studies by Spector and Biederman (1976), until a resurgence of interest was created by two influential papers. One of these by Allport, Styles, and Hsieh (1994) extended the Jersild paradigm, performing a series of experiments that cast serious doubt on the assumption that task switching involved attentionally demanding executive processes. The second influential paper by Rogers and Monsell (1995) extended the range of methods applied to the analysis of task switching, concluding that there was an executive attentionally demanding contribution. These studies stimulated extensive new research, resulting in a growing body of highly detailed analysis and modeling of the hypothetical processes involved in switching (see, for example, Allport & Wylie, 1999; Meiran, 1996; Rubinstein, Meyer, & Evans, 2001).

Our own involvement in the area was concerned to develop a switching task that was simple and robust enough to be performed by patients suffering Alzheimer's Disease. This ruled out many of the elegant new developments that were appearing, and encouraged us to stay relatively close to the original Jersild paradigm. The task we chose involved presenting the subject with a column of single digits. In one condition, subjects were required to add one to each digit and write down their answer. To ensure that there was no ambiguity, this condition always followed each digit with a plus and equals sign. A second condition was equivalent except that it contained minus signs, while the third and crucial condition involved alternating plus and minus signs. Performance was timed over columns of twenty items by stopwatch. Young, normal elderly, and AD subjects all showed a clear switching cost, but while the cost was significantly greater for the AD patients than the elderly, age did not appear to increase switching time.

This lack of an age effect surprised us, since there are reports of age effects in task switching in the literature. However, as Salthouse, Fristoe, McGuthry, and Hambrick (1998) point out, many of these come from a comparison between performance on the two forms of the Trails Test. In form A, the response sheet has an array of circles each containing a number on one sheet or a letter on the other. Subjects are instructed to join the circles starting with number 1, going on to 2, 3, etc., or starting with A then B then C, etc. In form B of the test, both numbers and letters are present in the array, and subjects are instructed to start with A then move to 1, then to B, then to 2, etc. Form B is reliably slower than A, a difference that is typically attributed to switching cost. There are however, other variables involved such as the need to keep in mind the more complex instructions in B while performing a visual search task. Given that there does appear to be an age deficit in visual search, it may be the interaction between the two variables that causes the deficit. In an attempt to investigate this further, Salthouse et al. (1998) presented their young and elderly subjects with a range of tasks, some of which were assumed to require task switching. They concluded that there was evidence of a common switching component, but that when other concomitant variables were statistically controlled, that task switching appeared to be relatively insensitive to the effects of age. We decided to investigate this in two further experiments, concentrating on the effect of age rather than AD.

The first experiment was a replication and extension of our arithmetic switching task. In a series of experiments aimed at investigating the role of working memory in task switching Baddeley et al. (2001) studied the effects of a verbal version of the traits task on the simple arithmetic task described previously. While performing the arithmetic tasks, young subjects were required to recite days of the week or months of the year in canonical order, a task that was assumed to disrupt the operation of the phonological loop. In a more demanding condition that itself involved switching, subjects were required to alternate between days and months (e.g. Friday June Saturday July Sunday August etc.). When the plus and minus signs were provided on the arithmetic response sheets, only the more demanding alternating task caused a differential increase in switching time. When the signs were not present, forcing the subjects to "remember" whether to add or subtract, even suppression had a major decremental effect, which was significantly increased by the requirement to alternate days and months. We concluded that when signs were absent, both the phonological loop and the central executive played in role in performing this task.

In the Baddeley et al. (2001) studies just described, only young subjects were used. We therefore decided to replicate using 18 young and 18 elderly volunteers from the Bristol University subject panel. Our first experiment involved presenting subjects with the same material as we had used for our patient study, with plus and minus signs present. We tested our subjects performing the task alone, and while reciting the days of the week or months of the year, (the articulatory suppression condition), or the while alternating the days and months (an additional executive load). Our results are shown in Figure 12.3. Analysis of variance showed significant main effects of age, task switching (blocked vs. alternating), and secondary task, but no interaction between switch condition and age. Thus, despite the presence of arithmetic signs, we obtained a clear switching deficit. Both the concurrent tasks significantly reduced speed of performance, but there was no suggestion of an interaction between age and the effects of either switching or concurrent task effect. The pattern of errors was consistent with this picture. Our results are therefore broadly in line with those of Salthouse et al. (1998).

However, Spector and Biederman (1976) have argued that the presence of plus and minus signs changes the nature of the switching arithmetic task

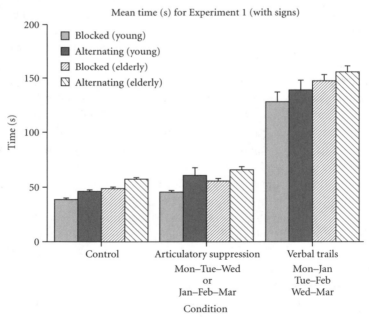

Fig. 12.3 Performance of young and elderly subjects on a blocked and alternating arithmetic task in which plus and minus signs are included. The additions and subtractions are blocked, or alternated, and are tested under three levels of concurrent load.

sufficiently to make it atypical of most switching paradigms. We therefore carried out a second study which was identical, except that these signs were omitted. The results are shown in Figure 12.4. The most dramatic change from the previous result stems from the magnitude of the secondary task effect, with even simple recitation of days or months clearly slowing performance.

Analysis of variance indicated significant effects of presence of switching, secondary task, and age. The interaction between condition and secondary task was highly significant, with both the articulatory suppression and central executive tasks greatly increasing switching costs. Once again however, although there was a main effect of age, it did not interact with the cost of alternation, or of the secondary task.

All three of our experiments therefore show that the simple requirement to alternate between adding and subtraction has a marked and robust impact on performance. All three show overall age effects on latency, but none shows any evidence of an interaction between age and switching. Our evidence therefore suggests that task switching *per se* is not particularly vulnerable to age effects, although it does decline under Alzheimer's Disease. In drawing this conclusion however, it should be borne in mind that it is far from obvious that the concept of switching reflects a single coherent underlying process; indeed, it seems highly unlikely that the deficit that leads to perseveration when patients with frontal lobe damage perform the Wisconsin Card Sorting Test is the same as that involved in our simple alternating task (see Baddeley et al. 2001;

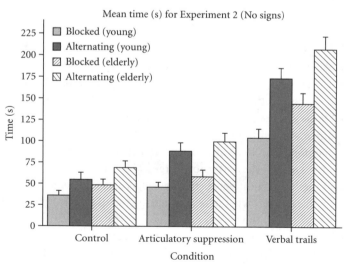

Fig. 12.4 Tasks switching and concurrent activity for young, elderly, and AD subjects on block or alternating addition and subtraction when plus and minus signs are omitted.

Rubenstein et al. 2001 for further discussion). The study of task switching is currently an area of great theoretical and experimental activity which will no doubt in due course clarify this issue.

The working memory—LTM interface

A fourth crucial function of the central executive, was proposed to reflect its capacity to form an intelligent interface with long-term memory (Baddeley, 1996). The concept of an episodic buffer was proposed to give an account of the link between long-term and working memory (Baddeley, 2000). The episodic buffer is assumed to comprise a multi-dimensional storage system of limited capacity that is capable of providing an interface between the visuo-spatial and phonological subsystems, and between working memory, perception and long-term memory. It is assumed to have limited storage capacity, and to be dependent upon executive control. It is also assumed to act as one means of binding together information into integrated chunks. Initial attempts to develop the concept have concentrated on studying the role of attentional capacity in binding. One way of manipulating this variable has been to study the comparative performance of young and elderly subjects, and patients suffering from AD, three groups who are assumed to differ in focused attentional capacity. Our first study concerned the question of how immediate verbal serial recall is supported by information from semantic and syntactic knowledge, information that appears to facilitate the binding of successive words into chunks (Miller, 1956).

One problem in addressing this question using normal prose is that of equating degree of knowledge across subjects. Hambrick and Engle (2002) tackled this problem by using a closely specified area of knowledge, namely baseball. They selected young and old subjects varying widely in their knowledge of the subject, going on to test retention of a baseball commentary. They also measured the working memory span of their participants. They obtained large effects on recall of level of knowledge of baseball. There was also a significant tendency for younger subjects, and those with greater working memory span to recall more, although effects were relatively modest, compared with the effect of knowledge. The crucial question, however, concerned the interaction between knowledge, age, and span. More specifically, would greater knowledge *reduce* age and span effects by providing an extra boost, or would the extra knowledge *increase* the advantage enjoyed by the young and/or high span subjects, an outcome they term "the rich get richer hypothesis." This proved to be the case; the young and high span subjects benefited more from specialist knowledge, although these interaction effects were small compared to major influence of baseball expertise.

We ourselves chose to tackle the problem of differential knowledge by simplifying and constraining the material used. Our constrained sentences were made up from a very limited set of nouns, verbs, adjectives, and adverbs. This limited set of items was permuted so as to generate meaningful but bland sentences all syntactically simple, active, and declarative, whose length could be varied by the addition of adverbs and adjectives. A typical sentence might be "The elderly lawyer rapidly sold the old red bicycle to the happy teacher." Memory span for such material is about seven or eight items, consistently better than the same items in scrambled order, (five to six items), but substantially less than sentences taken, for example, from a newspaper (12–16 items). We are currently in the process of studying the characteristics of our constrained sentence span task, but in the meantime have carried out one study in which age and AD are involved.

Luzzi and Baddeley (unpublished) tested 20 young Italian subjects, 20 controls, and 20 patients diagnosed as suffering from AD. Figure 12.5 shows the mean memory span of these subjects when tested for immediate recall of constrained sentences or of the equivalent words in scrambled order. We obtained significant effects of both material (F1, 57 = 313.21, $p < .001$) and group (F2, 57 = 79.53, $p < .001$). Importantly, the group × material interaction was also significant, whether considered overall (F2, 57 = 20.17, $p < .001$), or when broken down so as to look separately at the effects of age and disease. When the patient group is excluded, a significant interaction of material with age is found (F1, 38 = 10.69, $P < .01$), and when the young group is excluded there is a significant interaction between material and disease (F1, 38 = 10.69, $P < .01$). Our data like that of Hambrick and Engle supported the "rich get richer" hypothesis. The young appear to be able to make better use of the semantic and syntactic constraints than the elderly, while the elderly gain more advantage than AD patients.

A possible objection to our analysis is that we should have used percentage change as our measure. I myself regard such percentage measures as

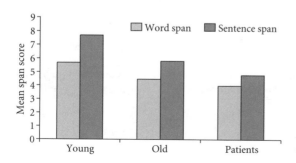

Fig. 12.5 Immediate serial recall for scrambled words and constrained sentences in young, elderly, and AD subjects.

inappropriate. They tend to reduce the differential effect for whatever group or condition performs most highly. In the case of accuracy scores it is a matter of convention whether performance is scored in terms of number of items correct or number wrong. A score based on correct responses will reduce the percentage change for a younger higher performing group, while a score based on errors will have exactly the opposite effect. As the same data can produce two opposite conclusions, this form of analysis would seem to be invalid.

A possible way out of the dilemma is to use Z scores, expressing in the current case, the advantage gained by the presence of semantic context in terms of the standard deviation in performance in the random word group. Expressed in this way, semantic coding improves the performance of the young by 3.14 standard deviation units, the elderly by 2.90 units, and the AD patients by 2.39 units. Hence, although our conclusions at this point must remain tentative, the data tend to suggest that, although the provision of extra information from long-term memory will aid immediate memory span in the elderly as well as the young, the elderly gain less benefit. There are of course a number of possible reasons for this, including reduced attentional capacity, and possible greater susceptibility to proactive interference.

Conclusions

The results of our studies are summarized in Table 12.1. The capacity to focus attention, and to utilize long-term knowledge in immediate recall both appear to be impaired by age. In contrast, the capacity to divide attention and to switch between tasks seem to be relatively preserved, at least as measured by the tasks we selected. In the case of AD patients however, all four aspects of attentional control that were studied showed clear impairment.

The study of aging is clearly of enormous practical and theoretical significance. It also offers a potential way of understanding normal function by means of the fractionation techniques that have proved so valuable in neuropsychology. The complications of dealing with change and multiple collineararity however, make it a much more difficult field for providing simple and relatively unequivocal

Table 12.1 Summary of results of our studies on attentional control in aging and Alzheimer's Disease

	Focussed capacity	Division of attention	Attention switching	Interface with LTM
Elderly	—	0	0	—
AD patients	—	—	—	—

0 = No clear deficit attributable.   — = Deficit.

dissociations. Double dissociations are rare, and robust single dissociations not open to obvious alternative interpretations are far from common. I am however, currently optimistic enough to believe that evidence of the type just described, in conjunction with converging evidence from other sources, may contribute to our general understanding of cognition, as well as helping us understand in more detail the ways in which cognitive function changes as we grow older.

So thank you Patrick for making the process of cognitive aging as intriguing as it is inevitable. And thank you editors for allowing my hoard of aging data finally to see the light of day; if it is all nonsense, blame Pat.

References

Allport, A., Styles, E. A., & Hsieh, S. (1994). Shifting attentional set: Exploring the dynamic control of tasks. In C. Umilta & M. Moscovitch (Eds.), *Attention and performance XV*. Cambridge, MA: MIT Press.

Allport, A., & Wylie, G. (1999). Task-switching, stimulus-response bindings, and negative priming. In S. Monsell and J. Driver (Eds.), *Attention and performance XVIII*. Cambridge, MA: MIT Press.

Anderson, N. D., Craik, F. I. M., & Naveh-Benjamin, M. (1988). The attentional demands of encoding and retrieval in younger and older adults: Evidence from divided attention costs. *Psychology and Aging, 13*, 405–423.

Baddeley, A. D. (1996). Exploring the central executive. *Quarterly Journal of Experimental Psychology, 49A*, 5–28.

Baddeley, A. D. (2000). The episodic buffer: A new component of working memory? *Trends in Cognitive Sciences, 4*, 417–423.

Baddeley, A. D. (2003). Double dissociation: Not magic but still useful. *Cortex, 39*, 129–131.

Baddeley, A. D., Bressi, S., Della Sala, S., Logie, R., & Spinnler, H. (1991). The decline of working memory in Alzheimer's disease. *Brain, 114*, 2521–2542.

Baddeley, A. D., Chincotta, D. M., & Adlam, A. (2001). Working memory and the control of action: Evidence from task switching. *Journal of Experimental Psychology: General, 130*, 641–657.

Baddeley, A. D., Della Sala, S., Gray, C., Papagno, C., & Spinnler, H. (1997). Testing Central Executive functioning with a pencil-and-paper test. In P. Rabbitt (Ed.), *Methodology of frontal and executive functions* (pp. 61–80). Hove, UK: Lawrence Erlbaum Associates.

Baddeley, A. D., Gathercole, S. E., & Papagno, C. (1998). The phonological loop as a language learning device. *Psychological Review, 105*, 158–173.

Baddeley, A. D., & Hitch, G. J. (1974). Working memory. In G. A. Bower (Ed.), *Recent advances in learning and motivation* (Vol. 8, pp. 47–89). New York: Academic Press.

Baddeley, A. D., Logie, R., Brereton, N., & Nimmo-Smith, L. (1985). Components of fluent reading. *Journal of Memory and Language, 24*, 119–131.

Baltes, P. B., & Lindenberger, U. (1997). Emergence of a powerful connection between sensory and cognitive functions across the adult life span: A window to the study of cognitive aging? *Psychology and Aging, 12*, 12–21.

Brinley, J. F. (1965). Cognitive sets, speed and accuracy of performance in the elderly. In A. T. Welford & J. E. Birren (Eds.), *Behavior, aging and the nervous system.* Springfield, IL: Thomas.

Burke, D. M., MacKay, D. G., Worthley, J. S., & Wade, E. (1991). On the tip of the tongue: what causes word finding failures in young and older adults? *Journal of Memory and Language, 30*, 542–579.

Cerella, J. (1985). Information processing rates in the elderly. *Psychological Bulletin, 89*, 67–83.

Cerella, J. (1994). Generalized slowing in Brinley plots. *Journal of Gerontology: Psychological Sciences, 49*, 65–71.

Craik, F. I. M. (1968). Short-term memory and the aging process. In G. A. Talland (Ed.), *Human Aging and Behavior* (pp. 131–168). New York: Academic Press.

Craik, F. I. M. (1986). A functional account of age differences in memory. In F. Klix & H. Hagendorf (Eds.), *Human memory and cognitive capabilities* (pp. 409–422). Amesterdam: Elsevier.

Craik, F. I. M., Morris, R. G., & Gick, M. L. (1990). Adult age differences in working memory. In G. Vallar & T. Shallice (Eds.), *Neuropsychological impairments of short-term memory.* Cambridge University Press.

Craik, F. I. M., & Salthouse, T. A. (1992). *The handbook of aging and cognition.* Hillsdale, NJ: Erlbaum.

Daneman, M., & Carpenter, P. A. (1980). Individual differences in working memory and reading. *Journal of Verbal Learning and Verbal Behavior, 19*, 450–466.

Della Sala, S., Baddeley, A. D., Papagno, C., & Spinnler, H. (1995). Dual task paradigm: A means to examine the central executive. In K. J. Grafman & F. Boller (Eds.), *Structure and functions of the human prefrontal cortex* (pp. 161–190). New York: Annals of the New York Academy of Sciences.

Fienberg, S. E. (1971). Randomization and social affairs: The 1970 draft lottery. *Science, 171*, 251–261.

Fisk, A. D., & Fisher, D. L. (1994). Brinley plots and theories of aging: The explicit, muddled, and implicit debates. *Journal of Gerontology: Psychological Sciences, 49*, 81–89.

Foster, J. K., Black, F. E., Buck, B. H., & M. J., Bromskill. (1997). Aging and executive functions: A neuroimaging perspective. In P. Rabbitt (Ed.), *Methodology of frontal and executive function* (pp. 117–134). Hove, UK: Psychology Press.

Greene, J. D. W., Hodges, J. R., & Baddeley, A. D. (1995). Autobiographical memory and executive function in early dementia of the Alzheimer type. *Neuropsychologia, 33*, 1647–1670.

Hambrick, D. Z., & Engle, R. W. (2002). Effects of domain knowledge, working memory capacity and age on cognitive performance: An investigation of the knowledge-is-power hypothesis. *Cognitive Psychology, 44*, 339–387.

Hasher, L., & Zacks, R. T. (1988). Working memory, comprehension and aging: A review and a new view. In G. Bower (Ed.), *The psychology of learning and motivation* (Vol. 22, pp. 193–225). New York: Academic Press.

Henson, R. (2001). Neural working memory. In J. Andrade (Ed.), *Working memory in perspective* (pp. 151–174). Hove, UK: Psychology Press.

Jersild, A. T. (1927). Mental set and shift. *Archives of Psychology, Whole No. 89.*

Light, L. L. (1992). The organization of memory in old age. In F. I. M. Craik & T. A. Salthouse (Eds.), *The handbook of aging and cognition* (pp. 244–272). Hillsdale, NJ: Erlbaum.

Lindenberger, U., & Pötter, U. (1998). The complex nature of unique and shared effects in hierarchical linear regression: Implications for developmental psychology. *Psychological Methods, 3*, 218–230.

Logie, R., Cocchini, G., Della Sala, S., & Baddeley, A. D. (in press). Is there a specific executive capacity for dual task co-ordination? Evidence from Alzheimer's disease. *Neuropsychology*.

Logie, R. H., Della Sala, S., Wynn, V., & Baddeley, A. D. (2000). Visual similarity effects in immediate serial recall. *Quarterly Journal of Experimental Psychology, 53A*, 626–646.

Luzzi, S., & Baddeley, A. D. Unpublished data.

May, C. P., Hasher, L., & Kane, M. J. (1999). The role of interference in memory span. *Memory and Cognition, 27*, 759–767.

Maylor, E. A., Godden, D. R., Ward, A., Robertson, I. H., & Baddeley, A. D. [Aging, selective attentions and the influence of modality]. Unpublished data.

Meiran, N. (1996). Reconfiguration of processing mode prior to task performance. *Journal of Experimental Psychology, Learning, Memory and Cognition, 22*, 1423–1442.

Miller, G. A. (1956). The magical number seven, plus or minus two: Some limits on our capacity for processing information. *Psychological Review, 63*, 81–97.

Miyake, A., & Shah, P. (1999). Toward unified theories of working memory: Emerging general consensus, unresolved theoretical issues and future directions. In A. Miyake and P. Shah (Eds.), *Models of working memory: Mechanisms of active maintenance and executive control* (pp. 28–61). Cambridge University Press.

Naveh-Benjamin, M., & Ayres, T. J. (1986). Digit span, reading rate and linguistic relativity. *Quarterly Journal of Experimental Psychology, 38*, 739–751.

Norman, D. A., & Shallice, T. (1986). Attention to action: Willed and automatic control of behaviour. In R. J. Davidson, G. E. Schwarts, & D. Shapiro (Eds.), *Consciousness and self-regulation. Advances in research and theory* (Vol. 4, pp. 1–18). New York: Plenum Press.

Parkin, A. J. (1997). Normal age-related memory loss and its relation to frontal lobe dysfunction. In P. Rabbitt (Ed.), *Methodology of frontal and executive function* (pp. 177–190). Hove, UK: Psychology Press.

Parkinson, S. R. (1982). Performance deficits in short-term memory tasks: A comparison of amnesic Korsakoff patients and the aged. In L. S. Cermak (Ed.), *Human memory and amnesia* (pp. 77–96). Hillsdale, NJ: Erlbaum.

Perfect, T. J. (1994). What can Brinley plots tell us about cognitive aging? *Journal of Gerontology: Psychological Sciences, 49*, 60–64.

Perfect, T. J., & Maylor, E. A. (2000). Rejecting the dull hypothesis: The relation between method and theory in cognitive aging research. In T. J. Perfect and E. A. Maylor (Eds.), *Models of cognitive aging* (pp. 1–18). Oxford University Press.

Posner, M. I., & Di Girolamo, G. J. (2000). Cognitive neuroscience: Origins and promise. *Psychological Bulletin*, 873–889.

Riby, L. M., Perfect, T. J., & Stollery, B. (2004). The effects of age and task domain on dual task performance: A meta-analysis. *The European Journal of Cognitive Psychology, 16*, 863–891.

Rogers, R. D., & Monsell, S. (1995). Costs of a predictable shift between simple cognitive tasks. *Journal of Experimental Psychology: General, 124,* 207–231.

Rubinstein, J., Meyer, D. E., & Evans, J. (2001). Executive control of cognitive processes in task switching. *Journal of Experimental Psychology: Human Perception and Performance, 27,* 763–797.

Salthouse, T. A., Fristoe, N., McGuthry, K. E., & Hambrick, D. Z. (1998). Relation of task switching to speed, age and fluid intelligence. *Psychology and Aging, 13,* 445–461.

Shallice, T. (1988). *From neuropsychology to mental structure.* Cambridge University Press.

Spector, A., & Biederman, I. (1976). Mental set and mental shift revisited. *American Journal of Psychology, 89,* 669–679.

Spinnler, H., Della Sala, S., Bandera, R., & Baddeley, A. D. (1988). Dementia, ageing and the structure of human memory. *Cognitive Neuropsychology, 5,* 193–211.

Stuss, D. T., & Knight, R. T. (2002). *Principles of frontal lobe function.* New York: Oxford University Press.

Welford, A. T. (1958). *Ageing and human skill.* London: Oxford University Press.

Wingfield, A., Stine, A. L., Lahar, C. J., & Aberdeen, J. S. (1988). Does the capacity of working memory change with age? *Experimental Aging Research, 9,* 185–189.

Zacks, R. T., & Hasher, L. (1988). Capacity theory and the processing of inferences. In L. L. Light and D. M. Burke (Eds.), *Language, memory and aging* (pp. 154–170). Cambridge University Press.

Chapter 13

The own-age effect in face recognition

Timothy J. Perfect and Helen C. Moon

Abstract

Previous research on face recognition has shown an own-age effect, such that older adults are more adept at recognizing faces of their own age than younger faces, with the reverse (or a null effect) for younger adults. This own-age effect is reminiscent of the well-established own-race effect; people are better at recognizing faces of their own race compared to other races. This latter effect has been attributed to differences in familiarity-based expertise leading to greater use of holistic processing for own-race faces. The strongest evidence for this is that the own-race effect is absent in recognition of inverted faces, where holistic processing is disrupted. The present study explored whether the own-age effect is similarly disrupted by inversion. Younger and older adults saw photographs of younger and older faces prior to a recognition test. At test, different photographs of the targets were presented, intermixed with an equal number of foils, with half of each presented upside down. Overall there was no effect of age on recognition, but there was a robust age × face age interaction, such that older adults were superior at recognizing older faces, and younger adults superior at recognizing younger faces. There was an interaction with inversion, but this acted so as to magnify the age × face age interaction. Consequently inversion does not disrupt the own-age effect in recognition, and thus the effect does not appear to have the same genesis as the own-race effect.

Introduction

If you want to spend an hour or two in the contemplation of the futility of the battle against the effects of getting older, I can do no better than suggesting that you type the words "face" and "aging" into an Internet search engine. You will be whisked into a world, ruled by plastic surgeons, in which the harsh realities of growing older are outlined, and often illustrated with alarming clarity. You will learn, as if you did not already know, that as we age, our hair starts to grey, or worse disappear from where it should be, instead sprouting where it should not. Our skin loses elasticity and starts to sag, wrinkles appear, bones thin, earlobes lengthen and bags appear under the eyes. In short, older adults appear different from their younger counterparts, both in terms of individual features (e.g. length of earlobes, hairiness of eyebrows), and configural properties of their faces (e.g. the distances between features are altered by sagging). Whilst the pages you will find on the Internet are dominated by a positivist approach, indicating what you can do to avoid the ravages of time (commonly featuring surgical interventions, or top-ten tips), the present pages are concerned with a different issue. The question of interest here is how well faces that differ in age are recognized by people of different ages.

Age differences in face recognition ability

Older adults are worse than younger adults at face recognition (e.g. Anstey, Dain, Andrews, & Drobny, 2002; Crook & Larrabee, 1992; Maylor, 1990). Given the known age deficits in memory and visual cognition this might not seem very surprising, or even perhaps very interesting. Like many other tests of recognition memory, older adults seem particularly prone to making false positive errors. That is they claim to recognize someone that they have not seen previously. (Support for this claim can be found in reviews of the verbal domain: Zacks, Hasher, & Li, 2000, and the face-recognition domain: Searcy, Bartlett, & Memon, 1999.) Whilst this may not be theoretically very interesting (since it mirrors work on recognition memory with verbal material), in itself may be of some practical importance, for example, in the area of eyewitness testimony. Until quite recently, older witnesses have received very little research attention, in contrast to the vast literature on child-witnesses. Happily, this situation is now being remedied (e.g. see work on older eyewitnesses by Memon and her colleagues; Memon, Gabbert, & Hope, 2004; Memon, Hope, Bartlett, & Bull, 2002; Searcy, Bartlett, & Memon, 1999). However, this chapter is not concerned with age-deficits in memory for faces *per se*, not least because a prolonged discussion of another example of poorer performance by older adults would not do justice to this volume. A much more interesting set of issues arise when one changes the question slightly. As Yarmey (1993) conceded, when considering the poorer performance of older eyewitnesses at identification tasks, there remains the possibility that the poorer performance seen by older witnesses might stem in part from their lack of familiarity with, or interest in, younger faces. Until fairly recently, the possibility of an own-age bias, akin to the own-race bias in face recognition (e.g. Meissner & Brigham, 2001), had not been explored. As it turns out, Yarmey was right, and there does seem to be evidence of an own-age bias, which makes understanding the face-recognition performance a lot more interesting than the early research suggested.

The own-age effect in face recognition

The own-age effect in face-recognition has received surprisingly little attention, in comparison to the widely studied own-race effect. For example, Meissner and Brigham (2001) conducted a meta-analysis of 35 studies on own-race bias, involving nearly 5,000 participants, whilst to the authors' knowledge, there are only a handful of studies that have explored younger and older adults' ability to recognize younger and older faces. We will begin by briefly describing these studies before turning our attention to a theoretical account of the effects of own-race effect previously reported, which has been applied to the own-age effect.

Bäckman (1991) reported the interactive effects of age and face–age on the recognition ability of adults. He compared four groups of adults (young, 19–27 years, young-old, 63–70 years, 76 year olds, and 85 year olds) on their face recognition ability. Participants saw 60 faces (classified as young or old) prior to a 20 minute retention interval and then a final old/new recognition test. The two oldest groups showed no age-bias, but were impaired relative to the other two groups. However, the young and the young-old groups showed a full cross-over interaction in their recognition abilities. That is the young were superior to the old at discriminating young-faces, but the old were numerically superior to the young for the older-faces.

A different pattern of results was reported by Bartlett and Leslie (1986) who compared younger and older adults in their ability to recognize faces across changes in pose and expression. Their younger sample were high school students aged 18, whilst their older sample were recruits from the local community, who averaged 74 years of age. The younger faces were in their twenties and thirties, whilst the older faces were aged between 40 and 80. Thus, neither age-group matched the age of the face stimuli, but nonetheless, there was an age by face–age interaction in the recognition data, as measured by nonparametric A'. On average, younger adults showed greater recognition ability for younger faces than older faces ($A' = 0.87$ and 0.79 for younger and older faces), but older adults showed no such age-bias ($A' = 0.80$ and 0.81 for the younger and older faces). This pattern, of age-bias in the younger sample only, was replicated in a second study in the same paper, and also seen in a study by

Mason (1986). That study showed younger (20 years) and older (75 years) female participants slides of younger and older adults. At test, participants made old/new judgments. In addition to an overall age effect on the recognition task, there was a marginally significant age × face age interaction. As with Bartlett & Leslie (1986), younger adults were more adept at younger faces than older faces, but older adults showed no age bias.

Recently, Perfect and Harris (2003) explored own-age bias in an eyewitness context, using lineup-identification as the final test criterion. Their main focus was on a phenomenon known as unconscious transference, which is the misidentification of a bystander as the perpetrator when that bystander appears in the lineup. Although the rationale for that work is not pertinent here, their design involved two face-recognition tests in which younger and older adults were given the opportunity to (mis)identify faces of different ages, and the results are germane. Additionally, their third experiment also included a standard lineup containing the perpetrator and so provided more standard assessments of recognition memory.

In their design, younger and older participants were initially exposed to a set of pictures of "perpetrators" and heard about the crimes they had committed. Later in the same test session, participants were presented with a series of "mug-shots" and asked whether any had been seen earlier in the session. In fact, all were new faces (innocent bystanders). One week later, participants returned and saw two lineups (one all male, one all female) each containing a bystander from the mugshots shown in the previous session. Experiment 1 used younger faces as stimuli, Experiment 2 replicated this with older faces as stimuli, and Experiment 3 used both younger and older faces. All three experiments compared younger (18–30 years) and older (65–80 years) adult volunteers. A number of findings are relevant.

The first test of recognition ability was the propensity to misidentify the mug-shots as people who had been seen earlier in the first experimental session. Across the three experiments, older adults were more likely to falsely identify a mug-shot as a previously seen perpetrator—whatever the age of the faces seen. In Experiment 1, younger bystanders were picked out 33.8% of the time by older participants, but only 7.5% of the time by younger adults. In Experiment 2, older bystanders were misidentified 22.9% of the time by older adults but only 12.8% of the time by younger participants. This pattern was replicated in a third experiment, albeit at a lower absolute level.

In contrast, the propensity to go on to mistakenly select one of the bystanders in the subsequent lineups showed an own-age bias effect. Older adults were more likely to select the younger bystander from the lineup in Experiment 1 than their younger peers. However, in Experiment 2, using older faces, no age-effect was apparent because younger adults now performed more poorly than they had in Experiment 1. This pattern was replicated in Experiment 3: older adults showed no age-sensitivity in their propensity to mistakenly identify a bystander, but younger adults were more likely to misidentify older faces than younger ones.

Just to complicate matters further, Experiment 3 also contained two lineups in which the true perpetrators did appear. Here also, own-age biases were apparent. However, unlike the bystander misidentification studies, here it was the older adults who were sensitive to the ages of the faces they had to identify. Younger adults were equally adept at identifying younger and older perpetrators (73% and 80% for younger and older faces), but older adults were particularly poor at picking out the younger perpetrators (37% and 83% for younger and older faces).

An eyewitness procedure was also used in another recent study of own-age bias. Wright and Stroud (2002) explored the ability of younger (18–25 years) and middle-aged (35–55 years) adults to make lineup decisions in target present (Experiments 1 and 2) and target absent (Experiment 2) test conditions. In Experiment 1, with a 1-day delay, 47% of younger adults successfully picked out the young perpetrator, compared to only 24% of the middle-aged participants. However, for the older perpetrator, only 37% of younger adults were successful compared to 47% of the middle-aged adults. This cross-over interaction was replicated in the target-present condition of Experiment 2, but was absent in the target-absent condition (where the correct response is "not in the lineup"), which showed no effects of age, and no age by face-age interactions at all.

One final study to explore the abilities of younger and older adults to recognize younger and older perpetrator was recently conducted by Memon, Bartlett, Rose, and Gray (2003). They used videos depicting older and younger criminals, and subsequently tested identification ability using target-present and target-absent simultaneous lineups. In line with the original face-recognition studies we reported at the start of the chapter, older adults were poorer overall, and particularly susceptible to false-alarm errors but there was no hint of an own age-bias in either age group, as has been found on other occasions. It is hard to know why this should be, although it must be acknowledged that in an eyewitness paradigm, each category of face–age is represented by relatively few individuals (2 in the Memon et al. case), and so atypical exemplars may particularly bias performance.

Clearly, across the few studies that have explored own-age bias in face-recognition, there are a number of inconsistencies. Whilst the majority have reported own-age bias effects, one has not, and where there are effects, the locus of these effects has differed across studies. On some occasions younger adults show age-sensitive effects, whilst on others older adults are age-sensitive. Unfortunately, with such a small literature to draw upon, in which the methods vary so widely, it is hard to draw sensible conclusions about why the different patterns may have occurred. Nonetheless, across the studies reported above, it seems reasonable to conclude that age-changes in face-recognition performance cannot be fully understood without reference to the age of the face-stimuli to be recognized. These findings are interesting for a number of reasons. From an applied perspective they are important in demonstrating the potential moderating effects of stimulus type on face-recognition performance in real world identification tasks. Thus, rather than simply testifying to the poorer memory performance of older witnesses (*cf.* the review of experts by Kassin, Tubb, Hosch, & Memon, 2001), it might be more appropriate to moderate this conclusion by reference to own-age effects. The results are also theoretically interesting, not least because full-cross over-interactions with superior performance by older adults are relatively rare, and when they occur they offer a strong refutation of the dull hypothesis (Perfect & Maylor, 2000), that older adults are simply worse at face recognition.

The overwhelming majority of researchers have tried to explain the presence of an own age effect in terms of an expertise based account, based upon familiarity (although see Bäckman, 1991 for a sceptical view on this). For example, Bartlett and Leslie (1986) argued that whilst younger adults have a preponderance of exposure to younger faces, older adults, through their lives have experience with both younger and older adults. A similar account was offered by Mason (1986). Such an account would explain why younger, but not older adults show an own-age bias, though it does make some untested assumptions about relative experience with faces of different ages, and the relative importance of recent and more distant experience.

Wright and Stroud (2002), found a full cross-over interaction between age and face age and conceded that it might be "premature to speculate on why the effect occurs" (p. 652), but nonetheless they likened the effect to the own-race effect, which, as we will see below, has been explained in terms of differential exposure. (And, interestingly, both full cross-over and asymmetric effects have been reported for the own-race effect.)

The own-race effect in face recognition

The existence of an own-race bias in eyewitness memory is a well-established empirical fact. In their meta-analytic review of the literature, Meissner and Brigham (2001) reviewed 35 studies involving nearly 5,000 participants, and covering a literature that spans 30 years, and reported a substantial overall effect. The theoretical explanation for the effect has at its core the notion of differential expertise in faces of one's own race vs. other races. This in turn is thought to lead to different methods of processing own-race and other-race faces. One recent version of this idea is the notion that people develop the use of configural (or holistic) processing of faces for those stimuli that is absent from recognition of other-race faces. There are a number of lines of evidence that support this line of argument.

Numerous studies have shown that recognition of upright own-race faces involves a configural element that makes face recognition "special" (e.g. Maurer, Le Grand, & Mondloch, 2002; Yin, 1969). In such studies, configural processing is demonstrated by showing an effect for upright intact faces that is absent (or much weaker) when processing either an inverted or scrambled face containing the same featural information. For example, Leder and Bruce (1998) tested participants' ability to detect changes in faces from encoding to test. They found that configural changes (shifting the relative positions of facial features) were more detectable for upright faces than inverted ones, whereas featural changes (replacing individual features with new ones) were equally detectable for upright and inverted faces. Young et al. (1987) presented participants with composites (the top half of one face with the bottom half of another face) of famous faces. These composites were either aligned (giving the impression of a new whole face) or misaligned (clearly giving the impression of two face halves). They found that naming of half a face was poorer when the two halves were aligned, compared to the mis-aligned condition, but once again, this effect only applied to upright faces. Similarly the part–whole effect (better recognition of face-parts when embedded within the appropriate whole-face context compared to an inappropriate context or no context) occurs only for upright faces (Tanaka & Farah, 1993). An entertaining demonstration of the effect of configural processing is the Thatcher Illusion (Thompson, 1980). In this illusion, Mrs Thatcher's image is distorted by inverting her eyes and mouth within her face. When presented upside down, the image does not look too grotesque, and the viewer is not always aware of what is wrong with the image. Once presented upright, the full grotesqueness of Mrs Thatcher's image is revealed.

The link between the holistic component and expertise has also been shown by studies of experts who demonstrate similar inversion effects for other material. Perhaps the most well known study is that by Diamond and Carey (1986) who showed that expert dog-judges were particularly impaired in their ability to recognize dog-exemplars when the stimuli were inverted. Nonexperts showed no effect of inversion in their ability to recognize particular examples of dogs.

The link between holistic processing and the cross-race effect has been demonstrated in a similar fashion. Participants are superior at recognizing faces from their own race, but this effect is much reduced, or removed entirely by inversion (e.g. Rhodes, Tan, Brake, & Taylor, 1989; Tanaka, Keifer, & Bukach, 2004). The inversion and cross-race effects have also both been associated with particular patterns of brain activation in ERP work. James, Johnstone, and Hayward (2001) showed that compared to upright own-race faces, inverted own-race faces and upright other-race faces were worse recognized, and both were associated with less activation in the N2 component of the ERP trace (thought to reflect extraction of structural information) but a greater N400-component (perhaps indicating that inverted faces and other race faces provide partial matches to many stored faces, thus requiring a process of selection). Thus, other-race recognition and inverted own-race recognition may share fundamental processing demands that lead to both showing impairment relative to upright, own-race face processing.

Recent work in computational modeling of face processing has also attempted to explain the experiential account of own-race bias in terms of differential exposure. Furl, Phillips, and O'Toole (2002) contrasted 14 different computational models in their ability to predict the own-race effect on the basis of differential exposure to different kinds of face. Only one class of models was entirely successful, namely developmental models which assume that early experience shapes the perceptual space used to classify faces. Thus, in this regard, own-race bias may resemble the age-of-acquisition effects seen for other materials.

Findings from the literature on verbal overshadowing (the impairment in recognition performance following the provision of a verbal description) also fit the holistic-expertise model. Verbal overshadowing effects are thought to operate by shifting participants away from holistic processing, toward featural processing (e.g. Dodson, Johnson & Schooler, 1997; Macrae and Lewis, 2002; Schooler, 2002; Westerman & Larssen, 1997). Two verbal-overshadowing findings are particularly pertinent here. Fallshore & Schooler (1995) showed that verbal overshadowing effects are absent for inverted own-race faces, but present for upright own-race faces. This fits the notions that verbal description causes reductions in holistic processing, and holistic processing is absent in inverted face recognition. Importantly, Fallshore and Schooler (1995) also showed that verbal overshadowing effects were absent for other race faces (both upright and inverted). They suggested that cross-race identifications are made on the basis of featural information only, and so such identifications are not impaired by shifting toward a featural processing mode. Interestingly, they also found that the verbal descriptions themselves were not subject to a cross-race effect—that is, the descriptions of other race faces are just as rich, and just as informative (to a naïve participant who uses the descriptions to make an identification) as descriptions of own-race faces. Thus the cross-race effect is not carried in the featural information described by the participant, but by the holistic, nonverbalizable aspect.

Given the evidence discussed above, it is it is easy to see why researchers exploring the own-age effect have likened that effect to the own-race effect. The theoretical account, based upon differential exposure, can readily be transferred to the own-age effect, with some minor tweaks to the assumptions. If one reasonably assumes that younger adults have more experience with younger faces, it would follow that they develop holistic processing for those faces, which they cannot apply to older faces. The converse would apply to older adults, with perhaps the added rider that they retain their previous holistic processing of younger faces (if one wishes to explain an asymmetric effect). One potential difficulty with transferring the account wholesale is that the computational models imply that the cross-race effect has to be established early. Clearly, older people were not born old, and did not have greater exposure to older adults in their childhood than the current cohort of younger adults. Differential early exposure cannot explain the own-age effect: the effect must surely stem from recent exposure. However, whilst there is an apparent similarity between the own-age bias and the own-race bias, we must not jump to premature conclusions. There is another own-group effect that is more difficult to explain in terms of differential exposure that might offer an alternative explanation of the own-age effect.

The own-sex bias in face recognition

The original study by Mason (1986), which explored the effects of age on face recognition ability, only tested female participants, but included both male and female test faces. In addition to the observed own-age bias, Mason (1986) also found that the female faces were better recognized ($d' = 2.45$) than male faces ($d' = 1.99$). Of course, this could have been an artefact of the faces selected, with male faces being less distinctive, but is suggestive of an own-sex bias. More recent work has tested both male and female participants on male and female faces. Lewin and Herlitz (2002) found a sex by sex of face interaction, which was asymmetric, with female participants showing superior recognition of female faces compared to male faces, but male participants showing no bias.

In contrast, Wright and Sladden (2003) reported a full cross-over interaction between sex and sex of face, thus demonstrating superior recognition of male faces by male participants, as well as the previously reported advantage seen for female faces by female participants. Additionally they contrasted a standard encoding condition with a condition in which witnesses saw faces with the hair excluded, and found that this attenuated the own-sex bias. They therefore concluded that a large proportion of the own-gender bias can be accounted for by differential usage of a feature-based cue—namely hairstyle.

The existence of sex by sex-of-face interactions in face recognition experiments is rather harder to explain in terms of differential exposure leading to differential use of holistic processing. In our society males and females of all ages see faces of both sexes equally. Whilst it may be possible to build an argument that more early experience is obtained for female faces (as the primary caregivers), there is no suggestion that this applies more to baby girls than baby boys. Thus, clearly, an own-group effect does not stem necessarily from greater exposure to one group, and might not imply greater use of holistic processing. Consequently applying the theoretical explanation of the own-race effect to the own-age effect might not be as straightforward as some previous authors have supposed, since the own-sex effect suggests a differential locus for the effect.

A second difficulty in transposing the holistic account of the own-race bias to the own-age effect is that other own-group effects have been seen on tasks that are clearly not holistic. Recall that Fallshore and Schooler (1995) found no own-race effect on verbal descriptions, and ascribed this to the featural (rather than holistic) nature of verbal descriptions. However, own-sex effects (Shaw & Skolnick, 1994, 1999; Yarmey, 1993) and own-age effects (Lindholm, 2005) have been reported on person descriptions tasks involving featural aspects of appearance, including clothing. Perhaps most compelling is that fact that Shaw and Skolnick (1994) found an own-sex effect on a person description task, but not on a face-identification task, when testing the same participants. Thus, the own-sex bias was apparent for the featural task, but not the holistic one. Following Fallshore and Schooler's logic, one must conclude that such own-group effects are not due to holistic processing.

Thus, there are two potential explanations of the own-age effect previously reported. The holistic processing account, which stems from the work on own-race effect, is that each age-group has developed a holistic processing bias for faces they are most often exposed to, which leaves them relatively impaired at recognizing unfamiliar faces of the opposite age. The featural processing account, which stems from the work on own-sex bias, is that each age group focuses on different features of a face, which are maximally useful for discriminating the faces of the most-encountered group (their own age) but less useful for discriminating faces of the other age. How are we to differentiate between these two accounts?

If we return to the literature on face-processing, a straightforward solution presents itself: inversion. Across a wide range of paradigms, the standard manipulation to impair holistic processing is to invert the faces, as we discussed above. A particular strength of this manipulation is that the general properties of the test stimulus remain unchanged after inversion (luminance, complexity, spatial frequency, etc.), and so any effects of such a manipulation are not due to such factors. Whilst we may anticipate an overall age-related impairment in face recognition, that might be related to these factors, or others, any age $\times$ inversion interaction cannot be explained away.

The own-race advantage is reduced by inversion (e.g. Rhodes et al. 1989), and so if the own-age effect is similarly reduced, it would suggest that younger and older adults do have a holistic processing bias that applies to their own age. The particular strength of this theoretical account is that the manipulation is predicted to impair most the condition in which the participants are the best. In the own-race effect, it is our own-race identification that is most impaired by inversion.

Since feature-based processing of faces is little impaired by inversion (e.g. Leder & Bruce, 1998), if the own-age effect is carried by differential reliance on different features, one might expect the own-age effect to survive the effects of inversion undiminished.

The study

Participants in this study initially saw a mixed list of 32 younger and older faces, presented one at a time. The photographs depicted head-and-shoulder shots facing full-on to the camera, in front of a plain white background. Younger faces ranged in age from 20–24, with a mean age of 22.2 years, whilst older faces ranged from 65–80, with a mean age of 73.4 years. These ages were known to us because all images used in this study were taken by the second author, who recruited volunteers at her local bingo hall. The photographs were taken using a digital camera, and printed A4 size on a colour laser printer for use in the study. Participants were presented with the photographs in a booklet, with the experimenter advancing the pages every 5 s. Participants were told that their memory for the faces would be tested, but were not instructed what the form of that test would take. Following an interval in which they completed a distracter task for 5 min, participants saw a second list consisting of 32 target faces and 32 new distracters. Half of the test items were younger faces and half were older faces, with half of each age presented upright, and half inverted. Which items served as targets and which as distracters was counterbalanced within each age group, as was the orientation of the test stimuli. As with the encoding stage, the faces were printed on A4 sheets in colour, and were presented in a booklet, with pages turned by the experimenter (to ensure that participants did not invert the page so as to return the faces to upright). Each page depicted a face viewed at 3/4 profile, using a different image to that presented at encoding. Participants were asked to indicate whether they had seen the face in the study phase and to indicate their confidence in each decision on a 10 point scale.

One hundred participants were individually tested. The younger group ($n = 50$), consisted of 41 females and 9 males, with a mean age of 20.2 (SD 2.1) years, whilst the older group ($n = 50$) consisted of 30 females and 20 males, with a mean age of 73.9 (SD 5.8) years. All were recruited in the local community, and were not acquainted with any of the people who had been photographed to create the test stimuli. All reported normal, or corrected to normal vision.

Results

Our interest was in whether an own-age bias had been seen in recognition, and whether older adults were particularly prone to false positive errors. Since we used an old-new recognition test, we first analysed hits and false alarms separately. Then, to determine that there is no overall response-bias effect driving any age interactions, we analyzed hits minus false positives.

Correct detections of targets

Overall, older adults correctly recognized fewer faces than their younger counterparts, (67% vs. 59%), $F(1, 98) = 8.71, p < 0.01$. There were also main effect of face age, $F(1, 98) = 13.37, p < 0.001$, such that younger faces were recognized less often (60%) than older ones (66%), and orientation, $F(1, 98) = 19.3, p < 0.001$, such that upright faces were recognized more often (67%) than inverted ones (59%). These main effects were qualified by a number of higher order interactions. Orientation did not interact with either age group $F(1, 98) = 1.39$, or face age, $F(1, 98) = 2.31$. However, there was a large interaction between face-age and age group, $F(1, 98) = 86.3, p < 0.001$, such that younger adults were better at younger faces than older faces (72% vs. 62%), whilst older adults showed the reverse pattern (48% vs. 70%). This in turn was modified by a significant three-way interaction between age group, orientation, and face age, $F(1, 98) = 6.29, p < 0.014$, which is illustrated in Figure 13.1.

Our interest was in testing the prediction that own-age bias would be removed by the effects of inversion. Thus the robust own-age effect reported

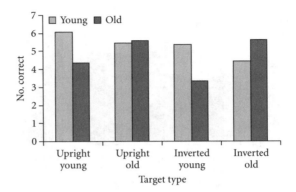

Fig. 13.1 The effect of target age and inversion on correct recognition of faces by younger and older adults.

above, and the presence of a three-way interaction with orientation is encouraging. However, Figure 13.1 makes clear that the effect of inversion is not to reduce the own-age effect. If anything, it appears to magnify this effect. We explored this three-way interaction with 2 two-way ANOVAs, looking at the interaction between age and face age separately for upright and inverted faces. As expected, for upright faces, there was a significant age group $\times$ face age interaction, $F(1, 98) = 29.4, p < 0.001$. However, contrary to our initial predictions, this interaction remained for the inverted faces, and if anything was even stronger, $F(1, 98) = 61.0, p < 0.001$.

False positive errors

The next analyses examined rates of false positive errors, using the same analytic approach as with hits. Previous research has suggested that older adults are particularly prone to false positive errors for younger faces. The question of interest here was whether such a pattern would be replicated, and whether the effect would be removed by inversion. Here there was no main effect of age group, $F(1, 98) = 1.88$, with older adults making numerically fewer false positive errors (30%) than the younger adults (33%), contrary to expectations. However, younger faces caused more false positive errors (34%) than older faces (29%), $F(1, 98) = 4.67, p < 0.05$, and inverted faces caused more false positive errors (39%) than upright faces (24%), $F(1, 98) = 66.0, p < 0.001$.

These main effects were once again qualified by higher order interactions. Whilst there was no interactions between orientation and either face age, $F < 1$, or age group, $F(1, 98) = 1.0$, there was a reliable face age $\times$ age group interaction, $F(1, 98) = 22.0, p < 0.001$. The means indicate a reliable own-age effect, since younger adults falsely identified 30% of the younger faces, but 36% of the older ones, whilst older adults falsely identified 37% of younger faces and only 23% of older faces. However, this two-way interaction was in

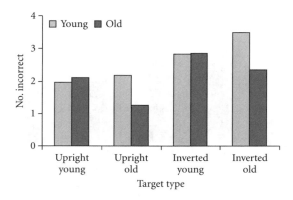

Fig. 13.2 The effect of target age and inversion on false identification of new faces by younger and older adults.

turn moderated by a three-way interaction that approached significance, $F(1, 98) = 3.31, p < 0.07$, which is illustrated in Figure 13.2.

As the three-way interaction was the critical test of our hypothesis that own-age effects would be ameliorated by inversion, we conducted follow up tests as before to test whether own-age effects in false positives were observable separately for upright and inverted faces. For the upright faces, the age group × face age interaction was significant, as predicted, $F(1, 98) = 8.10$, $p < 0.01$. For the inverted faces the effect was if anything larger, $F(1, 98) = 17.0, p < 0.001$, as before.

Hits minus false positives

To ensure that the patterns observed in the hits and false positive responses were not due to systematic shifts in the way the younger and older adults responded to the different kinds of items, we decided to run an analysis on hits controlling for false positives. The outcome was largely the same as the previous two analyses. There was only a marginal effect of age group, $F(1, 98) = 3.11, p < 0.08$, such that the corrected hit rate was 34% for younger adults, and 29% for older adults. There were also reliable effects of orientation $F(1, 98) = 72.2, p < 0.001$ (upright, 44%, inverted, 20%), and face age, $F(1, 98) = 15.6, p < 0.001$, (younger faces, 26%, older faces, 37%). Again, these main effects were qualified by higher order interactions. Consistent with the previous analyses, orientation did not interact with age group, $F < 1$, or face age, $F(1, 98) = 2.05$. However, as before there was a large age group × face age interaction, $F(1, 98) = 88.9, p < 0.001$. In line with the previous results, younger adults performed better with younger faces than older faces (42% vs. 26%), whilst older adults showed the reverse pattern (11% vs. 48%).

Once again, this two-way interaction was qualified by a three-way interaction between age group, face-age and orientation, $F(1, 98) = 6.29, p < 0.05$.

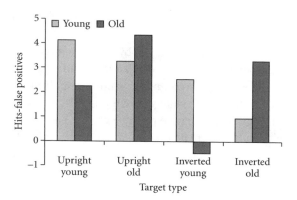

Fig. 13.3 The effect of target age and inversion on rate of hits minus false positive errors, for younger and older adults.

This interaction is illustrated in Figure 13.3. Follow-up tests conducted as before revealed the presence of reliable age × face age interactions for upright faces, $F(1, 98) = 39.4, p < 0.001$, and for inverted faces, $F(1, 98) = 68.5$, $p < 0.001$. Once again, the effects were if anything larger in the inverted condition, contrary to our initial expectations.

Inspection of Figure 13.3 shows that performance on inverted other-age faces was quite poor. The older adults were below chance on average, with false positives exceeding correct identifications. The younger adults only managed to correctly identify around one more inverted older face than they falsely identified, which although above chance, $t(49) = 3.16, p < 0.01$, is not very impressive. Clearly, our participants found recognition of other-age faces very difficult when they were presented upside-down at test. This was not because inverted faces are difficult *per se*, since those same pictures were recognized reasonably well by participants of the same age.

It is rare that one gets a data set that is as pleasingly clear cut, and compelling as the present one. Because of the nature of cognitive aging, normally one does not observe full cross-over interactions, and so one is left mulling over potential baseline differences in performance, and so explanations of age differences in terms of general factors such as difficulty, speed, intelligence, motivation, or visual acuity (see Perfect & Maylor, 2000 for a discussion of such issues). However, baseline differences are not a concern here. Whilst there was an overall main effect of age in hit rate, it was absent in false positives, and minimal for corrected recognition. In any case, this importance of this minor main effect is outweighed by the higher order interactions. If we consider Figure 13.3 again it is clear that the best performance by any group on any stimulus type is observed for the older adults with upright older faces—which numerically exceeds younger adults recognizing upright younger faces.

Clearly, these data do not conform to the dull hypothesis (Perfect & Maylor, 2000).

Before we discuss the age by face–age interactions, it is worth considering what we would have concluded if we had only used young faces as stimuli, as in the early face–recognition studies discussed above. We would have found that older adults were worse than their younger colleagues, and were also prone to making false positive errors. We would also have concluded that older adults were further impaired by the difficulty induced by inversion. We would have had no difficulty at all in integrating such a pattern into the literature on memory performance by older adults, and we would have supported the conclusions of the eyewitness experts (Kassin et al. 2001) who are prepared to testify to the poorer performance of older adults. However, what if we had only used older faces? In taking such an approach, we would have been entirely justified, since there is no *a priori* reason to select younger faces as stimuli, beyond their greater propensity to be engaged in criminal activity. If we had done that, we would have drawn *exactly the opposite conclusions*. We would have been forced to conclude that younger adults are poorer at face recognition, and particularly prone to false positive errors. Moreover, this apparently-memory-impaired group of younger adults were made worse by the factor of inversion. Clearly, such results would be harder to reconcile with the existing literature, and some might object to drawing conclusions based on the use of older faces alone. *But this is exactly the same logic as using only younger faces, and does not seem to have hindered researchers previously.*

Clearly there is something about the older faces that older adults find easy, and younger adults find hard, with the reverse being true for younger faces. There are two aspects to these data worthy of discussion: One is why a full cross-over was observed, and not the asymmetric effect reported previously (Bartlett & Leslie, 1986; Perfect & Harris, 2003). The second issue is the mechanism that is producing the effect.

One possible discrepancy between the present work demonstrating a full cross-over interaction between age and face age, and those previous studies showing asymmetric effects maybe the age of the older participants. Recall that Bäckman (1991) reported a cross-over interaction that was restricted to his youngest older group. Is that the case in the present study? Our older adults ranged in age between 65 and 84 years of age, thus spanning the range of young–old to older–old used by Bäckman. To explore whether the full interaction restricted to the younger of our older adults, we split our older sample into those aged less than 75 ($n = 27$), and those over 75 ($n = 23$), producing two groups with mean ages of 69 years and 79 years, respectively. The analysis of corrected recognition (hits minus false positives) between these two groups showed no overall age difference in performance between these two groups, and no significant interactions involving age and the factors of orientation and face age ($F < 1$ in every case). Thus, the age interactions observed in the whole sample appear to apply equally to both groups of older adults.

With regards the mechanism producing the effect, it is worth reiterating the point made by Bäckman (1991) with regards stimulus familiarity. The ability of participants to utilize prior expertise to bolster memory performance is well known. Thus, the amelioration of age-related deficits by means of using stimuli that favor the old is a well-known phenomenon. For example, Barrett and Wright (1981) showed that older adults were better able than their younger comparison group to recognize word lists consisting of dated terms such as *doily*. However, the explanation for such an effect is the greater conceptual knowledge of the material, enabling better encoding and retrieval processes. The advantage accrues because of the *prior* familiarity with the material leading to richer representations that can be used to support memory processing. But the materials used here are *not* familiar. This was not a test of recent and dated famous faces, but of unfamiliar faces, never seen before. The participants had no conceptual representation of these faces.

Therefore, what one must assume is that somehow the two age-groups process the two sets of faces in different ways. This might be because they attend to different sorts of features when studying a face, or making recognition decisions, or because they apply different kinds of representational templates to process the two kinds of face in differentially effective ways. On the basis of the own-race and own-sex literatures we hypothesized two possible mechanisms for the effect, but neither are fully supported by the data.

Of the two, the holistic account, based on the own-race effect fared worse. On the basis of prior work on cross-race identification we predicted that inversion would remove the own-age bias. Not only did this not happen, but the reverse was seen. If one accepts that inversion disrupts configural processing then it must follow that the bias present in the recognition of inverted faces cannot be due to configural processing. This in turn puts serious doubt on whether configural processing is the root of the own-age effect in upright face recognition.

The featural account, based on the own-sex effect fared better. Here we predicted that inversion would have no effect on the own-age effect. Thus, whilst we might have expected the observed own-age effect in inverted faces, this view would not have predicted the observed exaggeration of the effect.

There is a simple descriptive account that can explain why the own-age effect gets larger with inversion. If one assumes that recognition of other age faces is difficult, and that recognition of inverted faces is difficult, then one can readily predict that recognition of other-age inverted faces should be particularly difficult. There are two problems with this account: first it does not psychologically explain *why* other age faces are hard to recognize, and second, the same argument does not seem to apply to other-race faces. Recall, for other race faces, recognition does not get much worse with inversion—rather it is the own-race recognition that gets worse (Fallshore & Schooler, 1995; Rhodes et al. 1989). Thus, one is left with the same problem of explaining why other-age faces are difficult, and how this difficulty is different to the difficulty people have with other-race faces.

In the introductory section to this chapter we contrasted the own-age effect with the own-race effect and the own-sex effects. Given that we used equal numbers of male and female faces, we decided that it was worth exploring whether an own-sex effect was present in the current data set, notwithstanding the imbalance in the genders across the two age groups. Whilst we found that female faces were better recognized than male faces, $F(1, 98) = 7.35$, $p < 0.01$, this did not interact with the gender of the participants, $F < 1$, and there was no three-way interaction with orientation, $F < 1$. Thus, whilst our participants demonstrated a robust own-age effect, they showed no hint of an own-sex effect in their face-recognition performance.

There is an interesting social–psychological explanation that may be worthy of further exploration, although it must be admitted that it runs into some of the same difficulties as the cognitive explanations we have focused on here (for fuller discussion, in relation to the own-race effect, see Levin, 2000; Sporer, 2001). This theory has been used to explain the presence of own-race bias in identification, but in principle could be applied to any own-group bias, and does not rely upon prior exposure. The theory builds upon experimental social psychology research on the in-group heterogeneity and out-group homogeneity effects. These effects are as follows: when given individuals to classify, people are motivated to discriminate between those that belong to their own social group, but treat as similar those who belong to another social group. So, even using the minimal group paradigm, in which participants are notionally assigned to one team or another, leads people to view their own team as a more individuated, and the other team as more similar. Clearly, such a view can be applied equally to classifications of people based on race, age, or gender, and hence to all the recognition biases discussed above. This perspective has a particular advantage in the current context because it can offer an explanation of why we saw an own-age effect, but no own-sex effect in the present data set. Our participants were recruited to an aging study, in which they were informed that they would be tested for their memory for younger and older faces. Thus the relevant category in the present study was age, and not sex. If sex was not a salient dimension to our participants, they may not have classified other sex faces as the outgroup.

Levin (2000) has applied this theoretical position to the case of cross-race identifications. His position is not that people *cannot* holistically process other race faces, (as would be implied by cognitive model in which superior processing for own-race faces stems from richer or more discriminable representations), but that they *do not*. The reason that they do not process other race faces fully is that instead they focus on the factor that rules them out of the ingroup—namely race. Clearly it is a small step to apply such ideas to people of different ages. Perhaps our younger and older adults did not fundamentally differ in terms of how they process faces—in either featural or holistic terms—but they chose to classify the faces as "like them" or "not like them." Those that were like them, by virtue of their age, received further processing, whilst those who were not like them, received less processing and so were less well recognized, particularly in the difficult inverted test condition.

Clearly, such an account is speculative, and we do not have the data to address this idea yet. For now, we must be satisfied with the demonstration that older adults are not merely poorer at face recognition than their younger peers, as many eyewitness experts believe (Kassin et al. 2001). Instead we have observed an ecologically moderated effect, in which older adults are better than their younger colleagues on a task that is more relevant to the older adults lives—recognition of older faces.

References

Anstey, K., Dain, S., Andrews, S., & Drobny, J. (2002). Visual abilities in older adults explain age-differences in Stroop and fluid intelligence but not face recognition: implications for the vision-cognition connection. *Aging, Neuropsychology and Cognition, 9*, 253–265.

Bäckman, L. (1991). Recognition memory across the adult life span: the role of prior knowledge. *Memory and Cognition, 19*, 63–71.

Barrett, T. R., & Wright, M. (1981). Age-related facilitation in recall following semantic processing. *Journal of Gerontology, 36*, 194–199.

Bartlett, J. C., & Leslie, J. E. (1986). Aging and memory for faces versus single views of faces. *Memory and Cognition, 14*, 371–381.

Crook, T. H., III, & Larrabee, G. J. (1992). Changes in facial recognition memory across the adult life span. *Journal of Gerontology: Psychological Sciences, 47*, P138–P141.

Dodson, C. S., Johnson, M. K., & Schooler, J. W. (1997). The verbal overshadowing effect: why descriptions impair face recognition. *Memory and Cognition, 25*, 129–139.

Diamond, R., & Carey, S. (1986). Why faces are and are not special: an effect of expertise. *Journal of Experimental Psychology: General, 115*, 107–117.

Fallshore, M., & Schooler, J. W. (1995). Verbal vulnerability of perceptual expertise. *Journal of Experimental Psychology: Learning, Memory and Cognition, 21*, 1608–1623.

Furl, N. Phillips, P. J., & O'Toole, A. J. (2002). Face recognition algorithms and the other-race effect: computational mechanisms for a developmental contact hypothesis. *Cognitive Science*, **26**, 797–815.

James, M. S., Johnstone, S. J., & Hayward, W. G. (2001) Event-related potentials, configural encoding and feature-based encoding in face recognition. *Journal of Psychophysiology*, **15**, 275–285.

Kassin, S., Tubb, V. A., Hosch, H. M., & Memon, A. (2001). On the general acceptance of eyewitness testimony research: a new survey of the experts. *American Psychologist*, **56**, 405–416.

Leder, H., & Bruce, V. (1998). Local and relational aspects of face distinctiveness. *Quarterly Journal of Experimental Psychology*, **51A**, 449–473.

Lewin, C., & Herlitz, A. (2002). Sex differences in face recognition—Women's faces make the difference. *Brain and Cognition*, **50**, 121–128.

Levin, D. T. (2000). Race as a visual feature: using visual search and perceptual discrimination tasks to understand face categories and the cross-race recognition deficit. *Journal of Experimental Psychology: General*, **129**, 559–574.

Lindholm, T. (2005). Own-age biases in verbal person memory. *Memory*, **13**, 21–30

Macrae, C. N., & Lewis, H. L. (2002). Do I know you? Processing orientation and face recognition. *Psychological Science*, **13**, 194–196.

Mason, S. (1986). Age and gender as factors in facial recognition and identification. *Experimental Aging Research*, **12**, 151–154.

Maurer, D., Le Grand, D., & Mondloch, C. J. (2002). The many faces of configural processing. *Trends in Cognitive Sciences*, **6**, 255–260.

Maylor, E. A. (1990). Recognizing and naming faces: aging, memory retrieval and tip of the tongue state. *Journal of Gerontology: Psychological Sciences*, **45**, P215–P226:

Meissner, C. A., & Brigham, J. C. (2001). Thirty years of investigating the own-race bias in memory for faces: a meta-analytic review. *Psychology, Public Policy and Law*, **7**, 3–35.

Memon, A., Bartlett, J., Rose, R., & Gray, C. (2003). The aging eyewitness: effects of age on face, delay and source-monitoring ability. *Journal of Gerontology: Psychological Sciences*, **58B**, P338–P345.

Memon, A., Gabbert, F., & Hope, L. (2004). The ageing eyewitness. In J. Alder (Ed.), *Forensic psychology: Debates, concepts and practice* (pp. 96–109). Willan: Forensic Psychology Series.

Memon, A., Hope, L., Bartlett, J., & Bull, R. (2002). Eyewitness recognition errors: the effects of mugshot viewing and choosing in young and old adults. *Memory and Cognition*, **30**, 1219–1227.

Perfect, T. J., & Harris, L. (2003). Unconscious transference and false identification in younger and older adults. *Memory and Cognition*, **31**, 570–580.

Perfect, T. J., & Maylor, E. A. (2000). Rejecting the dull hypothesis: The relation between method and theory in cognitive aging. In T. J. Perfect & E. A. Maylor (Eds.), *Models of Cognitive Aging* (pp.1–18). Oxford University Press.

Rhodes, G., Tan, S., Brake, S., & Taylor, K. (1989). Expertise and configural encoding in face recognition. *British Journal of Psychology*, **80**, 313–331.

Schooler, J. W. (2002). Verbalization produces a transfer inappropriate processing shift. *Applied Cognitive Psychology*, **16**, 989–998.

Searcy, J. H., Bartlett, J. C., & Memon, A. (1999). Age differences in accuracy and choosing in eyewitness identification and face recognition. *Memory and Cognition, 27*, 538–552.

Shaw, J. I., & Skolnick, P. (1994). Sex differences, weapon focus and eyewitness reliability. *Journal of Social Psychology, 134*, 413–420.

Shaw, J. I., & Skolnick, P. (1999). Weapon focus and gender differences in eyewitness accuracy: Arousal versus salience. *Journal of Applied Social Psychology, 29*, 2328–2341.

Sporer, S. L. (2001). Recognizing faces of other ethnic groups: an integration of theories. *Psychology, Public Policy and Law, 7*, 36–97.

Tanaka, J. W., & Farah, M. J. (1993). Parts and wholes in face recognition. *Quarterly Journal of Experimental Psychology, 46A*, 225–245.

Tanaka, J. W., Kiefer, M., & Bukach, C. M. (2004). A holistic account of the own-race effect in face recognition: evidence from a cross-cultural study. *Cognition, 93*, B1-B9.

Thompson, P. (1980). Margaret Thatcher—a new illusion. *Perception, 9*, 483–484.

Westerman, D. L., & Larssen, J. D. (1997). Verbal-overshadowing effect: evidence for a general shift in processing. *American Journal of Psychology, 110*, 417–428.

Wright, D. B., & Sladden, B. (2003). An own gender bias and the importance of hair in face recognition. *Acta Psychologica, 114*, 101–114.

Wright, D. B., & Stroud, J. N. (2002). Age differences in lineup identification accuracy: people are better with their own age. *Law and Human Behavior, 26*, 641–654.

Yarmey, A. D. (1993). Adult age and gender differences in eyewitness recall in field settings. *Journal of Applied Social Psychology, 23*, 1921–1932.

Yin, R. K. (1969). Looking at upside-down faces. *Journal of Experimental Psychology, 81*, 141–145.

Young, A. W., Hellawell, D., & Hay, D. C. (1987). Configural information in face perception. *Perception, 16*, 747–759.

Zacks, R. T., Hasher, L., & Li, K. Z. H. (2000). Human Memory. In F. I. M. Craik & T. A. Salthouse (Eds.), *The handbook of aging and cognition* (2nd ed. pp. 293–358). Mahwah, NJ: Lawrence Erlbaum Associates.

Section 4

Real-world cognition

Chapter 14

Cognitive ethology: giving real life to attention research

Alan Kingstone, Daniel Smilek,
Elina Birmingham, Dave Cameron, and
Walter F. Bischof

Abstract

Studies of attention, often conducted in artificial laboratory experiments, may
have limited validity when performance in the natural world is considered.
For instance, for over two decades investigations of "reflexive" and "volitional"
attention have tended to be grounded in methodologies that do not capture
the demands of attention in everyday life. Recent studies suggest these laboratory investigations have lost touch with real life contexts and accordingly
they may generate fundamental misunderstandings regarding the principles
of human attention and behavior. We identify the basic assumptions of
laboratory research that has led to this state of affairs, and suggest a new set of
assumptions that lead to a new research approach, which we call "cognitive
ethology." The implication is that if one is to understand human attention in
everyday life then research needs to be grounded in the natural world and not
in experimental paradigms.

Introduction

Patrick Rabbitt has never been one to accept the status quo. None of his
students escaped this strong part of his personality, and for many of us, it
helped to define who we became. One of Pat's most enduring lessons centered
around the idea that the models in psychology are largely "snapshots" of

This work was funded by the Natural Sciences and Engineering Research Council of Canda,
and the Michael Smith Foundation for Health Research. Thank you also to Patrick Rabbitt
for the wonderful years spent in his lab, and to Peter McLeod for his insightful comments on
an earlier version of this chapter.

idealized static cognitive sytems. Pat often punctuated this point by noting that experimental psychologists routinely throw away the first set of trials in an experiment as "practice trials." As Pat was fond of saying, these initial trials routinely produce the largest performance changes that will be found in a study. And yet, these initial trials are discarded and left unanalyzed because researchers desire stable systems that can be controlled, manipulated, and modeled.

This issue raised by Pat has plagued me over the years because seeded deeply within it was the notion that experimental psychologists were not really getting it right, nor were they going to get it right doing research the way they were doing it. That is, research in the pursuit of stability and control was not going to tell us what we really want to know—how people function in real life where things are highly variable and often outside the domain of experimental control. The present chapter represents an initial attempt by my lab to take on Pat's challenge to get things right and to learn how people function in real life. Our particular area of interest is human attention.

A laboratory paradigm for studying attention

We begin by closely considering one of the most well known laboratory paradigms for studying attention: The Posner cueing paradigm (Posner, 1978, 1981). In this paradigm, a central fixation dot that is flanked by two boxes is presented at the center of a computer screen. The task is simply to press the spacebar on a computer keyboard as quickly as possible when a visual target object appears inside one of the boxes. This target object is preceded by an attentional cue, which is either a brief peripheral flash surrounding one of the two boxes or a central arrow pointing toward one of the boxes (see Figure 14.1(a) and (b)). The standard and highly robust finding is that a target is detected fastest when it appears in the box that was cued by the peripheral flash or central arrow. On the assumption that the brain processes attended items more quickly than unattended items, it is concluded that target detection time was speeded for a target at the cued location because attention had been committed to the box that was cued.

Countless studies of this sort have led to the conclusion that there are two categories of attention, exogenous (reflexive) attention and endogenous (volitional) attention, both of which can be manipulated and measured by the Posner paradigm. When one of the two boxes is flashed briefly, as depicted in Figure 14.1(a), attention is considered to be oriented reflexively to the box that brightened. This attention shift is thought to be reflexive because people are faster to detect a target in the cued box even when flashing the box does

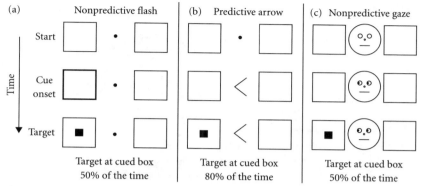

Fig. 14.1 Variations of the Posner paradigm. Each panel presents three stages of a typical trial (start, cue onset, and target onset); in these examples, the target (a small black square) appears at the cued box. In one variation of the paradigm (a), at the start of each trial, a central fixation dot is flanked by two squares (boxes). The left or right box is cued by a brief flash (illustrated by the thick black line), and then a target (the black square) is presented. The task is to press a key as quickly as possible when the target appears. The target appears in the cued (flashed) box 50% of the time and in the uncued (not flashed) box 50% of the time. Thus, the cue does not predict where the target will appear. In another variation (b), the left or right box is cued by an arrow pointing toward it, and the target appears in the cued box 80% of the time and in the uncued box 20% of the time. Thus, the cue predicts where the target will appear. In a third variation (c) the left or right box is cued by eyes looking toward it, and the target appears in the cued box 50% of the time and in the uncued box 50% of the time. Thus, the cue does not predict where the target will appear.

not predict where the target will occur (e.g. the target appears in the cued box 50% of the time and in the uncued box 50% of the time). Attention can also be oriented volitionally. When a central arrow points toward one of the two boxes, as depicted in Figure 14.1(b), attention is thought to be oriented volitionally to the box pointed at by the arrow. This attention shift is considered volitional because people are thought to be faster to detect a target in the cued box only when the arrow predicts where the target will occur (e.g. the target appears in the cued box 80% of the time and in the uncued box 20% of the time).

The Posner paradigm and reality

It is perhaps instructive at this point to compare the displays used in the Posner paradigm, which are shown in Figure 14.1, with the type of scenes encountered outside the laboratory, examples of which are shown in

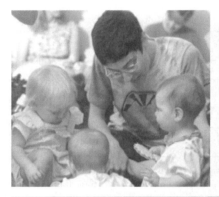
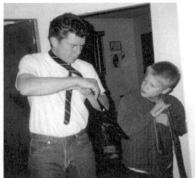
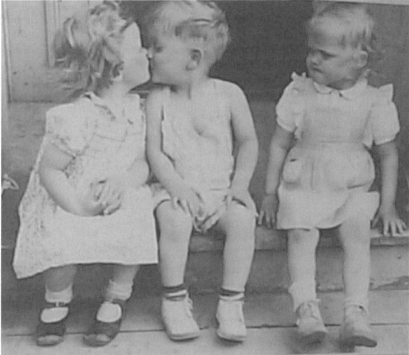

Fig. 14.2 Prototypical examples of everyday scenes that occur in life.

Figure 14.2. Even a cursory comparison begs the following type of question: To what extent does the simple, impoverished and highly artificial experimental task of detecting a light within a cued or uncued box have to do with the many complex, rich real-life experiences that people share? In other words, what does the cuing paradigm have in common with everyday situations such as children playing under the supervision of an adult, a father teaching a son how to tie and tie, or a little girl watching another two friends kiss? On the face of it, not very much.

Even a cursory look at the naturalistic scenes shown in Figure 14.2 yields many hypotheses regarding attention that are unlikely to ever be generated from laboratory studies of attention. For instance, inspection of the scenes suggests that people's direction of gaze might be a critical cue, perhaps even a reflexive one, for orienting attention in the real world. In 1998, Chris Friesen and I tested this idea by modifying the Posner paradigm in two important ways. First, arrows pointing to the left and right were replaced by a schematic face that looked left or right. Second, the predictive value of the central cue was eliminated; that is, eye direction did not predict where a target item would appear (see Figure 14.1(c); also Friesen & Kingstone, 1998). Note that because the eyes were centrally located and spatially nonpredictive, the traditional line of thinking predicted that they would not lead to shifts of attention. The result was that, contrary to this prediction, eye gaze did trigger shifts of attention, with all types of responses (target detection, target localization, and target identification) being enhanced almost immediately for targets that appeared at the gazed-at location. This rapid onset of an attention effect, and the fact that it occurred in response to a spatially nonpredictive stimulus, demanded the conclusion that the attentional shift was reflexive (Cheal & Lyon, 1991; Jonides, 1981; Müller & Rabbitt, 1989).

This conclusion, that centrally nonpredictive eye-gaze can direct trigger reflexive shifts of attention, led us to reconsider the fundamental notion that arrows only direct attention when they are spatially predictive, that is, the shifts are volitional in nature. Since a classic study by Jonides (1981, experiment 2), which failed to find positive evidence that nonpredictive central arrows will trigger a shift in attention, researchers have assumed that arrows do not produce a shift in attention unless they predict where an item will appear. We considered the possibility, for the first time, that central arrows might be much like eyes and that they might orient attention even when they are not predictive. We tested this possibility by replacing spatially nonpredictive eyes with spatially nonpredictive arrows (Ristic, Friesen, & Kingstone, 2002). The results were unequivocal. People attend to where arrows point even when they know that the arrows do not predict where a target will appear. In other words, like eyes, arrows produce a reflexive shift in attention to the cued location. This result has been confirmed by several investigators (Friesen, Ristic, & Kingstone, 2004; Hommel, Pratt, Colzato, & Godign 2001; Tipples, 2002) establishing that attention can be directed reflexively to locations indicated by nonpredictive arrows. The failure of Jonides (1981) to obtain this significant outcome may be attributed to several factors, including his arrow cue being hard to discriminate (it was flashed for only 25 ms) and his study lacking sufficient experimental power (fewer than 10 participants were tested and RTs at the cued location were based on less than 20 trials).

We believe that the recent experiments on eye gaze and nonpredictive central arrows have important implications for laboratory studies of attention. Specifically, the findings indicate that the Posner cuing paradigm is fundamentally flawed. Central cues such as eyes and arrows, which were assumed to tap volitional attention, actually do not engage volitional orienting. Thus, what was taken as a fundamental truth turned out to be completely in error. How could this mistake happen? How could this error be overlooked for over 20 years of research? We believe that the answer rests with the fact that laboratory research in the field of attention is based on two crucial assumptions—both of which are problematic.

Assumptions underlying laboratory research

Studies of attention in the laboratory are grounded on two basic assumptions. One is that human attention is subserved by processes that are stable across different situations. For example, the processes that are studied in the lab are assumed to be the same as the processes that are expressed in the real world. Second, one can maximize analytical power of a process by minimizing all variability in a situation save for the factor being manipulated. Note that the first assumption enables one to lay claim to processes in the real world without ever leaving the lab. And the second assumption demands that the laboratory situation be as controlled as possible. Ironically, the combination of these two assumptions has the effect of driving researchers further away from real life situations into highly contrived and artificial laboratory environments, all the while seducing the investigators into the belief that they are getting closer and closer toward a true understanding of how attention operates in real life.

While the assumptions of process-stability and situational-control are commonly held and readily applied in studies of attention, adopting them comes with a high degree of risk. The assumption of stability, for example, eliminates any need or obligation by the scientist to confirm that the factors being manipulated and measured in the lab actually express themselves in the real world. The field does of course check routinely that the effects being measured are stable *within the lab environment*, by demanding that results in the lab be replicable. Unfortunately, a result that is stable within a controlled laboratory environment does not necessarily entail that it is stable outside the lab. Indeed, there are many examples within the field of human attention indicating that even the most minor changes *within* a laboratory situation will compromise the replicability of an effect (e.g. Kingstone & Klein, 1993; Soto-Faraco, Morein-Zamir, & Kingstone, in press). Indeed, the fragility of laboratory findings whereby small changes in an experimental situation results in radically different experimental outcomes, should perhaps not be particularly surprising. There is now a growing body of literature indicating that "process stability" is tied intimately to the specifics of a situation, with brain re-configurations occurring continuously in response to even subtle environmental changes. Neisser (1976) referred to the dynamic reconfigurations as "schemata," Monsell (1996) referred to them as "task-set reconfigurations," and Di Lollo et al. (2001) have referred to them as "configurable input filters." Thus, while the assumption of process stability is remarkably convenient because it allows one to think that the work in the lab has some relevance to real world situations, the fact is that there is a very real risk, indeed a high likelihood, that the process being studied in the lab will not exist outside the lab.

Associated with the above is the fantastic risk of wasting many years and dollars conducting research that is replicable but which has little, if anything, to do with cognitive processes beyond the lab in real life environments. This follows because by simply assuming a process is stable across situations—specifically from the lab to real life—means that one never has to check whether the results in the lab are at all relevant to real life performance. This seems to be the reason why for more than 20 years researchers failed to notice that the Posner cuing paradigm, while producing results that were highly replicable, did not measure what people believed it was measuring. It was only after considering the results derived in the Posner paradigm against real life situations (e.g. how eye-gaze might influence attention) that this error was detected (Kingstone, Smilek, & Ristic, 2003).

The problem gets even worse, however, because it is often the case that attempts to test the first assumption of stability against real life situations are immediately met with apparently insurmountable obstacles. These obstacles arise from the second assumption of experimental control. The first obstacle is that processes in the lab often become defined by the experimental controls that were used to examine them. In addition, if this obstacle were somehow overcome and the controls that define a phenomeon were reproduced in the real world, a researcher is immediately posed with the challenge of making the case that the data collected in a real life situation are in fact a manifestation of the process that was measured previously in the lab. This is a daunting, and perhaps ultimately impossible, obstacle to surmount. This is because data that are attributed to a particular process in the lab can always be re-attributed to other factors that were left free to vary in a real life situation.

We believe that these two obstacles actually reflect a more fundamental problem that arises from the assumption of control when it is applied to nonlinear systems like human cognition and attention. While experimental control can be effective at revealing basic characteristics of simple linear systems, general systems theory has established that experimental control is unlikely to be effective at revealing important characteristics of complex, nonlinear systems such as the human attention system. This is because certain characteristics of complex systems are only revealed, or emerge, when several variables vary together in highly specific ways (see Ward, 2002; Weinberg, 1975). This is precisely what is not allowed to occur in highly controlled laboratory situations.

Considered together, it appears that there are both practical and principled reasons to question whether selecting tasks based on the assumptions of stability and control is likely to inform us about cognitive processes as they are expressed in real life situations. Moreover, it is sobering to contemplate the fact that these two assumptions can lead researchers to unwittingly and unthinkingly commit their lifetime to studying processes that may be expressed only within artificial lab situations.

Cognitive ethology: moving towards a different way of studying attention

In light of these considerations our most recent work has begun to move away from studying human attention in standard artificial laboratory paradigms. While we are still conducting laboratory-based investigations, we have sought to conduct studies that remove as many constraints on the behavior of our participants as possible. Thus rather than making causal claims about fundamental processes, our goal initially is simply to *observe* and *describe* behavior as it occurs. As such, our new approach, what we call *cognitive ethology*, is characterized by giving up the assumptions of stability and control for the scientific and objective study of human behavior under natural conditions. Our laboratory tasks, though not identical to real world tasks, have increased substantially in their ecological validity (see Hutchins, 1995; Koch, 1999; Neisser, 1976). Our hope is that by using this new cognitive ethological approach we might uncover new aspects of attention that have eluded researchers wedded to standard laboratory-based paradigms.

In our first attempts to move in this new direction we sought to study a task that individuals appear to engage in effortlessly every day—that of inferring where other people are attending. Our specific aim was simply to get a feeling for the types of cues that people use when they infer the attentional states of others. In our study two groups of participants viewed photographs that

(a)

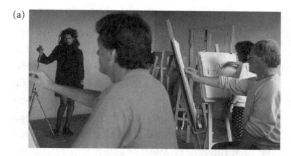

(b)

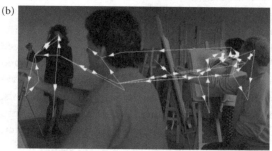

(c)

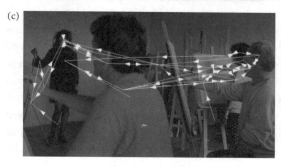

Fig. 14.3 Aggregate eye movement data from one of the scenes we presented to participants. (a) Depicts the original scene presented to participants; (b) shows data from participants who were asked to "describe the picture"; (c) shows data from participants who were asked: "Where are people in the picture directing their attention, and how do you know?". The arrows depict transitions between regions that occurred more often than would be expected by chance.

depicted one or more individuals involved in everyday behaviors, such as painting or playing basketball. An example of a picture used in the study is shown in Figure 14.3(a).

One group of participants (the "inference" group) was required to view the picture and then answer the following question: Where are the people in the picture directing their attention, and how do you know? Another group (the "describe" group) was required to view the pictures and simply describe each picture. Our goal was not to make inferences about underlying cognitive mechanisms but to simply observe and describe behavior as it occurred. We observed and described what information participants used to infer the attentional states of the individuals in each picture using a combination of *objective* (third-person) and *subjective* (first-person) measures. The objective measure involved monitoring participants' eye movements and examining the patterns of eye fixations that emerged as they viewed each picture. We reasoned that participants would fixate the information that they considered to be important for either making inferences about attentional allocation in the picture or for describing the pictures. In addition to observing the third-person eye fixation data we also measured the first-person reports that participants provided after they viewed each image. Of particular interest were the subjective reports of those participants who inferred where the individuals in the pictures were allocating their attention and who also reported what information they used to make such inferences. We thought that participants' subjective reports might provide a valuable insight into the cues that they used when making inferences about the attentional states of others.

As our approach did not involve controlling behavior, we were challenged with how to effectively analyze the complex patterns of behavior that emerged as participants engaged in our open-ended investigation. To examine the eye-movement data we divided the scenes into regions of interest (e.g. the eyes, heads, and bodies of people in the picture). Once a scene was divided into regions, we evaluated both the static fixation patterns (e.g. fixation frequency, fixation duration) for each region, as is done in most studies of scene viewing (e.g. Antes, 1974; Buswell, 1935; Henderson & Hollingworth, 1999), as well as the transition-patterns between various regions (see Liu, 1998). The regions were comparable across the two groups of participants, which then allowed us to directly compare how the patterns of eye fixations among these regions differed as a function of whether participants were inferring attentional allocation in the picture or merely describing the picture.

Figure 14.3(b) and (c) provides an illustration of the type of performance patterns we obtained. Figure 14.3(b) represents the eye movement data that occurred in the describe condition, and Figure 14.3(c) shows the data for the inference condition. The white arrows indicate transitions between different regions that occurred more often than would be expected by chance.

The data in Figure 14.3(b) and (c) suggest that individuals were primarily fixating the faces of the individuals in the picture, the drawings of the artists, and the tripod held by the model. Thus, the eye movement data suggest that people use information from faces and the actions that the people in the picture are performing both to describe the picture and to make inferences about where the people in the picture are directing their attention. A comparison of the eye movement data for the inference group to the eye movement data for the describe group revealed some particularly interesting findings. First, observers who inferred the attentional states of people in the picture fixated on the eyes of these people more frequently than observers who described the picture. That is, relative to the total number of fixations, observers in the inference group fixated the eyes of the model and artists more often than observers in the describe group. Second, this effect was specific to the eyes. When other body regions (such as the head, torso, arms, and legs) were analyzed, the inference and describe groups showed no difference in fixation frequencies. Thus, there appears to be a specific increase in the use of eye gaze information when observers are inferring the attentional states of others.

Examination of the transitions suggests that while there are some significant transitions from people's faces to the objects that the people are attending, this certainly did not occur for all of the faces. It seems that significant transitions mirroring gaze paths of the people in the picture only occurred in situations where direction of gaze was ambiguous, such as the direction of gaze of the model. A comparison of the significant transitions across the describe and inference conditions is also revealing. One striking observation that can be made by comparing the pictures in Figure 14.3 is just how similar the fixation areas and the significant transitions are across the two conditions. We think these findings are interesting when compared with the findings of Yarbus (1967) who reported that scan patterns differ substantially when participants are given different viewing instructions. The similarity in scan paths between the describe and inference conditions in our study suggests the tentative hypothesis that when participants view pictures with the purpose of describing them, they might actually be inferring the attentional states of the individuals in the picture.

Importantly, this is precisely what was indicated by the subjective reports. Moreover, the subjective report data provided an interesting insight into the cues that people use to infer attention that would not be expected either from an analysis of the eye-movement data alone or from previous studies of attention. Notably, when participants were asked how they knew where people in the picture were directing their attention, participants reported using cues such as the body orientation of the people in the picture and what appeared to be the focus of the scene, for example, the model in the painting scene. In addition to these observations, it is worth noting that many of the subjective reports echoed what was suggested by the eye movement data. For instance, participants reported that direction of gaze of the people in the scene was an important indicator of where people appeared to be attending.

Although the findings that we are reporting here merely represent our first, preliminary steps in a new research direction, they have already revealed several interesting points worthy of further investigation. For example, are people always inferring attentional states of others when first perceiving scenes? Importantly we expect that performance differences will emerge not only with changes in the task that participants are asked to perform, as demonstrated here, but also with the type of scene that is shown to participants and with the type of participant that is viewing a scene. In keeping with our new approach, the challenge is not to eliminate this variance by imposing experimental control, but rather to observe, describe, and finally understand it.

The ultimate goal: studying attention in the real world

Although it is difficult to leave the comfortable confines of a controlled laboratory setting, our ultimate goal is to study attention outside the laboratory as individuals perform everyday tasks in their natural environments. Rather than being constrained by our laboratory settings and their associated paradigms, we are moving in the direction of exploring how people behave as they function within the environment one ultimately intends to understand—the real world as it exists outside the laboratory. Of course, such an approach involves studying what people actually do in everyday life, how they appear to be doing it, what they think that they are doing, how they feel about what they are doing, and so forth, and looking for ways of understanding these performance outcomes.

We believe that a central component to studying attention in the real world is to become comfortable with giving up the assumptions of process stability and situational control, as we have begun to do in the study described briefly above. The goal of this approach is to simply observe and describe the complex patterns of behavior that people produce as they engage in complex everyday tasks, in order to ultimately gain a true understanding of human attention and performance.

A *Nature* publication by Land and Lee (1994) provides another excellent illustration of this approach. These investigators were interested in understanding where people look when they are steering a car around a corner. This simple issue had obvious implications for human attention and action, as well as for matters as diverse as human performance modeling, vehicle engineering, and road design. To study this issue, Land and Lee monitored eye, head, and steering wheel position, as well as car speed, as drivers navigated a particularly tortuous section of road. Their study revealed that drivers rely on a "tangent point" on the inside of each curve, seeking out this point 1–2 seconds before each bend and returning to it reliably. This finding was new to the field, and interestingly, the drivers themselves were unaware of the fact that they were searching for and applying a tangent point when navigating curves.

The study conducted by Land and Lee illustrates elegantly that meaningful research can be conducted without falling into the standard experimental assumptions of stability and control. By stating that one is interested in understanding how an individual performs a particular task in the real world, like driving around a corner, one is implicitly acknowledging that this task may be unlike any other task that one performs within the specific domain of driving; and indeed, it may have no counterpart in any other cognitive domain. Thus it is neither claiming to be a model task for other situations, nor is it assuming that there is a model task that can speak to this particular driving situation. In other words, a real world research approach rejects the assumption of process stability. In doing so it assumes that processes may be contextualized to the situation within which they occur. As noted previously, there is a wealth of evidence, ranging from Neisser's "schemata" to Di Lollo's "configurable input filters," indicating that this is precisely the case.

The Land and Lee study is also important because by choosing to measure performance as it occurred naturally in the environment, they were rejecting the standard *a priori* assumption that any variance that is not manipulated experimentally is something to be controlled and minimalized. This alternative way to deal with variance, to let it occur naturally and measure it, requires the assumption that variance may reveal key characteristics of cognitive processing. In other words, it requires the assumption that variance is part of the cognitive signal and as such it must be understood. Interestingly, this assumption dovetails with the most basic tenet of general systems theory, that complex systems are only revealed when several variables are permitted to co-occur. In sum, the real world approach rejects the standard of assumptions of stability and control, and in their place we find a commitment to understanding the situation, and the variance within that situation. According to the real world approach, the initial job of the researcher is simply to observe and measure what people do in the situation of interest. Of course, this approach is unlikely to be of much value in artificial laboratory situations where human behavior is typically highly constrained. For example, in a typical attention experiment people are only allowed to move one finger to press one key, with all other movements being banned including even minor movements of the eyes. Yet observation of real world behavior is very different. As Koch puts it "*description* is no lowly or easy task; it is in fact the very basis—indeed, the flesh—of nonspurious knowledge" (Koch, 1999, p. 27). In other words, description of attentional behavior in the real world is intrinsically valuable because it is grounded in what people really do and as such the questions related to it can be both anchored and meaningful rather than abstract and trivial.

Just as there were practical problems for the assumptions of stability and control when they are applied to understanding real world phenomena, one finds that there are also practical problems for the assumptions of situation and variance. The key problem is quite simply that it is very hard to do research at the real world level. It is hard for several reasons. First, it is difficult because there are no "off the shelf" model-tasks to use when one conducts research in this way. Hence, one cannot, for instance, simply manipulate the Posner cuing paradigm (Hunt & Kingstone, 2003) or the visual search paradigm (Eastwood, Smilek, & Merikle, 2001; Fecteau, Enns, & Kingstone, 2001; Smilek, Eastwood, & Merikle, 2000) or the attentional blink paradigm (Giesbrecht, Bischof, & Kingstone, 2003), and believe that one is gaining new insights into how people allocate their attention in everyday life. Instead, one has to spend a good deal of time simply observing and describing what people appear to be doing with their attention. And because one cannot control what people do, one finds that there is a tremendous amount of variation in the behavior that people produce, not only between people but for the same person at different times. It is also very difficult because there is very little data in the literature on how people actually allocate their attention in the real world rather than in artificial laboratory environments. This means that what questions and approaches are most interesting and likely to bear fruit are largely unknown. It also means that there may be little or no previous work performed on how to go about analyzing the data one collects, and therefore, one is often having to create new tools to understand the data that have been collected.

We would argue, however, that these problems can be viewed as exciting opportunities for researchers interested in discovering how attention is really allocated in the world. All the data one collects, all the questions that one explores and answers, provide a foundation for future investigations and a benchmark against which all other studies will need to be measured.

Summary and concluding comments

The goal of attention research is, and has always been, to understand how human attention operates as people behave in their everyday lives. As we have noted, however, in practice, the current laboratory-based research approach does not seem to be reaching this goal, and in fact, it may be moving the field further away from it. Our discussion of the underlying assumptions of the standard laboratory-based research approach—the assumptions of stability and control—brings to light both principled and practical reasons for why the laboratory-based approach is unlikely to reach its goal of understanding how attention is allocated in everyday life.

We have articulated what we believe to be an alternative approach to the standard lab-based methodology. This alternative approach replaces the assumptions of stability and control with the assumptions related to understanding individuals as they behave unconstrained in their natural environments and the variance that emerges with it. These latter assumptions are polar-opposites to the traditional assumptions of stability and control.

The present chapter also suggests principled and practical ways to focus attention research and to identify research questions that are meaningful. It is often the case that research questions are paradigm-driven or perhaps driven by a set of informal introspections of the researcher. In contrast to this usual way of generating research questions, we suggest that research might benefit by being grounded in systematic observations of real-world behavior, and that research concepts might best be grounded in what people really do objectively and what they perceive themselves to be doing. Indeed, William James clearly identified lay understanding as the starting point for attention research in his much quoted statement "everyone knows what attention is." Ironically, although many researchers use this quote when attempting to define attention, the field has rarely committed its research effort to determining what people think attention is and how they allocate it in everyday life. To be clear, we are not suggesting that attention research simply be more *applied*. Though it might focus on applied problems, such as driving cars and flying planes, attention research ultimately needs to study *every* aspect of attention as individuals define it and as it is used in real life settings. Pure research on the nature of real cognitive practices is needed.

In this chapter we have emphasized an approach that we call cognitive ethology. By observing and measuring what people really do in their natural environments one can begin to define the problem space in a manner that becomes grounded in real life situations and not contrived laboratory environments. This means that subsequent laboratory investigations can be protected from pursuing behavior and questions that are merely paradigm-driven and paradigm-specific. It also means that one is free to ask questions that are meaningful and relevant to real life rather than being constrained by, and limited to, artificial laboratory environments. Our hope is that our cognitive ethological research approach will lead to pure research that will ultimately expand and deepen our understanding of human cognition.

References

Antes, J. R. (1974). The time course of picture viewing. *Journal of Experimental Psychology*, **103**, 62–70.

Buswell, G. T. (1935). *How people look at pictures*. University of Chicago Press.

Cheal, M. L., & Lyon, D. R. (1991). Central and peripheral precuing of forced-choice discrimination. *Quarterly Journal of Experimental Psychology: Human Experimental Psychology*, **43A**, 859–880.

Di Lollo, V., Kawahara, J., Zuric, S. M., & Visser, T. A. W. (2001). The preattentive emperor has no clothes: A dynamic redressing. *Journal of Experimental Psychology: General*, **130**, 479–492.

Eastwood, J. D., Smilek, D., & Merikle, P. M. (2001). Differential attentional guidance by unattended faces expressing positive & negative emotion. *Perception and Psychophysics*, **63**, 1004–1013.

Fecteau, J. H., Enns, J. T., & Kingstone, A. (2001). Competition-induced visual field differences in search. *Psychological Science*, 11, 386–393.

Friesen, C. K., & Kingstone, A. (1998). The eyes have it! Reflexive orienting is triggered by nonpredictive gaze. *Psychonomic Bulletin and Review*, 5, 490–495.

Friesen, C. K., Ristic, J., & Kingstone, A. (2004). Attentional effects of counterpredictive gaze and arrow cues. *Journal of Experimental Psychology: Human Perception & Performance*, 30, 319–329.

Giesbrecht, B., Bischof, W. F., & Kingstone, A. (2003). Visual masking during the attentional blink: Tests of the object substitution hypothesis. *Journal of Experimental Psychology: Human Perception and Performance*, 29, 238–258.

Henderson, J. M., & Hollingworth, A. (1999). High-level scene perception. *Annual Review of Psychology*, 50, 243–271.

Hommel, B., Pratt, J., Colzato, L., & Godign, R. (2001). Symbolic control of visual attention. *Psychological Science*, 12, 360–365.

Hunt, A., & Kingstone, A. (2003). Inhibition of return: Dissociating attentional and oculomotor components. *Journal of Experimental Psychology: Human Perception and Performance*, 29, 348–354.

Hutchins, E. (1995). *Cognition in the wild*. Cambridge, MA: MIT Press.

Jonides, J. (1981). Voluntary versus automatic control over the mind's eye's movement. In J. B. Long & A. D. Baddeley (Eds.), *Attention and performance. Part IX* (pp. 187–203). Hillsdale, NJ: Erlbaum.

Kingstone, A., & Klein, R. M. (1993). What are human express saccades? *Perception & Psychophysics*, 54, 260–273.

Kingstone, A., Smilek, D., & Ristic, J. (2003). Attention, researchers! It is time to take a look at the real world. *Current Directions in Psychological Science*, 12, 176–180.

Koch, S. (1999). *Psychology in human context: Essays in dissidence and reconstruction*. University of Chicago Press.

Land, M. F., & Lee, D. N. (1994). Where we look when we steer. *Nature*, 369, 742–744.

Liu, Andrew (1998). What the driver's eye tells the car's brain. In G. Underwood (Ed.), *Eye guidance in reading and scene perception* (pp. 431–452.) Oxford, England; Elsevier Science Ltd.

Monsell, S. (1996). Control of mental processes. In V. Bruce (Ed.), *Unsolved mysteries of the mind: Tutorial essays in cognition* (pp. 93–148). Howe, Sussex: Erlbaum (UK) Taylor & Francis.

Müller, H. J., & Rabbitt, P. M. (1989). Reflexive and voluntary orienting of visual attention: Time course of activation and resistance to interruption. *Journal of Experimental Psychology: Human Perception & Performance*, 15, 315–330

Neisser, U. (1976). *Cognition and reality*. Principles and implications of cognitive psychology. San Francisco: Freeman.

Posner, M. I. (1978). *Chronometric explorations of mind*. Hill sdale, NJ: Lawrence Erlbaum Associates.

Posner, M. I. (1981). Cognition and neural systems. *Cognition*, 10, 261–266

Ristic, J., Friesen, C. K., & Kingstone, A. (2002). Are eyes special? It depends on how you look at it. *Psychonomic Bulletin and Review*, 9, 507–513.

Smilek, D., Eastwood, J. D., & Merikle, P. M. (2000). Does unattended information facilitate change detection? *Journal of Experimental Psychology: Human Perception and Performance, 26,* 480–487.

Soto-Faraco, S., Morein-Zamir, S., & Kingstone, A. (in press). On audiovisual spatial synergy: The fragility of the phenomenon. *Perception & Psychophysics.*

Tipples, J. (2002). Eye gaze is not unique: Automatic orienting in response to uninformative arrows. *Psychonomic Bulletin and Review, 9,* 314–318.

Ward, L. M. (2002). *Dynamical cognitive science.* Cambridge, MA: MIT Press.

Weinberg, G. M. (1975). *An introduction to general systems thinking.* New York: Wiley.

Yarbus, A. L (1967). *Eye movements and vision* (B. Haigh, Trans.). New York: Plenum Press. (Original work published 1965).

Chapter 15

Are automated actions beyond conscious access?

Peter McLeod, Peter Sommerville,
and Nick Reed

Abstract

Extensive practice leads to both expertise and automation of actions. Expertise implies knowledge of a skill but automation implies loss of conscious control. So, does practice lead to more or less ability to describe how the skill is performed? We show that despite their greater expertise at the skill, adults are less able than children to describe how they tie their shoelaces or to recognize the method that they use. Adults know the goals but not how they are achieved. We also show that adults are not able to explain how they know where to go to catch a ball, nor, in some cases, to describe what they are doing as they catch one. Expertise leads to some actions becoming beyond conscious access.

Introduction

Building on the observations by Bryan and Harter (1899) of the changes that took place as people developed the skill of telegraph operation (i.e. transcribing Morse code into words and vice versa), Fitts (1964) proposed that as a skill is practiced, control of the actions involved passes from a cognitive representation to an autonomous one. The same idea was described by Shiffrin and Schneider (1977) as the shift, following practice with a consistent mapping between stimulus and response, from controlled processing to automatic processing. The idea appears again in the model of cognitive skill acquisition proposed by Anderson (1982) as the shift in control, with practice, from declarative to procedural. In all these descriptions the final stage of skilled performance is automated. Well-learnt patterns of behaviour can be executed without the need for conscious control. This conforms to common experience. Novice car drivers have to think carefully about what they are doing and can do little else at the same time. The experienced driver no longer need attend to the basic elements of driving such as changing gear or maintaining lane position, and so, provided nothing unusual is happening, can carry on a conversation, tune the radio or make a call on a mobile phone while driving.

It may be generally agreed that skilled performance does not *require* conscious control when the task is in a routine phase, but are the actions of the skilled performer really *beyond* conscious access? The common sense answer might seem to be No—the more skilled you are, surely, the more you know about what you are doing. If you want a golf lesson do you go to an expert or a novice for advice? Despite the apparently obvious answer to this question we will demonstrate situations in which novices can describe what they are doing but experts cannot. Further we will show that experts sometimes claim to be doing one thing when in fact they are doing something quite different. The expert knows what the goals of his skill are but does not necessarily have conscious access to how he achieves them.

The idea that the control of behaviour can be outside conscious access has a long history in Psychology. For example, Freud described his patient Anna O. who refused to drink. Under hypnosis she recalled a memory of a dog slobbering over a glass of water and then someone drinking from it. Freud believed that the patient found this memory so traumatic that it had been suppressed and could no longer be consciously accessed, and yet it exerted control over the patient's choice of behaviour. More recently, Reason's study of errors in everyday life (Slips of Action) has demonstrated that well-learnt routines can be executed without conscious control (Reason, 1979). He found that a common pattern was for an error to occur when someone was distracted as they reached a choice point in a well-learnt sequence of behaviour where a variety of continuations were possible. They would realize some time later that although they had started out on the intended sequence they had not been following the originally chosen continuation from the choice point. For example, one of Reason's subjects reported that he had intended to "change into something comfortable for the evening." He went to his bedroom, took his clothes off, and then realized that he had put his pyjamas on. The "put pyjamas on" routine starts in the same way as the "changing clothes" routine—go to the bedroom and take your clothes off—and only diverges after clothes have been taken off. The "put pyjamas on" routine had run successfully without the actor being aware of what he was doing.

One reason why well-learnt patterns of behaviour might be expected to run outside conscious control comes from consideration of efficient system design. If a specific response pattern should always be used in a particular situation it is inefficient to use high level cognitive processes to run the pattern each time it is needed. It is more efficient to delegate the execution of the response to a dedicated, independent low-level process and save the high level decision making capacities to deal with things that only they can do, such as responding to an unexpected event. This might explain why well-learnt patterns *can* run outside conscious control. But it is not clear whether this level of representation would continue to be accessible to conscious introspection or not.

Tying shoelaces

At an intuitive level tying shoe laces is an example of a skill which matches Fitts's description of skill learning. The child is told how to tie its laces. Initially the task is performed slowly and effortfully with each stage of the process carefully monitored. Eventually, after performing the sequence thousands of times the adult has the impression that at a conscious level he makes the decision to initiate the program and the appropriate sequence of movements then runs off with little attention to, or awareness of, the individual actions that achieve the goal. Initially the child could presumably describe the actions it was performing because it had to remember them to perform the task. Do skilled adult performers still know what actions they are performing or only the goal they wish to achieve?

Experiment 1(a)

First we need to check whether shoe lace tying is more automated for adults than for children.

Participants. These were 15 children aged 5–6 years who had learnt to tie their shoelaces within the previous year and 18 university students.

Procedure. Each participant was timed tying a shoelace on a shoe on their foot, first with their eyes open, then with their eyes shut.

Results

Figure 15.1 shows the mean time taken by the adults and the children, with eyes open and shut. Not surprisingly, the adults were much faster at tying their shoe laces than the children. A more significant result is that shutting the eyes affects children but not adults. (Several children could not tie their shoelaces with their eyes shut and were dropped from the analysis.) The children were slower to tie their shoelaces with their eyes shut (17.1 s vs. 12.6 s, $t(14) = 4.4, p < 0.01$) but with adults it made no difference (5.2 s vs. 5.1 s, $t(17) = 0.3$, ns).

This supports the idea that the program used by the children who have recently learnt to tie their laces is still under closed-loop control—progress is monitored using visual feedback. Presumably it is still, therefore, to some

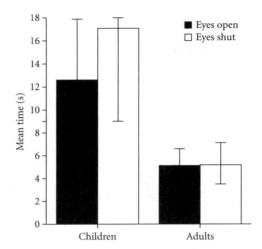

Fig. 15.1 The mean times in seconds (and SDs) for children and adults to tie their shoelaces with their eyes open and shut.

extent, under conscious control. Adults, on the other hand, no longer use visual control. They execute an open-loop sequence without visual monitoring. This is consistent with the idea that the adult shoelace tying program is automated but the children's is not.

Experiment 1(b)

The aim of this experiment was to determine whether the adults, who are highly practised at tying their laces, know more or less about what they are doing than the children, who have recently acquired the skill.

The first two operations most people make when tying their shoelaces are to put one lace over then under the other to form a half-knot, and then to make a loop on one side of the half knot. Pilot studies showed that there are four common ways in which people make this first loop (some people making it on the left and some on the right). Figure 15.2 shows these methods for the loop on the right side of the half-knot. It can be seen that in all methods both hands are used to form the loop.

Participants. These were 15 female and 6 male children aged 5–6 years who had learnt to tie their shoelaces within the last year and 13 male and 7 female university students.

Procedure. Participants were asked to tie their shoelaces and were filmed as they did so, to see which method they used. All used one of the methods shown in Figure 15.2. Then they were told to clasp their hands together (to prevent motor-rehearsal) and asked to describe how they tied their laces. They were then asked two specific questions about their method: "On which

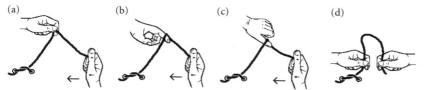

Fig. 15.2 The four principal ways that the first loop is formed on the right: (a) by holding the lace at the top of the loop; (b) by wrapping the lace around the first finger; (c) by wrapping the lace around the thumb; (d) by holding the lace at the bottom of the loop and putting the hands together. The same loop can also be made on the left side, using the mirror images of methods (a)–(d).

side do you make the first loop?" and "To make the first loop do you use your left hand, your right hand or both hands?" They were then shown the four methods in Figure 15.2 as well as a fifth way involving the formation of the first loop with one hand. Each way was demonstrated on a lace, the demonstrations being performed slowly and in a spatially exaggerated way. They identified which method they thought was closest to the one they used.

Results

All the children said that the first thing they did was to make a half-knot and then to form a loop. They all reported the side on which they made the loop correctly. Out of the 21, 13 said that they used two hands to make the first loop, the rest maintaining (incorrectly) that they used one hand. Like the children, all the adults said that they first made a half-knot and then formed a loop. All but one correctly indicated which side they formed it on. However, only 6 out of the 20 adults said that they used two hands to make the first loop, the remaining 14 claimed (incorrectly) that they used one hand. The children were reliably more accurate than the adults at reporting whether they used one hand or two to form the first loop ($z = 2.05, p < 0.05$).

The multiple-choice question tested whether participants could select the method they used from the five methods demonstrated. Chance performance was 20%. Twelve of the 21 children (57%) were correct; 4 of the 20 adults (20%) were correct. Children were above chance ($z = 2.1, p < 0.05$); adult performance did not differ from chance.

Given that Experiment 1(a) showed that adults do not use visual feedback when tying their laces perhaps it is not surprising that they are unable to recognize which method they use. But it might be argued that the adults' performance was so poor because the demonstration they had to recognize was of someone else tying a shoelace rather than the view they would get if they tied it themselves. So four videos were made from the point of view of someone tying their own laces using methods A and C, either on the right or the left. The 16 adults who used one of these methods were then shown the four videos and asked to choose which one was their own method. Only five correctly identified the video clip that mirrored their performance. This proportion does not differ significantly from chance ($z = 0.39$, $p = 0.69$).

Discussion

The children who had recently acquired the skill were mostly able to describe how they achieved the first key goal of tying laces. The adults, who had far more practice at the skill, were no longer able to do this. The majority were unaware that they used both hands to form the first loop, and, as a group, were no better than chance at recognizing how they did it.

This result is consistent with the predictions of the Fitts model of change in the control of skill with practice—control passes from the cognitive (and reportable) to the autonomous (and unreportable). If you wish to achieve the same goal repeatedly, you develop a program to do this. There is no need for conscious access to the individual actions embedded in the program and so it is more difficult for the expert to report what he does than for the novice. But there is another possibility. Maybe conscious control is actively harmful to a well-learnt act. You would not do it as well if you thought about it. The adult inability to report what they do may indicate conscious control being actively inhibited. Evidence consistent with this interpretation comes from a second series of experiments.

Catching balls

Tying shoelaces is an example of the sort of taught skill that matches Fitts' description of skill acquisition. A child is originally given a set of verbal instructions about how to perform the task. Gradually, as the skill is acquired, he thinks less and less about how to perform the task and the correct action sequence unfolds without conscious thought. But there are other skills that are not taught. The learner knows the goal that has to be achieved and gradually, with practice, acquires the ability to achieve the goal without ever being taught the required actions. What happens when such a skill is learnt? Is the performer able to describe what he has learnt?

A classic example of such a skill is learning to catch a ball. Children are not taught how to catch a ball because no one knows how it is done (apart from the select group who have read McLeod, Reed, & Dienes, 2003). The child is just told to "watch the ball." Some balls fall out of its reach and some land in its arms. An as yet unknown learning mechanism finds some central tendencies from the experiences of watching the balls that land in the arms and those which do not. Gradually the child develops an interception strategy and starts to move to try and reach the interception point before the ball hits the ground.

There are some simple and consistent patterns which occur if you watch an object thrown toward you depending on whether the ball will hit you or not. For simplicity we will just consider balls coming directly toward the observer. Figure 15.3 shows α, the angle of elevation of gaze above the horizontal from observer to ball, as a stationary observer watches a ball thrown toward him from a few metres away. The ball will either go overhead (far or close), hit him in the eye, or fall in front of him (close or far). In all cases the angle of gaze rises initially as the ball goes up in the air but as ball starts to fall the observer's experience depends on where the ball will land. If it is going overhead the angle of gaze continues to increase, accelerating as the ball approaches. If it is going to fall short the angle of gaze stops increasing, drops to zero and then becomes negative. But if the ball is going to hit the observer in the eye there is a unique pattern—the angle of gaze continues to increase throughout the flight, reaching its maximum value just as the ball hits the observer.

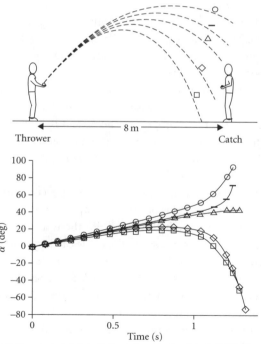

Fig. 15.3 Upper: balls thrown toward a stationary observer. Lower: how the angle of elevation of gaze from fielder to ball changes as the ball approaches the observer.

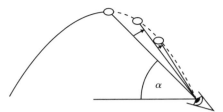

Fig. 15.4 If the ball is going to hit the observer in the eye the angle of elevation of gaze from observer to ball increases throughout the flight.

Many people find it hard to believe that the angle of gaze to a ball that will hit you goes up continuously. They imagine the ball from the point of view of an observer watching someone else catch a ball (as in the upper part of Figure 15.3). For the external observer it is true that as the ball goes up and then down his angle of gaze as he follows it goes up and down too. But for the catcher this is not so. Although the ball is falling throughout the second half of its trajectory it is also approaching him. If it is going to hit him in the eye, the angle of gaze rises continuously. This can be intuited from Figure 15.4. At whatever part of the flight the line of gaze from observer to ball is drawn, the ball's next position will be above that line. Therefore the angle of gaze as the observer follows the ball will increase throughout the flight, reaching a maximum value just as it hits him. The proof of this comes from considering that an object on a ballistic trajectory is accelerating downwards (under gravity) and decelerating forwards (because of wind resistance). If its vertical and horizontal velocity are such that at time $t + 1$ it is below the line of gaze from observer to ball at time t (and therefore α decreases) it can only fall further below the line of gaze at time t as the flight progresses (because it is accelerating down and decelerating forward). Thus it will not hit the observer in the eye. So, if the ball hits the observer in the eye at the end of the flight, α must have increased continuously throughout the flight.

When someone runs to catch a ball they have to try and generate a collision with an object that was not originally on a collision course. People appear to use the unique pattern of information about a ball that will hit them to try and achieve this collision. Every study that has measured the angle of elevation of gaze to the ball as people run has shown that they run in such a way that α increases at a decreasing rate as they run (see McLeod, Reed, & Dienes, 2001, 2004). The strategy that fielders appear to follow is to run so that they generate the information that they would have got if they had been stationary and the ball was going to hit them. This strategy guarantees interception (McLeod & Dienes, 1996; McLeod, P., Reed, N., & Dienes, Z. (in press).) (provided, of course, the fielder can run fast enough to implement it. If the ball is going to land too far away from the fielder for him to catch it, he will not be able to keep the angle of gaze rising as he runs.)

Experiment 2

We asked people to imagine what would happen to their angle of gaze when they watched a ball which they caught at eye level and then asked them to report what happened to their angle of gaze just after they had caught a ball at eye level.

Participants. These were seven university students, with ages ranging from 19 to 31.

Procedure. Angle of elevation of gaze was explained graphically and examples given of the way it would change as they watched an object such as a rocket rising in the air or a parachutist descending to the ground. First (the pre-catch condition) they were asked to imagine how their angle of gaze would change if they were watching a ball thrown toward them from about 10 metres away which would have hit them in the eye had they not caught it. Then (the post-catch condition) they caught a series of balls thrown toward them. They were asked to concentrate on how their angle of gaze changed during each trial while the ball was in flight and encouraged to catch the balls at eye level. They were allowed to move forward or backward up to 1 m from their start position to make it more likely that some balls could be caught at eye level. After each trial, they were asked to describe how their angle of gaze changed as they watched the ball until it landed in front, went overhead or was caught.

In both pre- and post-catch conditions the subjects were asked to give a confidence rating in their judgement on a scale from 0 (complete guess) to 10 (certain).

Recording of α. A video camera recorded the trials at 25 frames a second from a side-on position in which the ball's flight and the catcher's head were within the field of view. The ball and catcher's eye position were measured from the film so that the value of the angle of elevation of gaze from catcher to ball could be obtained at 40 ms intervals.

Results

Pre-catch. The descriptions of what they thought would happen to their angle of gaze if they watched a ball, which they caught at eye level are given in Table 15.1. Six of the seven subjects (all except number 3) believed that their angle of gaze would go up and down in a roughly symmetrical fashion. This is fundamentally incorrect. The angle of gaze only goes up and then down symmetrically if the ball falls to the ground. Thus most of the participants reported what they would have seen had they watched someone else catch a

Table 15.1 The Statements of the subjects in Experiment 2[a]

Subject	Pre-catch
1.	Up and then back down to zero. (8)
2.	Angle starts at less than 0°, then increases to maximum height, then decreases back to 0° when caught. (8)
3.	Slow increase to constant. (10)
4.	Increases with flight of ball to around 30° and then decreases in the same fashion. (8)
5.	Increase to about 45° then follow ball down to about 10°. (6)
6.	Initial increase then gradual decrease as the ball gets nearer. (8)
7.	Begins at 0°, increases to about 40°, then decreases back to zero at the same rate. (7)

Subject	Post-catch
1.	Up a little then down a little. (6)
2.	Start below 0°, increased to maximum height, then decreased to just greater than 0°. (8)
3.	Increases to constant. (10)
4.	Followed ball up and then down to 0°. (8)
5.	Increased to 15° then constant. (7)
6.	Increased all the time. (7)
7.	Increased then remained constant. (8)

[a] In the pre-catch condition they described what they thought would happen to their angle of gaze as they watched a ball that they could catch at eye level. In the post-catch condition they described what they had just experienced as they caught the ball. (The angle of gaze that they actually experienced is shown in Figure 15.5 with subject 1 at the top.) In both cases the correct answer is that their angle of gaze goes up continuously. The confidence judgement on a scale of 0 (guess) to 10 (certain) is given after each statement.

ball (as in the upper part of Figure 15.3), not what they would see if they caught a ball themselves. Despite the inaccuracy of these judgements they were made with considerable confidence. The median confidence rating of the six fundamentally incorrect statements was 8 on a scale with a maximum of 10. The statements were not guesses—the participants were confident about their judgements.

Post-catch. For each participant the catch was selected where the fielder had caught the ball closest to eye level. Figure 15.5 shows the value of α experienced by each subject throughout the catch. α increased continuously throughout the flight except for fielders 1 and 7 where α was constant for the last 80 ms before the ball was caught.

Their statements about how α had changed for these flights are given in Table 15.1. One subject, number 6, gave a correct description of his experience. Arguably subject 7 gave an accurate description. Three of them (1, 2, and 4) still maintained that their angle of gaze went up and then down. Although overall this is more accurate than the pre-catch descriptions, for several of the

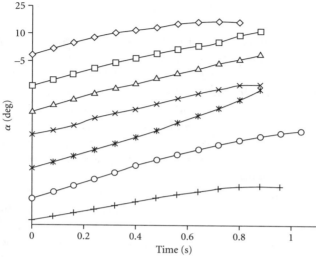

Fig. 15.5 Values of α experienced by subjects as they caught a ball at eye height. The original estimates of α from the frame-by-frame analyses were smoothed by replacing the value of α for each frame with half its original value for that frame plus a quarter of the value from each of its nearest neighbors. The top line shows subject 1, with successive lines showing the other subjects. The scale is shown in degrees for subject 1. The same scale, displaced, is used for the other subjects. That is, they all experienced an initial α between $-5°$ and $0°$, and a terminal α between about $20°$ and $40°$.

catchers the erroneous preconception that as the ball goes up and down, their gaze must do so as well, appears to be more salient than the information they got from monitoring their angle of gaze as they moved to catch the ball. The participants' confidence in their judgements was little changed from the pre-catch judgements. The three subjects whose judgements remained fundamentally inaccurate (1, 2, and 4) showed no change in confidence (median 8 in both conditions). The three participants whose accuracy improved after taking a catch (5, 6, and 7) showed no change in confidence with a median of 7 in both conditions.

Discussion

These experiments demonstrate the separation between people's ability to perform a skilled action and their ability to describe what they have done. The modal model of skill acquisition (Anderson, 1982; Fitts, 1964; Shiffrin & Schneider, 1977) predicts that this might happen as a result of practice. As a skill is acquired, control passes from a cognitive representation to an autonomous one. In consequence the actions that are performed to achieve the goal become less accessible to conscious report.

The shift from declarative to procedural knowledge was demonstrated with people tying their shoelaces. The actions required could be described and recognized by children who had just acquired the skill but not by adults who had far more practice. Adults knew the goal to be achieved (form a loop) but could neither describe how they did it nor recognize the action they used when it was shown to them. The inability of experts to describe what they are doing was also demonstrated in the studies of ball catching. Six out of seven participants were unable to describe what strategy they used. This conclusion is not surprising for a skill that is acquired implicitly—no one can explain what they do when they ride a bicycle, for example. However, the lack of knowledge went deeper than simply not being able to explain their strategy. Immediately after they had taken a catch they were asked what their experience had been, and it would often be misreported. The failure was not just "I do not know" but was a report that their experience had been one that, if it had happened (I followed the ball up and then down to 0°) would have led to them *failing* to catch the ball. This is the experience they have had every time they have failed to catch a ball and never when they have caught it. How can they confuse these two experiences when the outcomes are so different?

Initially the idea that experts cannot describe what they are doing may sound implausible. If you ask a skilled driver how to do a hill start, surely he could tell you? But perhaps what he would tell you would be a high-level goal description—"do not release the handbrake until the clutch has begun to bite" rather than how to achieve this. To judge by the difficulty many people have in learning how to balance the accelerator and clutch so that the car neither slides back or jerks forward when the brake is released, it is not easy to describe how this skill is performed.

Our observations of a dissociation between the ability to act and the ability to describe the action fit with other studies of the control of action. Milner and Goodale (1993) reported a patient (DF) who suffered severe brain damage following carbon monoxide poisoning. She showed a complete dissociation between her ability to respond to a visual stimulus and her ability to report the visual signal she was acting on. If shown a slit she could not report its orientation. But if given an object and asked to push it through the slit she could do this accurately, adjusting the orientation of the object correctly as it approached the slit. She could use visual information to control her action but she could not describe what she based the action on. This was interpreted by Milner and Goodale in terms of the anatomical and functional separation of pathways in the brain, with a visual projection to the temporal lobe underlying the ability to report the visual basis for an action and a visual projection to the parietal lobe underlying the ability to perform the action. This separation is apparent in DF as a result of severe brain damage. But perhaps the separation in Milner and Goodale's patient does not require such an extreme state of affairs. Our subjects also showed a dissociation between an ability to act and an ability to report that act.

One curious aspect of the results with people catching balls was that they often reported what they would have seen if they had watched someone else performing the act rather than the experience they had themselves. This may reflect the salience of the apparently obvious, but erroneous, belief that since the ball goes up and down and you watch the ball, your gaze must go up and down too. And as we know from the Einstellung effect (Luchins, 1942) a salient but unhelpful pattern of thought can block a better one. An alternative possibility is that the report is influenced by a "mirror neuron" representation which was involved in acquisition of the skill. Rizzollati and Arbib (1998) found neurons in the macaque brain that fired both when the animal performed a motor act (such as grasping a peanut) and also when it watched someone else perform the same act. Such cells are a possible neural basis for imitation. Acquiring skills like ball catching that cannot be taught verbally because the teacher does not know how to do it may involve imitation of someone who already has the skill. When you watch someone else catch a ball you will indeed watch the ball go up and watch it come down and that fact may become part of the mirror neuron representation of the skill. A possible implication of our results is that when asked to report what you observed yourself, you use the mirror neuron representation of the skill that was involved in learning it. What happens when you watch someone else perform the task and when you do it yourself are different so you end up making an incorrect report.

There is a further possibility. Freud's analysis of his patients whose overt behaviour was controlled by an experience to which she no longer had conscious access, suggests a brain in which the subconscious is in control, only allowing the conscious part access to information which it is capable of using effectively. Perhaps this is an appropriate model of the acquisition of implicit skills. Low level neural networks are good at discovering the regularities in the relations among sensory experience, action, and outcome that lead to us learning how to run to catch a ball or to move our postural adjustment muscles in such a way that we stay on a bicycle. However, this low-level, subconscious part of the system also knows that the high-level, conscious part of the system would come up with its own theories about how to do these tasks. These theories might be inappropriate as with our fielders who believed that they watch the ball up and then down when they catch it. So, rather than let the high-level system interfere with the low level, the low level allows the high level to have its theories, but does not allow it access to or control over the low level mechanisms that perform the task.

References

Anderson, J. R. (1982). Acquisition of cognitive skill. *Psychological Review, 89*, 369–406.

Bryan, W., & Harter, N. (1899). Studies on the telegraphic language: The acquisition of a hierarchy of habits. *Psychological Review, 6*, 345–375.

Fitts, P. M. (1964). Perceptual-motor skill learning. In A. W. Melton (Ed.), *Categories of human learning* (pp. 243–285). New York: Academic Press.

Luchins, A. S. (1942). Mechanization in problem solving—the effect of Einstellung. *Psychological Monographs, 54*, 95.

McLeod, P., & Dienes, Z. (1996). Do fielders know where to go to catch the ball or only how to get there? *Journal of Experimental Psychology: Human Perception and Performance, 22*, 531–543.

McLeod, P., Reed, N., & Dienes, Z. (2001). Towards a unified fielder theory: What we do not yet know about how fielders run to catch the ball. *Journal of Experimental Psychology: Human Perception and Performance, 27*, 1347–1355.

McLeod, P., Reed, N., & Dienes, Z. (2003). How fielders arrive in time to catch the ball. *Nature, 426*, 244–245.

McLeod, P., Reed, N., & Dienes, Z. (in press). The generalised optic acceleration cancellation theory of catching. *Journal of Experimental Psychology: Human Perception and Performance.*

Milner, A. D., & Goodale, M. A. (1993). Visual pathways to perception and action. In T. P. Hicks, S. Molotchnikoff, & T. Ono (Eds.), *Progress in brain research* (Vol. 95, pp. 317–337). Amsterdam: Elsevier.

Reason, J. (1979). Actions not as planned. In G. Underwood & R. Stevens (Eds.), *Aspects of consciousness.* London: Academic Press.

Rizzolatti, G., & Arbib, M. A. (1998). Language within our grasp. *Trends in Neurosciences, 21*, 188–194.

Shiffrin, R. M., & Schneider, W. A. (1977). Controlled and automatic human information processing: Part II. Perceptual learning, automatic attending and a general theory. *Psychological Review, 84*, 127–190.

Chapter 16

Operator functional state: the prediction of breakdown in human performance

G. Robert J. Hockey

Abstract

The problem of predicting increased risk and skill breakdown is a major issue in complex work environments. It is examined in this paper through the application of an operator functional state framework, based on assessment of the cognitive-energetical potential for sustained performance in skilled operators in relation to task goals and priorities. A concern with overall system efficiency, rather than with single task effectiveness, allows us to better understand performance changes in relation to task-related decision making, and the constraints and costs of control activity. Maintenance of primary task outputs requires the operation of a compensatory process that acts to protect vulnerable cognitive goals from competition, particularly from (stronger) emotional and biological goals. While primary performance goals are typically maintained under stress the presence of compensatory activity means that there are often decrements in secondary or auxiliary components of performance, and markers of strain (effort, fatigue, increased sympathetic activation, and EEG changes). These "latent decrements" are likely to have implications for breakdown in primary performance, especially if it can be established that the compensatory process is near its limit. Although there is, at present, no direct way of determining this critical state, the paper will summarise ongoing research using new methods of performance breakdown analysis that is beginning to address the problem.

Introduction

This paper takes a new look at an old problem—understanding the origins of decrement in human performance. A clear understanding of the term "(human) performance" is central to this undertaking. In the motivational control approach adopted here, when a task goal is in place, task-related actions are assumed to be controlled by reference to internal standards or set points, and modifed through negative feedback until overt performance matches goal targets. This process allows the goal to be maintained, and purposive behaviour promoted (e.g. Carver & Scheier, 1982; Hyland, 1988; Schönpflug, 1985). Indicators of performance are assumed to reflect but one aspect of the complex self-regulatory activities that are the normal mode of human–environmental interaction in the context of goal management. Because of the need to adapt to changing environmental conditions, there is always competition for access to the executive control mechanism, and the regulatory activity required to maintain performance on the specified task involves activity in systems other than those directly implicated in the task— effectively "costs." Therefore, a valid assessment of decrement needs to take account of these auxiliary processes, and must be considered in relation to all goal management behaviour.

Central to this is the assumption that individuals are able to operate adapt- ively with respect to task demands, and change the settings of mental processes in order to maintain effective performance. The origin of this idea in my own work is Pat Rabbitt's insightful work on adaptive control in the management of speed and error in sequential responding (Rabbitt, 1981), which signalled a paradigm shift in research on human performance. The present paper will attempt to take this further by using an operator functional state (OFS) frame- work to examine a number of issues relating to the detection of performance decrement in more complex tasks, and show how this approach is being used in current work on adaptive automation.

Operator functional state

The problem of predicting increased risk and skill breakdown is a major issue in complex work environments. It is examined in this chapter through the application of an OFS framework. OFS refers to the cognitive-energetical capacity for sustained performance, in relation to task goals and priorities and their attendant physiological and psychological costs (Hockey, 2003; Wilson & Russell, 2003). Specifically, OFS is a function of: (a) current operator back- ground factors (as induced by conditions such as sleep loss or fatigue); (b) the mode of interaction with task goals (priorities, effort, control); and (c) stable operator characteristics (skill, coping style).

The concept of OFS is central to current applied approaches to the problem of managing complex performance (particularly in safety-critical work such as aviation and process plant operation), where breakdown of task control may have serious consequences, though the general principles can be applied to the performance of any goal-directed activity. The OFS framework recognizes the inherently adaptive nature of performance—as a response not only to current task demands, but also to prevailing conditions and constraints imposed by biological and personal needs—both long- and short-term. Furthermore, a state theory of performance degradation such as OFS demands a system-level analysis, rather than one considering only task performance. This means assessing patterns of human/task/environment interaction, involving multi-level indicators of both direct and indirect behaviour, as well as the costs of goal management.

The central assumption of OFS is that valid inferences about the capacity of operators to perform tasks effectively need to be based on analysis of the functional state of the broader cognitive-energetical resources of the system (Hockey, 1986, 1997, 2003). This requires a concern not only with what operators can do, but also what they cannot do; not just with task performance, but also physiological processes serving adaptive behaviour, and metacognitive indicators of state—anxiety, effort, and fatigue; not just with short-term responses to current demands, but also longer-term maintenance of effectiveness; not just with primary performance measures, but also secondary tasks and changes in strategic behaviour. The paper will consider the nature of performance goals in relation to other goals, and show how a compensatory control process is necessary to help maintain performance in the face of these competing attentional objectives. It will summarize evidence on indirect (latent) degradation—predicted by the theory, and a necessary part of the broader picture of decrement—and outline some current work on the development of OFS methods in the assessment of performance decrement.

A system context for assessing performance changes

Most human performance testing is based on the assessment of limited behavioural responses to highly specified task goals. Unlike, say, assessment of the performance of a chemical plant or a railway or an office, it does not typically imply a broader concern with competence of the overall system, or with the state of auxiliary factors that help to determine the effectiveness of end-point actions. Whereas it is routine to consider the energy used in meeting industrial output targets, or environmental and maintenance costs of a modified transport system, analysis of human performance is rarely concerned with the emotional and psychophysiological costs of maintaining overt task criteria.

A system perspective enables us to make a distinction between *effectiveness* and *efficiency* (Hockey, 1997; Schönpflug, 1983). Efficiency is a major requirement for industrial processes—success but only with acceptable costs. By far the majority of studies that use performance methods to assess the effects of task conditions are concerned only with effectiveness—how well specific output targets are achieved. A concern with system efficiency means taking into account the costs to the system as a whole of achieving these outputs. This is particularly relevant when comparing conditions in which manifest performance does not differ, since it may imply that success in maintaining the required standard is achieved at the expense of disruption to other (currently less important) processes. We refer to these spill-over effects as "latent decrement," since they reflect a compromised system state that may impose constraints on adaptive responses in the face of further demands.

Of course, performance tasks are not used just to measures effects of stressors. Their more widespread use is to provide a window on underlying mental processes. However, even here, researchers sometimes fail to fully appreciate the rationale for the use of performance methods. From the investigator's point of view, the rationale is clear: tasks are designed to provide external indicators of the functional level of underlying mental operations. If a process is predicted to operate less well (say, because of competition from other mental operations) relevant task measures are expected to show a decrement. However, this procedure has a questionable validity, assuming a rather unusual level of compliance on the part of the "performer." From his or her perspective, the task represents an externally-imposed set of goals, requiring them to direct behaviour toward the achievement of specified target outputs and maintain this goal state over the duration of the session. This means maintaining task goals in memory, selectively attending to task information, avoiding distraction from competing (more relevant, long-term) goals, and suppressing affective responses such as frustration, boredom, or fatigue. It is clear that the performer often fails to do this (by becoming distracted, losing motivation, or just deciding that other goals are more important). What then can we justifiably infer about the operation of underlying mental processes from an observed reduction in task output or an increase in errors?

The nature of performance decrement

Problems in detecting decrement

The essence of the problem of understanding decrement is that it is not easy to tell whether an operator is capable of carrying out a task under demanding conditions simply by examining the overt level of performance achieved. This is because performance may be "protected" by a compensatory reallocation process so that it appears normal. However, the apparent stability may hide genuine problems of task management. Use of more sophisticated performance analysis and OFS methodology usually reveals latent decrements (Hockey, 1997), in the form of increased effort and strain, errors in (less critical) secondary tasks, or increased activation and disturbances in the physiological systems driving effort and task engagement.

The same kinds of adaptive mechanisms have been identified both under high workload, and in the response to stress and difficult working conditions, such as loud noise, sleep deprivation, and shift work. Skilled, highly motivated operators in real life safety critical tasks normally maintain overt performance criteria very effectively, even under severe demand and stress (Hockey, 1997). Where breakdown does occur, it is typically characterized by a "graceful degradation" (Navon & Gopher, 1979) rather than catastrophic failure. From a practical viewpoint, the problem is that, for a period before manifest degradation is observed, the operator is likely to be in a state of limited functional competence, being able to manage only predictable routine task demands, or produce bursts of effortful control. If we could monitor the development of such states, and predict work phases when operations may be at risk, we would be in a much better position to prevent serious consequences of performance breakdown.

The relativity of performance goals

A second problem with the logic of performance assessment is that laboratory tasks are not the only thing that people have to do. Many users of performance measures appear to ignore (or at least have lost sight of) the essential biological context of behaviour. The emphasis on regulatory control means that the behaviour involved in carrying out performance goals needs to be considered an integral part of the overall adaptive behaviour of the individual, competing for control of action not only with other cognitive goals but also with fundamental emotional, biological, and motivational needs. This is particularly relevant since emotional goals are typically more potent in capturing attention than cognitive goals (Öhman, Flykt, & Esteves, 2001). This is probably because of their greater overall relevance for system priorities (e.g. requirements for self-preservation, eating, or protection of young). Emotion-based goals (particularly those activated by adverse or threat signals) are enduring and self-energising, and sustained by powerful biological events (Taylor, 1991). These can arise both from the external environment and internal bodily processes such as the patterning of hormonal and neurotransmitter activity. They appear to be under automatic control, and only partly accessible by direct regulatory action. In contrast, cognitive goals are more transient, arbitrary and context-specific, and more controllable directly. They are also likely to be vulnerable to disruption by inputs relevant to the stronger bodily goals. Under some circumstances, cognitive goals may not even be as relevant as transient emotional needs such as feeling calm, avoiding strain, or relaxing.

Mechanisms of goal disturbance

Two broad kinds of disruption to performance goals may be identified; displacement and loss of activation (essentially equivalent to the problems of selective and sustained attention). Cognitive goals may be displaced by other competing goals (as in the familiar effects of intrusion from distracting events in dichotic listening and visual attention studies), but such effects may also occur with intrusion from emotional or bodily events, such as the involuntary orienting response to peripheral threat signals during cognitive work (Oatley & Johnson-Laird, 1990), or the more sustained distraction associated with powerful states such as hunger or strong emotion (Taylor, 1991).

In the second form of disruption, loss of activation may occur simply as a function of time, with increasing difficulty of sustaining attention on the task. The recent renewal of interest in the vigilance problem (e.g. Grier et al. 2003) suggests that the classic decrement over time occurs because of a problem in maintaining effortful attending. On this view, even simple monitoring requires active control, and may suffer from a failure of executive function (Shallice, 1988). Loss of attention in the absence of overtly competing task events could occur either as a passive loss of activation, or through the operation of an active inhibition process. In fact, loss of goal activation may be the same process as that underlying displacement if it is assumed that competition for control of action in the latter case comes from an underlying motivational requirement for rest (or change of goal). I will come back to this possibility later, in discussing the role of fatigue in performance decrement. For the moment it serves the purpose of identifying the requirement for goal maintenance as a likely source of performance decrement.

The pre-emptive control potential of emotional states ensures that effective emergency responses to environmental changes are readily available. By further preventing fixation on short-term or low-level goals, even in the absence of strong alternatives, such a mechanism ensures flexibility of shifts in goal orientation, allowing novel events to be investigated and other cognitive needs considered. Despite all this, human performance can be extraordinarily resistant to disruption. Kahneman (1971) pointed out that attentional selectivity was very effective, showing little disturbance under a very wide range of demanding conditions. How is this achieved? One possibility is that the hypothesised vulnerability of cognitive goals may, paradoxically, serve an adaptive function. Maintaining cognitive goals in focal attention requires active protection, invoking the special purpose mechanism of selective attention. Such protection is effortful, however, and places increasing demands on executive mechanisms under demanding conditions. One of the clearest consequences of this is an increase in regulatory costs, as evidenced by activity in relevant behavioural and physiological systems (Hockey, 1997; Kahneman, 1973; Teichner, 1968). Before considering performance protection directly, however, we need to briefly review the literature on the identification of stress effects.

Performance under stress: a brief review

Rather surprisingly, stressors appear to have relatively small effects on performance. In general, apart from transient effects, the extensive early research on performance of visually-based tasks under noise and other "distractors" regularly failed to show any clear effects (see Kryter, 1970), even when marching bands were introduced to the classroom in one study. Only with the intensive programme of work carried out in the 1950s and 1960s (notably at the Applied Psychology Unit in Cambridge) were such effects observed, using stressors such as noise, sleep deprivation, prolonged work and drugs, primarily as a result of developing a range of stress-sensitive tasks. Broadbent and his colleagues (see Broadbent, 1971) recognized that effects may be masked or compensated by the built-in redundancy and strategy options available to the system (e.g. working faster between momentary disruptions), and designed tasks that challenged this regulatory process, for example, by presenting information rapidly, in unpredictable locations, and without breaks (serial reaction), or by making critical events rare and unpredictable (vigilance). The effects observed were, however, rather subtle, and generally small. For example, rather than reducing overall response speed, stressors caused more errors or an increase in the number of occasional delayed responses.

Patterns of stressor effects

The general view of stress effects presented here is that stressors pose a general threat to task goals that may be overcome by adaptive behaviour on the part of the performer. However, stressors also appear to pose specific threats for different information processing tasks. The analysis of stress effects on performance carried out by Hockey and Hamilton (1983) found somewhat different patterns of decrement for different groups of stressors across a range of indicators: speed, accuracy, memory, selectivity, and alertness, which may be seen as profiles of the expected kinds of information processing problems for specific stress conditions, in the absence of effective compensatory regulation.

The most general pattern of decrement is associated with conditions such as noise, danger, and conditions that give rise to anxiety. This may be regarded as the modal stress state, involving a subjective state of high activation, high selectivity of attention, a preference for speed over accuracy, and reduced effectiveness of working memory (Hockey & Hamilton, 1983). Decrements are more common on tasks of long duration, especially where the use of working memory (WM) is central to maintaining the flow of the work. Selective attention is normally very effective, unless response is required to a number of different events or sub-tasks, in which case only the most important may be maintained. A familiar effect of such stressors is narrowed attention, in which high priority features of tasks are maintained and secondary aspects neglected. Such an effect has been observed for a wide range of stress states, including noise, threat of shock, danger, and test anxiety (Baddeley, 1972; Broadbent, 1971; Hockey, 1979; Hockey & Hamilton, 1983). Other stressors are associated with different kinds of changes. For example, memory appears unaffected by heat or with extended work periods. In all cases, however, it has become clear that we cannot separate underlying effects on cognitive processes from those relating to changes in performance goals or strategies. An increase in reliance on one kind of process may be the result of a strategic reduction in the use of another. Because of this, patterns of stressor effects cannot be discussed without reference to an understanding of what the performer is trying to do when carrying out a task, and of what conflicts exist between different goals.

An interesting observation is that any decrements are more likely to occur in laboratory studies than in real-life work situations (Hockey, 1997). The reasons for this have not been formally addressed, though differences in skill level and motivation are likely to be important. Laboratory tasks are generally poorly learnt and provide the performer with goals that are private, transient, arbitrary, and trivial. Participants are encouraged to work as fast as possible, or without making errors (or both) for the duration of the task. Under stress, or when additional demands are imposed, there is little room for manoeuvre, and errors are more likely. By contrast, work tasks are (usually) meaningful and often executed in the public domain. They help to define us individually within the organization. They are also generally well-learnt and long-lasting. All these factors help to protect such tasks under stress or heavy environmental demand. The real-life context encourages the maintenance of task goals, and the use of sustained levels of effort, if required. Because work tasks are usually carried out well within the capacity of the individual, individuals are more likely to be able to increase effort when necessary. Finally, since work tasks are well-practised, more strategies are available for responding to disturbances and new demands, and more options are available about managing decrement.

Performance protection and state regulation

As I have already indicated, evidence from studies of performance under stress and high demands strongly supports Kahneman's claims for the effectiveness of attentional selectivity. I have argued that this is because performance is protected through the operation of a compensatory mechanism, ensuring that primary goals are maintained under executive control. Such a view was initially proposed by Teichner (1968). As in all control systems, the controlled variable (in this case, performance) is stabilized while the values of other (controlling) variables involved in the regulatory activity alter. Teichner takes the familiar case of body thermoregulation, and considers the fact that core temperature (the key variable) is effectively constant under a wide range of heat stress conditions. However, there are clearly a number of indirect indicators of heat stress associated with controlling variables (sweating, vasodilation, etc.) reflecting the activity of the regulatory process in achieving this stability. We would not wish to conclude that there was no problem of heat stress just because we could not observe a rise in core body temperature. Indeed, the effects on controlling variables are interpreted as indicating that continued exposure to extreme conditions may cause the control process to break down and core temperature to rise. With performance the same model can be applied: absence of a decrement in a primary task measure cannot be taken to mean that a stressor has no effect, or poses no threat to the long term stability of task activity. And changes in other relevant variables may mean that the risk of breakdown is increased.

Compensatory control model

Hockey (1997) developed a compensatory control model to incorporate these observations, and to account for a wide range of effects of stress and workload on performance. The model is based on a two-level control system, with lower level, routine regulation, and an upper level, effort-based regulation. A distinction between upper and low levels appears to be the minimum complexity needed to account for the data on effects of stress, attentional demands, and performance management (Broadbent, 1971; Hamilton, Hockey, & Rejman, 1977; Shallice, 1988) (though action theory approaches typically assume a multiple-level hierarchy of regulatory control; Frese & Zapf, 1994). Effective upper level control normally ensures the integrity of central aspects of task performance. However, if this is lacking or ineffective because of fatigue, changes in lower level processes would be expected to reveal the range of decrements indicated by Hockey and Hamilton's (1983) analysis.

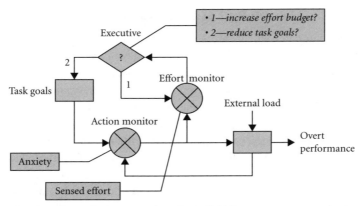

Fig. 16.1 The main features of Hockey's (1997) compensatory control model: see text for explanation.

For the purposes of the present chapter only an outline description is included here. The detailed operation of the model has been described in other places (see Hockey, 1997). From a control theory perspective, overt performance is assumed to be driven by task goals, with the help of feedback from current actions. Task goals determine the output criteria for performance (which events to respond to, how fast to work, how much accuracy is required, the sequencing of actions, and so on). As with all negative feedback systems, control is achieved, in principle, by comparing performance targets with current outputs (through the action monitor in Figure 16.1), and modifying the output until any discrepancy is removed (or kept within acceptable limits of goal tolerance). However, as Bandura (1996) has argued, formal control models can say very little about the wide variety of reactions people have to perceived negative discrepancies—whether they will respond with increased or decreased task motivation, and how performance will be affected. In our model effort regulation has the function of mediating between the experience of discrepancy and its effect on task goals.

Effort regulation

In the control model effort regulation is implemented through activity in a second, upper loop. The effort monitor is sensitive to increasing control demands in the lower loop (e.g. a failure to resolve a discrepancy, a slow rate of resolution, a high variance of outputs over time). As such it performs a similar role to that attributed to positive affect in the monitoring of progress toward goal attainment in Carver and Scheier's (1982) model of the metacognitive function of mood states. It is not necessary to agree with Kahneman's (1973) argument that effort is automatically increased to meet new demands. In the model presented here perception of the increased regulatory load causes control to be temporarily shifted to the higher level (the executive), where two control options are available—either an increase in effort to stabilize the task goal (and maintain performance), or a downwards adjustment of the goal to match what currently available effort can achieve (with a reduction in performance). Both have the effect of reducing the discrepancy, so allow the system to recover equilibrium, but with different effects on performance and regulatory costs.

In fact, two separate effort settings may be required for the upper control mechanism, both under the guidance of executive control. A lower set-point acts as a default for a given task environment (the working effort budget), based on the individual's anticipation of the task's attentional demands, their perceived level of skill, and strategic preferences (e.g. for speed-accuracy trade off settings; Rabbitt, 1981). The upper set point represents a working maximum for effort expenditure, based on individual tolerance criteria for task engagement. The difference between the two can be thought of as a "reserve effort budget" for meeting additional demands and unpredictable environmental changes. Any increase in demand can de dealt with by a resetting of the effort budget up to this upper limit, allowing regulatory control to continue routinely. We agree with Bandura (1996) that standard control models cannot explain why one person may choose to increase effort and so maintain performance on task goals (option 1 in Figure 16.1), and another reduce goal requirements instead (option 2). Indeed, the same individual may do one thing on one occasion, and the other on another. However, such questions can be addressed by including an evaluative, decision-making element in the model. The working hypothesis is that this choice is determined by factors such as long-term goals and standards, evaluation of costs and benefits of alternative actions, and current OFS variables such as effort expenditure and fatigue. (Bandura's self-efficacy approach is, in fact, very similar to this, though it is focused on belief systems rather than individual performance.)

Although we have not yet carried out formal experiments to test the two-level effort hypothesis, pilot studies with small groups of students are unequivocal in showing that individuals quite naturally distinguish between the two criteria. They are able to rate a set of five tasks appropriately in terms of "How much effort you would expect to have to allocate to be able to carry out the task well," giving high ratings to more difficult tasks (between 3 and 7 on a 10-point scale, with end points labelled "no effort at all" and "the most effort I could imagine being able to manage"). They also give higher (and less variable) ratings (7–9) of "How much effort you would be prepared to put into the task to maintain a high level of performance if conditions made it more difficult." Finally, students show steady increases in reported effort when demands are increased within specific tasks.

Full studies are being carried out at present to further investigate the metacognition of effort. They relate to the distinction that has sometimes been made (e.g. Mulder, 1986) between two kinds of effort; compensatory effort (for maintaining performance goals under stress) and computational effort (for meeting the demands of tasks). The two-level effort mechanism suggests a need for only one kind of effort, but with two levels or settings. The lower set point is equivalent to the computational effort associated with task demands, determined primarily by an assessment of processing requirements for specific tasks. As in the data summarized above, this is normally well below the assumed functional limits for effort expenditure, and likely to be quite stable for a given individual in a familiar task environment, though dependent on practice, experience and target criteria. The upper limit, by contrast, is more clearly motivational in origin, and more variable. It is hypothesized to be a function of individual differences in the perceived value of task goals, in the response to challenge, in the capacity for sustained work, and in the tolerance of aversive states associated with high levels of strain.

These predictions form part of the current experimental work in this area. The upper set point for effort allocation is also likely to change more under the influence of short-term factors such as fatigue (Holding, 1983; Meijman, Mulder, van Dormolen, & Cremer, 1992), self-control (Muraven, Tice, & Baumeister, 1998), and prevailing affective states (Ellis & Ashbrook, 1989; Hockey, Maule, Clough, & Bdzola, 2000) that may reduce the attractiveness of effort expenditure. There is also a clear link to Norman and Bobrow's (1975) distinction between data-limited (computational, lower limit) and resource-limited (compensatory, upper limit) constraints on performance. In terms of its compensatory function, the upper limit of the effort budget may be increased for activities that are more unpredictable or more critical in terms of outcomes. A high tolerance for effort enables an individual to respond with an increased work-rate to meet a newly imposed deadline, to maintain stable levels of performance in the presence of distractions, or to overcome fatigue to complete critical activities. Correspondingly, the upper limit on the reserve budget may be reduced when overall capacity has been compromised by fatigue, illness or chronic stress. This second level of effort allocation is more strongly associated with individual differences in patterns of performance degradation under stress and high workload. A small reserve budget will typically give rise to overt decrements under stress, while a larger budget is more likely to be associated with sustained performance and increased costs.

Latent decrement

The application of an OFS methodology allows us to examine performance decrement within a system-oriented framework, including both direct and indirect effects of operational conditions. In particular, measures of efficiency will usually provide a more sensitive and valid test of disruption than measures of effectiveness (how well set tasks are carried out). The compensatory processes involved in system regulation mean that, for detecting effects of performance disruption, we need to consider performance not only of primary (overt) task activity, but also of secondary tasks, and the costs of increased regulatory activity. Even where primary performance is maintained without loss, the increased strain of performance protection is expected to result in changes in other aspects of overall system performance. These may be classified as indirect decrements (or latent degradation), since the capacity for further response (e.g. to new emergencies) is likely to be compromised. Four more or less distinct forms of this latent degradation may be identified. Such effects are discussed in detail in other places (see Hockey, 1997) so are summarized only briefly here (Table 16.1).

Secondary task decrement

As observed in workload paradigms, effects of stress states may be detected more readily in less central components of behaviour. These effects are well established in paradigms where primary task activity may be impervious to increases in workload or demand (Wickens & Hollands, 1999). Effects of stressors on secondary tasks are fairly common, though not as well known because of a limited application of the methodology in this area. A well-established

Table 16.1 Types of latent decrements found under stress and high workload

Decrement type	Characteristics/examples
Secondary task decrements	Selective impairment of low priority task components *Neglect of subsidiary activities* *Attentional narrowing*
Strategy changes	Within-task shift to simpler strategies *Less use of working memory* *Use of responsive rather than proactive mode*
Regulatory costs	Strain of effortful control *Increased anxiety, mental effort, fatigue* *Sympathetic activation*
After-effects	Post-task preference for low effort strategies *Post-work fatigue* *Risky decision making, use of short-cuts*

example is that of attentional narrowing, effects being reported across a wide range of stressors; noise, deep sea diving, threat of shock, extended work, etc. (Baddeley, 1972; Hockey, 1979). This effect may also be considered to involve a strategic adjustment (as below), since the detailed pattern of performance depends on the manipulation of priority differences between task components.

Strategic adjustment

A second performance related decrement is the shift to a less demanding method of working, for example by reducing the reliance on working memory operations. One of the best known examples is Sperandio's (1978) demonstration that air traffic controllers responded to high workload by cutting back on the amount of individual routing of planes (in favor of a general strategy for all contacts). A similar result was found by Schönpflug and his colleagues (Schönpflug, 1983) in a simulated office management task. Participants made more use of external memory aids under noise and time pressure. In both these cases, the strategy change is adaptive because it reduces the mental demands of the task under the more difficult conditions, and maintains the main goal (safety, accuracy) at the expense of an increase in the time taken.

Regulatory costs

The third type of latent decrement refers to the generally observed increase in physiological activation and negative affective states under performance protection conditions. The effect is well illustrated by Lundberg and Frankenhaeuser's (1978), study of noise effects. In one study they found that effective arithmetic performance under noise, but increased levels of adrenaline and effort; in a second study an overt decrement was observed but no such costs. Veldman (1992) also found no effects of noise on a set of memory and search tasks, though this was accompanied by marked increases in heart rate and blood pressure.

After-effects

A fourth kind of latent decrement is associated with probe tests carried out after the main task has been completed. Such after-effects have not been widely studied (see Broadbent, 1979; Holding, 1983), though they are diagnostic of the long-lasting effects of fatigue associated with performance protection. The most characteristic finding is an increased reluctance to engage in effortful strategies on post-work tests (e.g. Holding, 1983; Meijman, van Dormelen, Mulder, & Cramer, 1992; Van der Linden, Frese, & Sonnentag,

2003) after extended periods of demanding work. The technique has not as yet been used within an OFS analysis of stressor effects, though it is strongly predicted to show the same kind of effects.

Current developments in the prediction of decrement

Over the past few years we have carried out an extensive programme of work to test aspects of the compensatory control model. This programme has adopted the OFS framework to provide a more systematic analysis of the nature of decrement in complex work under stress.

Cabin air management system (CAMS)

This approach makes use of a complex simulation task that allows performance to be assessed on sub-tasks having different levels of priority. High levels of task motivation and expertise are achieved by extended training and recruitment as "crew members" over a period of several months. The task adopted for this work was a complex, dynamic control task, the Cabin Air Management System (CAMS) (see Hockey, Wastell, & Sauer, 1998). This is a basic simulation of a life-support system for a closed system such as a space vessel or submarine. It is a multi-loop supervisory control system. In the inner loops, five life-support subsystems (oxygen, pressure, carbon dioxide, temperature, and humidity) are controlled automatically under fault-free operation; automatic controllers respond to sensed inputs by sending commands to open or close valves, switch-off heaters or air conditioning, etc. The higher-level supervisory control loop is closed by the operator, on the basis of monitoring of system state indicators and assessing overall operation state. When off-normal states are detected the operator is required to diagnose the fault and implement a sequence of recovery actions. The simulation also includes two secondary tasks. Alarm reaction time (ART) involved acknowledging (false) alarms occurring on the operator control panel (OCP) indicating that one of the system variables was out of range. System status check (SSC) was a prospective memory task requiring operators to make checks of oxygen and nitrogen tanks every two minutes. Duration of task sessions varied from 1–4 hours in different studies.

Perhaps surprisingly, operators have been found to be able to carry out this complex task equally well across a wide range of conditions, including noise, sleep deprivation, and increases in workload. As an example, consider the effects of sleep deprivation (Hockey et al. 1998), where primary performance showed no differences as a result of sleep condition. As predicted by compensatory control theory, however, there were clear indicators of latent decrement, in terms of secondary task, strategy changes, and affective state changes. Sceondary task decrements included delayed responses to alarms and increased errors in making system checks. Operators also used less demanding strategies when sleep deprived. Instead of the emphasis on active monitoring behaviour normally observed they tended to use a responsive mode, relying more on correcting the system by manual interventions once a variable had triggered an alarm. In addition, ratings of effort and fatigue were increased under sleep loss. Although subjective fatigue mainly reflects sleepiness in this situation, ratings were higher for those who protected task performance more effectively (by working harder to prevent sleep deprivation from reducing their commitment to task goals).

A current set of studies of workload and fatigue with Gareth Conway makes use of a version of CAMS in which faults cannot be corrected. Once an automatic controller for one of the five sub-systems becomes faulty the variable has to be controlled manually until the end of the task period. We are using a cyclic loading methodology in which the number of faulty sub-systems is increased from 2 to 5 in successive 15-min periods, then back down from 5 to 2, with faults reset before each. This allows us to investigate carry-over effects of fatigue from one period to the next, adopting the hysteresis methodology used in engineering to detect response lags and nonlinear response to change. Once again, there were no effects of load on primary task performance, during either the loading or unloading phase of the cycle, but strong effects of load, as well as hysteresis effects for secondary task measures. As Figure 16.2 indicates, both ART and SSC show impairment with increasing primary task load, and an increased decrement on the unloading phase of the cycle. We tentatively attribute this to a growth of fatigue during the loading phase, which limits the additional effort that may be allocated to these tasks. This is supported by analysis of subjective measures of fatigue and effort. Fatigue increased during loading, then remained at this high level during unloading, showing no sign of recovery. Effort increased with load and was higher overall during the unloading phase—for the protected primary task, but not for the two secondary tasks.

Adaptive automation

This cyclic loading methodology is being employed in our current programme of work on the identification of strain states that might predict performance breakdown. A major applied focus for such concerns is the design of automation in complex human-machine (H-M) systems, where the integrity of the system depends on the cooperation of human operators and computers. Despite the widespread benefits of automation, there are also well-documented problems

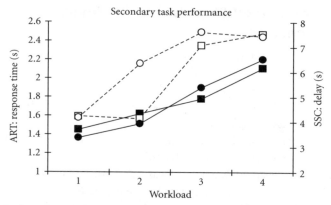

Fig. 16.2 Performance on the two secondary tasks as a function of cyclic loading (square symbols = ART, circles = SSC; full lines = loading phase; dashed lines = unloading phase).

for operator effectiveness (e.g. Parasuraman & Riley, 1997), often attributed to "clumsy automation," where humans are left only with the tasks that are too difficult (or too expensive) to automate. A reaction to this is found in recommendations for "human-centered" solutions (Billings, 1996), where the needs and responsibilities of operators are given priority. However, while generally effective, this approach has failed to take account of OFS-related constraints that make humans vulnerable to surges of demand and loss of capacity under stress. One possible solution to the dilemma is the application of OFS analysis methods in combination with recent developments in adaptive automation, or dynamic function allocation (Hancock, Chignall, & Lowenthal, 1985). The rationale for adaptive automation is that task functions are not fixed, but switched dynamically between human and machine in response to changing resources/needs of the two agents. These methods, first suggested over 20 years ago (Rouse, 1976), have become more practicable with technological advances, and are now widely regarded as an inevitable feature of the development of intelligent H-M systems. Most current applications are in aviation and transport, typically taking the form of computer aiding for the human when critical events occur (e.g. aborting take-off; ground proximity warning systems; sudden overload in air traffic control). However, there are strong indications that an adaptive automation solution may satisfy the two conflicting goals of complex H-M systems: (1) to maximize human involvement in task management; and (2) to protect system performance against the effects of a compromised operator state.

Application of the OFS paradigm for detecting high risk operator states

We are currently working with control engineers to design and build a system in which control may be switched between human and machine on the basis of measured changes in the underlying functional state of the human operator that predict episodes of performance breakdown. Until now, there has been no direct way of determining this critical strain state—when primary performance appears unimpaired but the compensatory process is at its limit, and is about to break down. In order to improve the validity and reliability of prediction we plan to include relevant physiological measures (both cardiovascular and EEG), and combine the indicators using fuzzy logic. We plan to force a breakdown in primary performance by progressive loading using a modified CAMS, then examine the state pattern that preceded (predicted) this breakdown. Because of their high bandwidth and rapid response, autonomic and EEG responses are particularly strong candidates for use as OFS indicators, in combination with primary and secondary task data and subjective measures of effort, fatigue, and anxiety. Secondary task indicators such as probe reaction time (RT) can reflect latent strain associated with the primary task. Cardiovascular (CV) indices, notably heart rate (HR) and heart rate variability (HRV), have been found to respond reliably to changes in workload and mental effort (Fahrenberg & Wientjes, 2000), particularly in operational settings where high-level problem solving is involved (Tattersall & Hockey, 1995). As with HRV, power spectrum analysis of the EEG is necessary to reveal effects of mental states, with the most sensitive markers based on ratios between the power observed in higher (β) and lower (α, θ) bands.

Sometimes overlooked in the adaptive automation literature is the need to distinguish between two kinds of high-risk state; low alertness and high strain/fatigue. Low alertness may be readily detected by the prevalence of low frequency activity in the EEG, and is used to trigger alerting devices in train drivers (Verwey & Zaidel, 1999). In constrast, as I have argued, strain is a high activation state, resulting from the sustained effort to maintain performance under high demands, and less readily identified using standard EEG and CV methods. Researchers at NASA-Langley labs (e.g. Pope, Bogarte, & Bartolome, 1995) have identified an "engagement index" $[\beta/(\alpha + \theta)]$, and used this to successfully trigger switches between manual and computer-aided control. Operators are switched to manual when engagement is low and back to automatic when it is regained. However, an adaptive system also needs to support the operator when engagement is too high (the strain state). In the other main current approach to adaptive automation, Wilson (e.g. Wilson & Russell,

2003) trains artificial neural networks (ANNs) to detect and classify multidimensional physiological patterns associated with different workload levels, and switch control away from the operator when "high workload" patterns are detected. However, the validity of this procedure is questionable. While a state of low alertness will always increase operational risk, a high workload profile *per se* may not be a threat in many situations, and may even indicate enjoyable engagement (Frankenhaeuser's (1986) "effort without distress") for professional operators. An intelligent solution would allow a period of rest from sustained manual control when strain is detected, but not force a switch back to computer control just because operators exhibit a high workload state (in the absence of strain).

Clearly, effective adaptive automation needs to be able to detect both risk states; low alertness and strain. In terms of physiological assessment, selection of EEG variables provides the major challenge. Wilson's ANN-based method provides an empirical solution but precludes the identification of underlying states. The NASA-Langley index does have a clear mapping onto an identifiable mental state, though this is inferred from EEG generalized across the cortex, so the term "general alertness" may be more appropriate than engagement (which implies specific task orientation). A more valid index of engagement may be derived from considering localised EEG changes. Gevins and Smith (1999) and others have inferred the operation of an executive (attention control) mechanism on the basis of increased power in the θ band (measured from frontal mid-line sites), with concomitant attenuation of α power. This dissociation of the two lower frequency bands (combined in the engagement index) promises an effective way of separating EEG indices of the intensity $[\beta/(\alpha + \theta)]$ and selectivity $[\theta/\alpha]$ of attentional processes, improving the diagnostic potential of EEG markers. This is central to the approach we are taking in our current work, making the assumption that different psychophysiological patterns provide information about different diagnostic features of high risk states. Reduced frontal-midline θ power may indicate either a strategic disengagement from executive processing or an unavoidable loss of selectivity with fatigue, dependent on convergent data from primary/secondary performance, general EEG alertness, cardiovascular strain, and subjective state.

Conclusions

The patterns of performance decrement observed under stress and high demand can be seen to reflect the adaptive response of the motivational control system to the changing requirements for goal priorities under environmental flux.

Maintenance of primary task outputs under difficult conditions can be achieved only through the operation of a compensatory process that acts to protect vulnerable cognitive goals from competition from (stronger) emotional and biological goals. While primary performance is often maintained under stress, this compensatory activity normally results in disruption to secondary or auxiliary components of overall system performance, and depletion of energetic resources. These may represent a source of latent degradation, only revealed as a breakdown in performance under critical conditions, such as sudden, unpredictable surges of load, changes of task priorities, or the requirement to sustain such control over long, unbroken periods. A concern with overall system efficiency, rather than with single task effectiveness, will allow us to understand performance changes in relation to the broader goals and priorities of human behaviour, and the implications of these patterned system changes for the management of both performance and well-being. Current work is focussed on applying these methods to the identification of sensitive markers of strain states for use in the development of adaptive automation systems.

References

Baddeley, A. D. (1972). Selective attention and performance in dangerous environments. *British Journal of Psychology, 63*, 537–546.

Bandura, A. (1996). Failures in self-regulation: Energy depletion or selective disengagement? *Psychological Inquiry, 7*, 20–24.

Billings, C. (1996). *Towards a human-centred approach to automation.* Englewood Cliffs, NJ: Erlbaum.

Broadbent, D. E. (1971). *Decision and stress.* London: Academic Press.

Broadbent, D. E. (1979). Is a fatigue test now possible? *Ergonomics, 22*, 1277–1290.

Carver, C. S., & Scheier, M. F. (1982). Control theory: A useful conceptual framework of personality-social, clinical and health psychology. *Psychological Bulletin, 92*, 111–135.

Ellis, H. C., & Ashbrook, P. W. (1989). The "state" of mood and memory research: A selective review. *Journal of Social Behavior and Personality, 4*, 1–21.

Fahrenberg, J., & Wientjes, C. W. J. (2000). Recording methods in applied environments. In R. W. Backs & W. Boucsein (Eds.), *Engineering psychology: Issues and applications,* London: Erlbaum.

Frankenhaeuser, M. (1986). A psychobiological framework for research on human stress and coping. In M. H. Appley & R. Trumbell (Eds.), *Dynamics of stress.* New York: Plenum.

Frese, M., & Zapf, D. (1994). Action as the core of work psychology: A German approach. In H. C. Triandis, M. D. Dunnette, & L. M. Lough (Eds.), *Handbook of industrial and organisational psychology.* Palo Alto, CA: Consulting Psychologists Press.

Gevins, A., & Smith, M. E. (1999). Detecting transient cognitive impairment with EEG pattern recognition methods. *Aerospace and Environmental Medicine, 70*, 1018–1024.

Grier, R. A., Warm, J. S., Dember, W. N., Matthews, G. Galinsky, T. L., Szalma, J. L. et al. (2003). The vigilance decrement reflects limitations in effortful attention, not mindlessness. *Human Factors, 45,* 349–359.

Hamilton, P., Hockey, G. R. J., & Reijman, M. (1977). The place of the concept of activation in human information processing theory: An integrative approach. In S. Dornic (Ed.), *Attention and performance VI.* New York: Academic Press.

Hancock, P. A., Chignall, M. H., & Lowenthal, A. (1985). An adaptive human-machine system. *Proceedings of IEEE: Man, Systems and Cybernetics, 19,* 627–629.

Hockey, G. R. J. (1979). Stress and the cognitive components of skilled performance. In V. Hamilton & D. M. Warburton (Eds.), *Human stress and cognition: An information processing approach* (pp. 141–177). Chichester, UK: Wiley.

Hockey, G. R. J. (1986). A state control theory of adaptation and individual differences in stress management. In G. R. J. Hockey, A. W. K. Gaillard, & M. G. H. Coles (Eds.), *Energetics and human information processing.* Dordrecht, The Netherlands: Martinus Nijhoff.

Hockey, G. R. J. (1997). Compensatory control in the regulation of human performance under stress and high workload: A cognitive energetical framework. *Biological Psychology, 45,* 73–93.

Hockey, G. R. J. (2003). Operator functional state as a framework for the assessment of performance degradation. In G. R. J. Hockey, A. W. Gaillard, & A. Burov (Eds.), *Operator functional state: The assessment and prediction of human performance degradation in complex tasks.* Amsterdam: IOS Press.

Hockey, G. R. J., & Hamilton, P. (1983). The cognitive patterning of stress states. In G. R. J. Hockey (Ed.), *Stress and fatigue in human performance.* Chichester, UK: Wiley.

Hockey, G. R. J., Maule, A. J., Clough, P. J., & Bdzola, L. (2000). Effects of negative mood states on risk in everyday decision making. *Cognition and Emotion, 14,* 823–855.

Hockey, G. R. J., Wastell, D. G., & Sauer, J. (1998). Effects of sleep deprivation and user-interface on complex performance: A multilevel analysis of compensatory control. *Human Factors, 40,* 233–253.

Holding, D. H. (1983). Fatigue. In G. R. J. Hockey (Ed.), *Stress and fatigue in human performance.* Chichester, UK: Wiley.

Hyland, M. E. (1988). Motivational control theory: An integrative framework. *Journal of Personality and Social Psychology, 55,* 642–651.

Kahneman, D. (1971). Remarks on attentional control. In A. F. Sanders (Ed.), *Attention and performance. Part III.* Amsterdam: North Holland.

Kahneman, D. (1973). *Attention and effort.* Englewood Cliffs, NJ: Prentice-Hall.

Kryter, K. D. (1970). *The effects of noise on man.* New York: Academic Press.

Lundberg, U., & Frankenhaueser, M. (1978). Psychophysiological reactions to noise as modified by personal control over noise intensity. *Biological Psychology, 6,* 55–59.

Meijman, T. F., Mulder, G., Dormolen, M. van, & Cremer, R. (1992). Workload of driving examiners: A psychophysiological field study. In H. Kragt (Ed.), *Enhancing industrial performance.* London: Taylor & Francis.

Mulder, G. (1986). The concept of mental effort and its measurement. In G. R. J. Hockey, A. W. K. Gaillard, & M. G. H. Coles (Eds.), *Energetics and human information processing* (pp. 175–198). Dordrecht, The Netherlands: Martinus Nijhoff.

Muraven, M., Tice, D. M., & Baumeister, R. F. (1998). Self-control as a limited resource: Regulatory depletion patterns. *Journal of Personality and Social Psychology, 74,* 774–789.

Navon, D., & Gopher, D. (1979). On the economy of the human information processing system. *Psychological Review, 86*, 214–255.

Norman, D. A., & Bobrow, D. (1975). On data-limited and resource-limited processes. *Cognitive Psychology, 7*, 44–64.

Oatley, K., & Johnson-Laird, P. L. (1990). Towards a cognitive theory of emotions. *Cognition and Emotion, 1*, 29–50.

Öhman, A., Flykt, A., & Esteves, F. (2001). Emotion drives attention: Detecting the snake in the grass. *Journal of Experimental Psychology: General, 130*, 466–478.

Parasuraman, R., & Riley, V. A. (1997). Humans and automation: use, misuse, disuse, abuse *Human Factors, 39*, 230–253.

Rabbitt, P. M. A. (1981). Sequential reactions. In D. H. Holding (Ed.), *Human skills.* New York: Wiley.

Rouse, W. B. (1976). Adaptive allocation of decision making responsibility between supervisor and computer. In T. B. Sheridan & G. Johansson (Eds.), *Monitoring behaviour and supervisory control.* Amsterdam: North Holland.

Schönpflug, W. (1983). Coping efficiency and situational demands. In G. R. J. Hockey (Ed.), *Stress and fatigue in human performance.* Chichester, UK: Wiley.

Schönpflug, W. (1985). Goal-directed behaviour as a source of stress: Psychological origins and consequences of inefficiency. In M. Frese & M. Sabini (Eds.), *Goal-directed behaviour: The concept of action in psychology.* Hillsdale, NJ: Erlbaum.

Shallice, T. (1988). *From neuropsychology to mental structure.* Cambridge University Press.

Sperandio, A. (1978). The regulation of working methods as a function of workload among air traffic controllers. *Ergonomics, 21*, 367–390.

Tattersall. A. J., & Hockey, G. R. J. (1995). Level of operator control and changes in heart rate variability during simulated flight maintenance. *Human Factors, 37*, 682–698.

Taylor, S. E. (1991). Asymmetrical effects of positive and negative events: The mobilization-minimization hypothesis. *Psychological Bulletin, 110*, 67–85.

Teichner, W. H. (1968). Interaction of behavioral and physiological stress reactions. *Psychological Review, 75*, 51–80.

Van der Linden, D., Frese, M., & Sonnentag, S. (2003). The impact of mental fatigue on exploration in a complex computer task: Rigidity and loss of systematic strategies. *Human Factors, 45*, 483–494.

Veldman, H. (1992). Hidden effects of noise as revealed by cardiovascular analysis. PhD thesis, University of Groningen.

Verwey W. B., & Zaidel D. M. (1999). Preventing drowsiness accidents by an alertness maintenance device. *Accident Analysis and Prevention, 31*, 199–211.

Wickens, C. D., & Hollands, J. G. (1999). *Engineering psychology and human performance* (2nd ed.). Upper Saddle River, NJ: Prentice-Hall.

Wilson, G., & Russell, C. A. (2003). Operator functional state classification using multiple psychophysiological features in an air traffic control task. *Human Factors, 45*, 381–389.

Index